STUDY GUIDE TO ACCOMPANY
BRUNNER AND SUDDARTH'S TEXTBOOK OF

Medical-Surgical Nursing TENTH EDITION

STUDY GUIDE TO ACCOMPANY
BRUNNER AND SUDDARTH'S TEXTBOOK OF

Medical-Surgical Nursing

TENTH EDITION

Mary Jo Boyer, R.N., D.N.Sc.
Coadjutant Nursing Faculty
Former Dean and Professor of Allied Health and Nursing
Delaware County Community College
Media, Pennsylvania

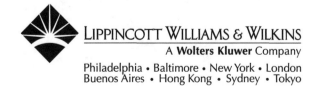

LIPPINCOTT WILLIAMS & WILKINS
A **Wolters Kluwer** Company

Philadelphia • Baltimore • New York • London
Buenos Aires • Hong Kong • Sydney • Tokyo

Ancillary Editor: Doris S. Wray
Composition: Peirce Graphic Services
Printer/Binder: Victor

10th Edition

ISBN: 0-7817-3215-8

The material contained in this volume was submitted as previously unpublished material, except in the instances in which credit has been given to the source from which some of the illustrative material was derived.

Any procedure or practice described in this book should be applied by the health care practitioner under appropriate supervision in accordance with professional standards of care used with regard to the unique circumstances that apply in each practice situation. Care has been taken to confirm the accuracy of information presented and to describe generally accepted practices. However, the authors, editors, and publisher cannot accept any responsibility for errors or omissions or for any consequences from application of the information in this book and make no warranty, express or implied, with respect to the contents of the book.

The authors and publisher has exerted every effort to ensure that drug selection and dosage set forth in this text are in accordance with current recommendations and practice at the time of publication. However, in view of ongoing research, changes in government regulations, and the constant flow of information relating to drug therapy and drug reactions, the reader is urged to check the package insert for each drug for any change in indications and dosage and for added warnings and precautions. This is particularly important when the recommended agent is a new or infrequently employed drug.

9 8 7 6 5 4

This book is dedicated to . . .

. . . My mother, *Eremelina,* who at age 83 continues to be a role model for educated and successful women

. . . My husband *Bill,* a trusted partner who has shared my life for 30 years

. . . My son *Brian,* my soul-mate, a philosopher and musician whose songs and writings have and will touch the minds and hearts of many

. . . My daughter *Susan,* my beautiful friend, whose happy heart, passionate determination, and athletic talents will shape the course of her life and enrich the lives of those she touches

Preface

The *Study Guide to Brunner and Suddarth's Textbook of Medical-Surgical Nursing, Tenth Edition,* was developed as a learning tool to help you, a nursing student, focus on content areas considered essential for understanding the concepts, techniques, and disease processes presented in the textbook. A Critical Thinking approach was used to present facts from a knowledge-based level (using multiple-choice, matching, fill-in and crossword puzzles) to the highest levels of analysis and synthesis (using comparison analysis, pattern identification, contradiction recognition, supportive argumentation, and critical analysis and discussion). The application of theory to practice is tested by having you complete nursing care plans, outline detailed patient teaching guides, and complete decision-making trees and critical clinical pathways. Case studies are offered at the end of most sections.

The answer to every question is presented in the Answer Key at the end of the book. Critical thinking, the nursing process, and a community-based focus to nursing care are incorporated throughout; information is tested from the viewpoint of nursing intervention. Some answers are derived from analysis and are implied. They may not be found specifically in the chapter. Pathophysiologic processes are included only if relevant to specific nursing actions.

It was my intent to present information in a manner that will stimulate critical thinking and promote learning. It is my hope that knowledge gained and reinforced will be used to provide competent nursing care to those in need.

Mary Jo Boyer, R.N., D.N.Sc.

Contents

UNIT 12
Integumentary Function   275

UNIT 13
Sensorineural Function   289

UNIT 14
Neurologic Function   299

UNIT 15
Musculoskeletal Function   321

UNIT 16
Other Acute Problems   339

UNIT 1
Basic Concepts in Nursing

1

Health Care Delivery and Nursing Practice

I. Interpretation, Completion, and Comparison

Multiple Choice. Read each question carefully. Circle your answer.

1. The definition of nursing has evolved over time. According to the American Nurses Association (ANA), registered nurses can and should:
   a. diagnose health alterations and prescribe specific nursing interventions.
   b. promote optimum levels of wellness and prevent illness.
   c. maintain health and assist patients with the dying process.
   d. do all of the above.

2. An underlying focus in any definition of nursing is the registered nurse's responsibility to:
   a. appraise and enhance an individual's health-seeking perspective.
   b. coordinate a patient's total health management with all disciplines.
   c. diagnose acute pathology.
   d. treat acute clinical reactions to chronic illness.

3. A Jewish patient who adheres to the dietary laws of his faith is in traction and confined to bed. He needs assistance with his evening meal of chicken, rice, beans, a roll, and a carton of milk. Choose the nursing approach that is most representative of promoting wellness.
   a. Nurse "A" removes items from the overbed table to make room for the dinner tray.
   b. Nurse "B" pushes the overbed table toward the bed so that it will be within the patient's reach when the dinner tray arrives.
   c. Nurse "C" asks a family member to assist the patient with the tray and the overbed table while the nurse straightens the area in an attempt to provide a pleasant atmosphere for eating.
   d. Nurse "D" prepares the environment and the overbed table and inspects the contents of the dinner tray. The nurse asks the patient whether he would like to make any substitutions in the foods and fluids he has received.

4. Using the concept of the wellness–illness continuum, a nursing care plan for a chronically ill patient would outline steps to:
   a. educate the patient about every possible complication associated with the specific illness.
   b. encourage positive health characteristics within the limits of the specific illness.
   c. limit all activities because of the progressive deterioration associated with all chronic illnesses.
   d. recommend activity beyond the scope of tolerance to prevent early deterioration.

5. To be responsive to the changing health care needs of our society, registered nurses will need to:

a. focus their care on the traditional disease-oriented approach to patient care, because hospitalized patients today are more acutely ill than they were 10 years ago.

b. learn how to delegate discharge planning to ancillary personnel so that RNs can spend their time managing the "high-tech" equipment needed for patient care.

c. place increasing emphasis on wellness, health promotion, and self-care, because the majority of Americans today suffer from chronic debilitative illness.

d. stress the curative aspects of illness, especially the acute, infectious disease processes.

6. The diagnosis-related groups (DRGs) legislation enacted in 1983 provides for:

a. a fixed rate of Medicare payment per diagnosis for hospital services.

b. a retrospective method of reimbursement based on a patient's length of stay.

c. all hospital and extended-care costs (such as nursing homes and home care) per diagnosis if the hospital participates with a peer review organization (PRO).

d. total reimbursement per diagnosis for as long as the patient requires hospitalization (as long as the patient is eligible for Medicare benefits).

7. Quality assurance programs created in the 1980s required that hospitals be accountable for all of the following except:

a. appropriateness of care related to established standards.

b. cost of services.

c. staff-patient ratios for nursing care.

d. quality delivery of services.

8. The primary focus of the nurse advocacy role in managing a clinical pathway is:

a. continuity of care.

b. cost-containment practices.

c. effective utilization of services.

d. a patient's progress toward desired outcomes.

9. Nursing practice in the home and community requires competence and experience in the techniques of:

a. decision making.

b. health teaching.

c. physical assessment.

d. all of the above.

10. Certification for registered nursing practice is:

a. mandatory for nurses working in specialty areas.

b. offered by the state boards of nursing at the time a graduate writes for licensure.

c. required in all states after a nurse has been practicing for 5 years.

d. suggested by the ANA as a way of validating expertise in clinical practice.

Fill-In. *Read each statement carefully. Write your response in the space provided.*

1. According to the Social Policy Statement of the ANA in 1995, nursing practice involves the *diagnosis and treatment of human responses to actual or potential health problems.* Choose three health problems, and write a human response to each that would require nursing intervention.

Health Problem	**Human Response Requiring Nursing Intervention**
a. Fractured right arm	Self-care limitations
b. COPD	Impaired ventilation
c. Ulcer, skin or stomach	pain
d. Sleep deprivation	confusion, Lethargy

2. It is expected that most nursing practice in the next 5 years will be in community and long-term care settings. This movement reflects legislative and sociologic changes consistent with:

Chronic illness ↑ in population over 65 yrs   shift from desease cure to health promotion

3. List Maslow's hierarchy of needs, and give an example for each need.

Need	Example
physiologic	food
saftey and security	Bed alarm, Financial
Belongingness and affection	companionship
Esteem and self respect.	Recognition by society
self actualization	achieved potienial in a area
Self fullfilment	creativity (painting)
Knowledge and understand.	information and understand.
Aesthetics	Attractive enviroment.

4. Health promotion efforts today target negative lifestyle behaviors such as:

stress	smoking, Drugs
improper diet	High risk behaviors
lack of exercise	sexual practices and poor Hygiene

5. Define the term *clinical pathway* as it relates to the concept of managed care.

Lists the sequencing of tests, treatments, activities, medications and so on, through which a patient must progress per Dx, within a set time period from Admiss. — discharge.

6. Explain when "care mapping" may be more beneficial than "clinical pathways" for managing care.

when a pt. has a complex condition or multiple underlying illness can be monitored for progress using phases and stages of a disease or condition rather than time frame.

7. Managed health care of the 1990s has resulted in declining pt. Hosp., shorter Hosp. stays, ↑ acuity of pts., and expansion of ambulatory care and explosion of community based care.

8. List four common characteristics of managed care (i.e., health maintenance organizations [HMOs]).

prenegotiated payment rates	utilization review
mandatory pre certification	Limited choice of provider
	Fixed price reinbursment.

9. List the purpose and goals of case management.
managing care for caseload of pts. and personnel who care for the pts. goals are quality care, appropriate and timely care delivery and cost reduction.

10. Explain the role of preferred provider organizations (PPOs).
allows consumers to choose hospitals and providers. reinbursment is on a fee for service basis.

II. Critical Thinking Questions and Exercises

Discussion and Analysis

1. As of 2001, it became obvious that the United States was entering a decade that would be known as the worst nursing shortage in history. It is predicted that by the year 2010, there will be significantly fewer nurses than needed. Describe three factors that you believe have influenced the nursing shortage.

Supporting Arguments

Read the paragraph below. Fill in the space provided with the best response.

Many recent changes in health care have significantly affected nursing care delivery and nursing education, including the aging population, increased cultural diversity, the rising cost of health care and technology growth, and federally legislated health care reform. Choose one factor that you believe has had *the most impact* on nursing care in the last 5 years, and support your argument with data (see pages 4–8 in the text).

The most important factor is: ↑ aging population

Supporting argument: With ↑ aging population and ↓ in nursing grads, care will be in jepordy.

Recognizing Contradictions

Rewrite each statement correctly. Underline the key concepts.

1. The <u>majority</u> of health problems in the ~~United States~~ today are of an ~~infectious and acute~~ **Chronic** nature.

2. A person with a chronic illness can ~~never~~ attain a high level of wellness, ~~because part of his or her health potential will never be reached.~~ if Pts. is successful in meeting his or her health potential within Limits of the chronic illness.

3. The World Health Organization's definition of health is ~~accurate, current, and comprehensive~~. restrictive not allowing for any variation in degree of illness or health.

4. It is predicted that by the year 2030, people older than 65 years of age in the United States will constitute about ~~35%~~ 20% of the total population.

5. The DRG legislation in 1983 created a tiered level of payment, per diagnosis, ~~allowing hospitals to extend days of care to the most needy.~~ restricting pts length of stay, to prescribed days based on each Dx.

6. The main focus of continuous quality improvement (CQI) is ~~that outcomes or products can be compared against a standard.~~ is on the processes that affect Quality.

7. Health care costs were about ~~11%~~ 15-22% of the U.S. gross domestic product (GDP) in the year 2000.

Examining Associations

1. Examine the progression of Maslow's hierarchy of needs in the figure that follows. Consider a recent clinical situation. Explain symptoms your patient exhibited that reflect one or more of the levels below.

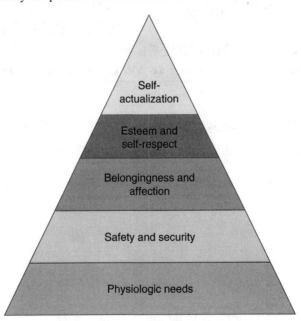

Self-actualization

Esteem and self-respect

Belongingness and affection

Safety and security

Physiologic needs

2. Using Figure 1–3, page 19 of the text, examine and explain the expected behaviors among the physician, patient, nurse, and ancillary personnel in the collaborative practice model.

Clinical Situations

Complete the following flow charts.

1. Klenner (2000) affirms the value of clinical pathway mapping as a tool to effectively chart a patient's response to illness or injury. Complete this clinical pathway to illustrate how one lifestyle habit (smoking) can result in illness.

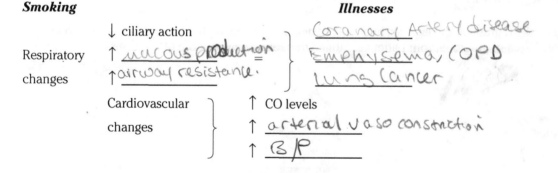

Smoking   *Illnesses*

↓ ciliary action   Coronary Artery disease

Respiratory   ↑ mucous production   Emphysema, COPD

changes   ↑ airway resistance.   lung cancer

Cardiovascular   ↑ CO levels

changes   ↑ arterial vaso constriction

                       ↑ BP

2. Continuous quality improvement (CQI) mandates the standardization of processes that are implemented and improved on a continuous basis. Complete the blank lines on the flow chart for the process of radial pulse assessment.

Radial Pulse Assessment

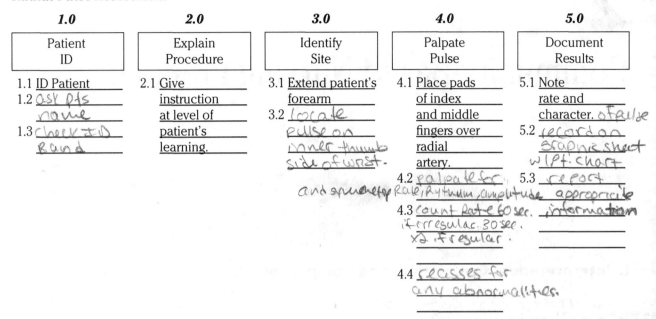

1.0	2.0	3.0	4.0	5.0
Patient ID	Explain Procedure	Identify Site	Palpate Pulse	Document Results
1.1 ID Patient 1.2 _ask pts name_ 1.3 _check ID Band_	2.1 Give instruction at level of patient's learning.	3.1 Extend patient's forearm 3.2 _locate pulse on inner thumb side of wrist. and sprineffp_	4.1 Place pads of index and middle fingers over radial artery. 4.2 _palpate for Rate, Rythum, amplitude_ 4.3 _count Rate 60 sec. if irregular. 30 sec. x2. if regular._ 4.4 _recisses for any abnormalitis._	5.1 Note rate and character. _of failse_ 5.2 _record on Graphic sheet w/ Pt. chart_ 5.3 _report appropriate information_

3. The Joint Commission on Accreditation of Healthcare Organizations (JCAHO) mandated in 1992 that health care organizations move toward implementation of CQI. A cause-and-effect diagram can illustrate potential causes of an effect so the cause can be examined and corrected. Complete the following diagram.

CQI Cause and Effect Diagram: Delayed Medication

Possible Causes

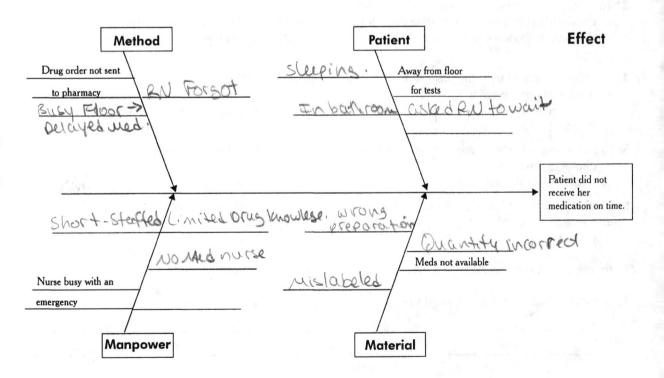

2

Community-Based Nursing Practice

I. Interpretation, Completion, and Comparison

Multiple Choice. *Read each question carefully. Circle your answer.*

1. The shift in health care delivery from acute care to community-based care is primarily the result of:
   a. alternate health care delivery systems.
   b. changes in federal legislation.
   c. tighter insurance regulations.
   d. the interfacing of all three conditions.

2. Choose an alternative health care delivery system that has dramatically reduced patient-care days in acute care settings.
   a. Health Maintenance Organizations
   b. Managed Health Care Systems
   c. Preferred Provider Organizations
   d. Each of the three is equally significant.

3. The most frequent users of home health services are:
   a. children with chronic, debilitating disorders.
   b. newborns who are sent home with apnea monitors.
   c. the frail and elderly who need skilled care.
   d. young adults on prolonged intravenous therapy.

4. Discharge planning from the hospital to home care begins when the:
   a. discharge order is written.
   b. nurse receives the physician's order for discharge.
   c. physician notifies the insurance company.
   d. patient is admitted to the hospital.

5. Nurses working in elementary schools are trained to deal with the leading health care problem of:
   a. dental disease.
   b. emotional problems.
   c. infections.
   d. sports injuries.

6. Nurses working in high schools expect to deal with the common health care problem of:
   a. anorexia.
   b. cancer.
   c. drug abuse.
   d. malnutrition.

Fill-In. *Read each statement carefully. Write your response in the space provided.*

1. List specific skills a nurse will need to function in community-based care.
   expert, independent decision makers, self directed, flexible, adaptab
   compotent in critical thinking, physical assessment, health edu
   and basic nursing care.

2. Distinguish between the terms "community-based nursing" and "public health nursing."

nursing care given to individuals and families in the community in which they live work and play and school. community health nursing. speciality area focused on total populations.

3. List several examples of "skilled" nursing services provided by home care.

IV therapy, injections, parenteral nutrition, venipuncture, catheter insertion, pressure ulcer and wound care, and ostomy care.

4. The first step in preparing for a home visit is for the nurse to:

Call pt to obtain permission for visit, scheduale visit and verify address.

5. Explain the purpose of the initial home visit.

The pt is evaluated and plan of care established.

6. List some examples of ambulatory health care settings.

Medical clinics, ambulatory care units, urgent care centers, cardiac rehab. programs, mental health and student health facilities

7. Name several subspecialties for nurse practitioners.

gerontology, midwifery, pediatrics, family planning, family, adult and women health.

8. Common chronic health problems of the homeless are:

DM, HTN, heart disease, Aids, and mental illness.

II. Critical Thinking Questions and Exercises

Discussion and Analysis

1. Describe a common clinical care situation for a patient outside the hospital. Determine whether the role, responsibilities, and suggested scope of practice are within the realm of community-based nursing or community health nursing.

2. Compare the educational preparation, job description, and expanded role of advanced practice nurses working in a clinic, an ambulatory care setting, an elementary school, and an industrial setting.

3. Compare and contrast three alternate health care delivery systems: health maintenance organizations, preferred provider organizations, and managed health care systems. Cite an example of how each system has contributed to reduced health care costs and affected health care services.

4. Distinguish between primary, secondary, and tertiary levels of preventive care and cite a clinical case example of each level.

Recognizing Contradictions

Rewrite each statement correctly. Underline the key concepts.

1. Community health nursing focuses on promoting and maintaining the health of individuals and groups. *or Public health nursing is focused on total populations*

2. Tertiary prevention is a level of community nursing practice that focuses on the early detection of disease.

3. The primary purpose of the initial home care visit is to give the patient and his or her family information about care and treatments. *Is for the nurse to establish a trusting relationship with the pt. and his/her family*

minimizing deterioration and improving the quality of life secondary focuses on early disease detection eg. mamograms.

3

Critical Thinking, Ethical Decision Making, and the Nursing Process

I. Interpretation, Completion, and Comparison

Multiple Choice. Read each question carefully. Circle your answer.

1. The least effective decision-making process used in critical thinking is:
   a. analyzing data.
   b. establishing assumptions.
   c. formulating conclusions.
   d. synthesizing information.

2. The term *metacognition* refers to the critical-thinking skill of:
   a. consultation.
   b. data analysis.
   c. self-reasoning.
   d. validation.

3. *Morality* is defined as:
   a. adherence to specific codes of conduct.
   b. commitment to informal, personal values.
   c. dependence on specified principles of behavior.
   d. an understanding of defined rules of behavior.

4. When an ethical decision is made based on the reasoning of the "greatest good for the greatest number," the nurse is following the:
   a. deontological theory.
   b. formalist theory.
   c. moral-justification theory.
   d. utilitarian theory.

5. Consider the ethical situation in which a nurse moves a confused, disruptive patient to a private room at the end of the hall so that other patients can rest, even though the confused patient becomes more agitated. The nurse's judgment is consistent with reasoning based on:
   a. "consequentialism," by which good consequences for the greatest number are maximized.
   b. "duty of obligation," by which an action, regardless of its results, is justified if the decision making was based on moral principles.
   c. "prima facie" duty, by which an action is justified if it does not conflict with a stronger duty.
   d. the "categorical imperative," by which the results of an action are deemed less important than the means to the end.

6. A hospital board of directors decided to close a pediatric burn treatment center (BTC) that annually admits 50 patients and to open a treatment center for terminally ill AIDS patients (with an expected annual admission of 200). This decision meant that the nearest BTC for children was 300 miles away. The board's decision was an example of ethical reasoning consistent with:

a. a formalist approach.
b. obligation or duty.
c. "the means justifies the end."
d. utilitarianism.

7. A terminally ill patient asks the nurse whether she is dying. The nurse's response is influenced by the moral obligation to:

a. communicate the patient's wishes to the family.
b. consult with the physician.
c. provide correct information to the patient.
d. consider all of the above measures before disclosing specific information.

8. A patient with a "Do Not Resuscitate" order requires large doses of a narcotic (which may significantly reduce respiratory function) for excruciating pain. After the patient requests pain medication, the nurse assesses a respiratory rate of 12 breaths per minute. The nurse's ethical decision should be to:

a. ask the patient to wait 20 minutes and reassess.
b. give half of the prescribed dose.
c. give the pain medication without fear of respiratory depression.
d. withhold the pain medication and contact the physician.

9. Choose the situation that most accurately represents a moral problem in contrast to a moral dilemma.

a. Three days after surgery, a patient requests narcotic pain medication every 3 hours. The nurse administers a placebo that reduces pain.
b. A 32-year-old father of three with advanced cancer of the lungs asks that everything be done to prolong his life, even though his chemo-therapy treatments are no longer effective.
c. A confused 80-year-old needs restraints for protection from injury, even though the restraints increase agitation.
d. A young patient with AIDS has asked not to receive tube feedings to prolong life because of intense pain.

10. Assessment begins with initial patient contact. Nursing activities during this component of the nursing process include:

a. interviewing and obtaining a nursing history.
b. observing for altered symptomatology.
c. collecting and analyzing data.
d. all of the above.

11. The end result of data analysis is:

a. actualization of the plan of care.
b. determination of the patient's responses to care.
c. collection and analysis of data.
d. identification of actual or potential health problems.

12. A therapeutic communication technique that validates what the nurse believes to be the main idea of an interaction is known as:

a. acknowledgment.
b. focusing.
c. restating.
d. summarizing.

13. An example of a medical diagnosis, in contrast to a nursing diagnosis, is:

a. fever of unknown origin.
b. fluid volume excess.
c. ineffective breathing patterns.
d. sleep-pattern disturbances.

14. In choosing the nursing action that illustrates planned nursing care prioritized according to Maslow's hierarchy of needs, a nurse would:

a. administer pain medication to an orthopedic patient 30 minutes before transportation to physical therapy for crutch-walking exercises.
b. discourage a terminally ill patient from participating in a plan of care, to minimize fears about death.
c. help a patient walk to the shower while the breakfast tray waits on the overbed table, because the shower area is vacant at this time.
d. interrupt a family's visit with a depressed patient to assess blood pressure measurement, because it is time to take the scheduled vital signs.

15. Consider the following nursing diagnosis: "Altered nutrition, less than body requirements, related to inability to feed self." An example of an immediate nursing goal is that the patient will:

a. acquire competence in managing cookware designed for handicapped people.

b. assume independent responsibility for meeting self-nutrition needs.

c. learn about food products that require minimal preparation yet meet individual needs for a balanced diet.

d. master the use of special eating utensils to feed self.

16. Registered nurses are responsible for delegating patient care responsibilities to licensed practical nurses (LPNs) and ancillary personnel. The most appropriate task to delegate to a nurse aide is:

a. assessing the degree of lower leg edema in a patient on bed rest.

b. making the bed of an ambulatory patient.

c. measuring the circumference of a patient's calf for edema.

d. recording the size and appearance of a bed sore.

Fill-In. *Read each statement carefully. Write your response in the space provided.*

1. Define the term critical thinking, according to Prideaux (2000). set procedures. that involve conscio multidemensional skill a cognative process. systematic, reflective, rational and goal oriented examination and analysis of al available information and ideas. The formulation of logical conclusions and decisio

2. Explain this statement: How a nurse perceives a situation and employs critical thinking skills depends on the "lens" through which she sees the situation. critical thinking is influenced by cultural, attitude, and experiences. of the individual, who sees the situation through the lens of his or her experien

3. List two types of "advance directives," or legal documents that specify a patient's wishes before hospitalization. a living will and durable power of attorney. they provide health care providers with info on pts. wishes for health care before illness accures

4. Explain the merit of having an "advanced directive." provide health care providers will info. on care for pt. before illness accurrs

5. Suggest an opening statement that a nurse can use during the interview process. Tell me what brought you here? What do you think your needs are? and tell me about your PMH?

6. Discuss how formulation of a nursing diagnosis and identification of collaborative problems differs from making a medical diagnosis. The nursing Dx identifies actual or potencial health problems. that are amenable to resolution by nursing action. Collaberative problems are physiologic complications that nurses monitor, in collaboration

7. Discuss the significance of using outcome criteria during the evaluation phase of the nursing process. Expected outcomes should be stated in behavioral terms and should be realistic as well as measurable. They serve as a measure of effectiveness of the nursing intervention.

Fill-In. *Read each statement below. Put "NO" in front of every nursing diagnosis and "CO" in front of every collaborative problem.*

1. _NO_ Anxiety related to impending surgery.

2. _NO_ Constipation related to altered nutrition.

3. _CO_ Potential complication: paralytic ileus secondary to postoperative inactivity.

with a MD, to detect onset changes in the pts status. A medical Dx Identifies diseases, conditions, or pathology that can be medically managed.

4. __CO__ Potential complication: sacral decubiti secondary to bed rest.

5. __NO__ Potential impairment of skin integrity related to prolonged bed rest.

6. __NO__ Ineffective breastfeeding related to fear of discomfort.

7. __CO__ Potential complication: hypoglycemia related to inadequate food intake.

8. __CO__ Potential complication: phlebitis related to intravenous therapy.

9. __NO__ Post-trauma response related to accident.

10. __CO__ Potential complication: oral lesions related to chemotherapy.

Matching. *Match the critical-thinking strategy in Column II with its associated nursing action listed in Column I.*

Column I	Column II
1. __e__ categorize information	**a.** assert a practice role
2. __g__ design a plan of care	**b.** formulate a relationship
3. __f__ determine assessment processes	**c.** generate a hypothesis
4. __d__ evaluate outcomes	**d.** provide an explanation
5. __a__ implement a standard plan	**e.** recognize a pattern
6. __c__ make a nursing diagnosis	**f.** search for information
7. __b__ manage collaborative problems	**g.** set priorities

Matching. *Match the definitions of ethical principles listed in Column II with their associated terms listed in Column I.*

Column I	Column II
1. __d__ autonomy	**a.** limiting one's autonomy based on the welfare of another
2. __e__ beneficence	**b.** similar cases should be treated the same
3. __b__ justice	**c.** the commitment to not deceive
4. __f__ nonmaleficence	**d.** freedom of choice
5. __a__ paternalism	**e.** the duty to do good and not inflict harm
6. __c__ veracity	**f.** the expectation that harm will not be done

II. Critical Thinking Questions and Exercises

Discussion and Analysis

Planning nursing care involves setting priorities and distinguishing problems that need urgent attention from those that can be deferred to a later time or referred to a physician. For each of the following patient care problems, circle the *initial priority of nursing care* from among the choices provided and write a rationale for your choice.

1. Activity intolerance, related to inadequate oxygenation:
   a. dyspnea SOB airway is first priority in nursing care
   b. fatigue
   c. hypotension

Rationale for choice: _____

_____

2. Alterations in bowel elimination: constipation, related to prolonged bed rest
   a. abdominal pressure and bloating
   b. palpable impaction *(circled)*
   c. straining at stool

Rationale for choice: _could be an obstruction in Intensfie if palpable_

_____

3. Altered oral mucous membrane, related to stomatitis
   a. erythema of oral mucosa
   b. intolerance to hot foods
   c. oral pain *(circled)*

Rationale for choice: _Keeping pain under control for pt to focus_
on eating or for relief.

Recognizing Contradictions

Rewrite each statement correctly. Underline the key concepts.

a distinct form of ethics because nursing is a separate profess...
1. Nursing ethics is considered ~~an applied form of medical ethics because nurses work only under physician direction~~

occurs when a clear conflict between one or more principles ex...
2. A moral dilemma, ~~in contrast to a moral problem, infers no conflict of moral~~ principle.

3. A nurse experiences moral uncertainty when he or she is prevented from doing what he or she believes is the correct action.

4. A nurse should always honor a terminally ill patient's request to withhold food and hydration if the patient is competent. *This action necessitates an evaluation of harm and may not be supported even for competent pts.*

5. By design, living wills are very prescriptive and are always honored as legally binding documents.
Living wills are not always honored because they change frequently with the pts. perspective as they become sicker.

Supporting Arguments

Read each situation. Offer logical supporting arguments for your response.

1. In vitro fertilization, based on sophisticated technology, has resulted in women in their 50s and 60s giving birth. Physicians argue that this is ethically sound if the woman meets the criteria that she is healthy and should live another 25 years. List three rationales to support this argument.

2. You are asked to defend the statement that "life support measures should never be used for anyone with a terminal illness." Develop three supporting arguments.

3. List two rationales to support the argument that age should be used as a criterion for determining the allocation of health care resources.

Clinical Situations

Read each nursing diagnosis. Write a specific outcome.

The planning phase of the nursing process incorporates documented expected patient outcomes for specific nursing diagnoses (ND). Write one outcome that indicates an improvement for each diagnosis.

1. ND: Activity intolerance, related to dyspnea

Outcome: _Pt. will be able to walk from room to nursing station_
every morning with respiratory rate within normal limits

2. ND: Impaired physical mobility, related to total hip replacement

   Outcome: Pt. will move from bed to chair on 2nd postoperative day w/ legs abducted.

3. ND: Fluid volume excess, related to compromised cardiac output

   Outcome: Pt. will achieve a balance between fluid intake and output with a wgt gain no greater than 1 lb/week.

4. ND: Altered nutrition: less than body requirements, related to anorexia

   Outcome: Pt. will eat 1800 cal/day to maintain a desired wgt of 135 lbs.

5. ND: Sleep-pattern disturbance, related to pain

   Outcome: Pt. will sleep 6-8 hours, without interruption, every evening.

CASE STUDY: Ethical Analysis

Read the following case study. Fill in the blanks below.

You are an RN and a board member of American Red Cross Disaster Relief Services. When a smallpox epidemic erupted among thousands in Washington, D.C., as a result of terrorist activity, the board was asked by the Office of Homeland Security to allocate limited resources. The board decided that those with the greatest chance of survival and those working for the government would be treated. Those individuals with preexisting or terminal conditions would not be treated. The decision resulted in multiple deaths while preserving the lives of those most likely to survive. The framework for decision making followed the utilitarian approach. Use the "Steps of an Ethical Analysis" (Chart 3–5, page 34 of the text) as a guide, and complete your decision-making process to determine whether you agree or disagree with the outcomes.

Assessment

1. List two possible conflicts between ethical principles and professional obligations.

   a. _____

   b. _____

2. People involved in the decision: Those affected by the decision:

   a. _____   a. _____

   b. _____   b. _____

   c. _____   c. _____

Planning

1. Treatment options: Medical facts:

   a. _____   a. _____

   b. _____   b. _____

2. Influencing information:

   a. _____

   b. _____

3. Ethical/moral issues: Competing claims:

   a. _____   a. _____

   b. _____   b. _____

Implementation

Compare the Utilitarian and the Deontological approaches.

Utilitarian	**Deontological**

1. Basis of ethical principles:

a. _____   a. _____

b. _____   b. _____

2. Predict consequences of actions:

a. _____   a. _____

b. _____   b. _____

3. Assign a positive or negative value to each consequence.

a. _____   a. _____

b. _____   b. _____

4. Choose the consequence, decision, or action that predicts the highest positive value.

a. _____   a. _____

b. _____   b. _____

Evaluation

1. The best, morally correct action is to:_____

_____

2. This decision is based on the ethical reasoning that:_____

_____

3. The decision can be defended based on the following arguments:

a. _____

b. _____

c. _____

4

Health Education and Health Promotion

I. Interpretation, Completion, and Comparison

Multiple Choice. Read each question carefully. Circle your answer.

1. Health education is:
   a. a primary nursing responsibility.
   b. an essential component of nursing care.
   c. an independent nursing function.
   d. consistent with all of the above.

2. Nursing responsibilities associated with patient teaching include:
   a. determining individual needs for teaching.
   b. motivating each person to learn.
   c. presenting information at the level of the learner.
   d. all of the above.

3. A nurse assesses that a patient is emotionally ready to learn when the patient:
   a. has accepted the therapeutic regimen.
   b. is motivated.
   c. recognizes the need to learn.
   d. demonstrates all of the above.

4. Nursing actions that can be used to motivate a patient to learn include all of the following *except:*
   a. feedback in the form of constructive encouragement when a person has been unsuccessful in the learning process.
   b. negative criticism when the patient is unsuccessful, so that inappropriate behavior patterns will not be learned.
   c. the creation of a positive atmosphere in which the patient is encouraged to express anxiety.
   d. the establishment of realistic learning goals based on individual needs.

5. Normal aging affects changes in cognition. Therefore, when teaching an elderly patient how to administer insulin, the nurse should:
   a. repeat the information frequently for reinforcement.
   b. present all the information at one time so that the patient is not confused by pieces of information.
   c. speed up the demonstration because the patient will tire easily.
   d. do all of the above.

6. The nurse reviews a medication administration calendar with an elderly patient. Being aware of sensory changes associated with aging, the nurse should:
a. print directions in large, bold type, preferably using black ink.
b. highlight or shade important dates and times with contrasting colors.
c. use several different colors to emphasize special dates.
d. do all of the above.

7. A nursing action that involves modifying a teaching program because a learner is not experientially ready is:
a. changing the wording in a teaching pamphlet so that a patient with a fourth-grade reading level can understand it.
b. contacting family members to assist in goal development to help stimulate motivation.
c. postponing a teaching session with a patient until pain has subsided.
d. all of the above.

8. A nurse identifies a patient's inability to pour a liquid medication into a measuring spoon. This diagnosis is part of the nursing process known as:
a. assessment.
b. planning.
c. implementation.
d. evaluation.

9. A nurse develops a program of increased ambulation for a patient with an orthopedic disorder. This goal setting is a component of the nursing process known as:
a. assessment.
b. planning.
c. implementation.
d. evaluation.

10. Outcome criteria are expressed as expected outcomes of patient behavior resulting from teaching strategies. An example is:
a. ability to climb a flight of stairs without experiencing difficulty in breathing.
b. altered lifestyle resulting from inadequate lung expansion.
c. inadequate ventilation associated with pulmonary congestion.
d. potential oxygenation deficit related to ventilatory insufficiency.

Fill-In. *Read each statement carefully. Write the best response in the space provided.*

1. List three significant factors for a nurse to consider when planning patient education:

_____, _____, and _____

2. Explain why health education is so essential for those with chronic illness.

_____

_____

3. Patient education is compehensive beyond an individual's right to and desire for information. Patient education is a strategy for: _____, _____, _____,

and _____

4. Define the term *adherence* as it relates to a person's therapeutic regimen.

_____

_____

5. Name several variables (factors) that influence a person's ability to adhere to a program of care.

_____

_____

6. Describe the nature of the teaching–learning process.

_____

_____

7. List at least six variables that make adherence to a therapeutic regimen difficult for the elderly:

a. _____ d. _____

b. _____ e. _____

c. _____ f. _____

8. Increased age affects cognition by decreasing:

a. _____ d. _____

b. _____ e. _____

c. _____ f. _____

9. Discuss how learner readiness affects a learner and the learning situation.

_____

_____

10. Discuss the relation between the nursing process and the teaching–learning process.

_____

_____

11. Two major goals from the *Healthy People 2010* publication are: _____

_____and _____.

12. Health promotion activities can be clustered around four active processes:

a. _____ c. _____

b. _____ d. _____

II. Critical Thinking Questions and Exercises

Recognizing Contradictions

Rewrite each statement correctly. Underline the key concepts.

1. Health education is a dependent function of nursing practice that requires physician approval.

2. The largest groups of people in need of health education today are children and those with infectious diseases.

3. Patients are encouraged to evidence compliance with their therapeutic regimen.

4. Evaluation, the final step in the teaching process, should be summative (done at the end of the teaching process).

5. Elderly persons rarely experience significant improvement from health promotion activities.

6. About 50% of elderly persons have one or more chronic illnesses.

Examining Associations

The health status of residents of the United States is a serious concern to individuals, health care practitioners, and health-promoton groups. A nation's health status can be measured by evaluating certain indicators. After reading *Healthy People 2010* (U. S. Department of Health and Human Services, 2000), complete the following chart. For each indicator listed, assign a rating score (1 = not relevant, 2 = important, 3= very significant) reflecting the degree to which the indicator affects an individual's health, the rationale for the score, and an activity to improve the score. The first row has been filled in as an example.

Indicator	Rating Score	Rationale	Improvement Strategy
Physical activity	3	Research has shown an increased percentage of inactivity among young adults over the last 10 years.	Increase time for physical activity in K–12 schools. Limit TV, video games, and computer time in the home.
Obesity			
Tobacco use			
Substance abuse			
Sexual behavior			
Mental illness			
Violent behavior			
Environmental pollution			
Lack of access to health care			

5

Health Assessment

I. Interpretation, Completion, and Comparison

Multiple Choice. Read each question carefully. Circle your answer.

1. The health history obtained by the nurse should focus on nursing's concern about
   a. a comprehensive body systems review.
   b. current and past health problems.
   c. family history.
   d. all of the above.

2. A patient has certain rights concerning data collection, such as the right to know:
   a. how information will be used.
   b. that selected information will be held confidential.
   c. why information is sought.
   d. all of the above.

3. Open-ended questions help persons describe their chief complaint. Choose the sentence that is *not* an open-ended question.
   a. "Describe the pain."
   b. "Tell me more about your feelings."
   c. "How did the accident happen?"
   d. "Is the pain sharp and piercing?"

4. The single most important factor in helping the nurse and physician arrive at a diagnosis is the:
   a. family history.
   b. history of the present illness.
   c. past health history.
   d. results of the systems review.

5. Choose the best question an interviewer would use to obtain educational or occupational information.
   a. "Are you a blue-collar worker?"
   b. "Do you have difficulty meeting your financial commitments?"
   c. "Is your income more than $20,000 per year?"
   d. "What college did you attend?"

6. An *inappropriate* interviewer response to the patient statement, "I will not take pain medication when I am in pain," is:
   a. "Is there another way you have learned to lessen pain when you experience it?"
   b. "Let a nurse know when you are in pain so you can be helped to decrease stimuli that may exaggerate your pain experience."
   c. "Refusing medication can only hurt you by increasing your awareness of the pain experience."
   d. "You have the right to make that decision. How can the nurses help you cope with your pain?"

7. All of the following are questions that will provide information about a person's lifestyle *except:*
   a. "Do you have any food preferences?"
   b. "Have you always lived in this geographic area?"
   c. "How many hours of sleep do you require each day?"
   d. "What type of exercise do you prefer?"

8. When obtaining a health history from an elderly patient, the nurse must remember to:
   a. ask questions slowly, directly, and in a voice loud enough to be heard by those who are hearing-impaired.
   b. clarify the frequency, severity, and history of signs and symptoms of the present illness.
   c. conduct the interview in a calm, unrushed manner using eye-to-eye contact.
   d. do all of the above.

9. On initial impression, the nurse assesses a patient's posture, stature, and body movements. This assessment is part of the physical examination process known as:
   a. auscultation.
   b. inspection.
   c. palpation.
   d. percussion.

10. An examiner needs to determine the upper border of a patient's liver. With the patient in the recumbent position, the examiner would percuss for a:
    a. dull sound.
    b. flat sound.
    c. resonant sound.
    d. tympanic sound.

11. During a physical examination, the nurse noted hyperresonance over inflated lung tissue in a patient with emphysema. The process used for this assessment was:
    a. auscultation.
    b. inspection.
    c. palpation.
    d. percussion.

12. A heart murmur was detected during a physical examination. The process used to obtain this information was:
    a. auscultation.
    b. inspection.
    c. palpation.
    d. percussion.

13. A waist circumference measurement can be useful in assessing excess abdominal fat. Women should try to maintain a waist circumference of _____ to remain healthy.
    a. 30–34 inches
    b. 35 inches
    c. 36–38 inches
    d. 39–41 inches

14. A serum albumin level of 2.50 g/dL indicates:
    a. a severe protein deficiency.
    b. low levels of serum protein.
    c. an acceptable amount of protein.
    d. an extremely high measurement of protein.

15. Several factors contribute to the altered nutritional status of the elderly. A *primary nutritional nursing consideration* during physical assessment is:
    a. altered metabolism and nutrient use secondary to an acute or chronic illness.
    b. decreased appetite related to loneliness.
    c. limited financial resources.
    d. the patient's ability to shop for and prepare food.

Fill-In. *Read each statement carefully. Write your response in the space provided.*

1. The role of the nurse in assessment includes two primary responsibilities: _____ and _____.

2. Describe how the nursing database differs from the physician's database.

_____

_____

3. Explain how mutual trust and confidence between the interviewer and the patient facilitate the communication process.

_____

_____

4. Define the term *chief complaint.*

_____

5. A number of diseases of first- or second-order relatives are significant when a nurse takes a patient's family history. List six diseases that are considered significant:

a. _____   d. _____

b. _____   e. _____

c. _____   f. _____

6. The three leading causes of death in the United States that are related in part to poor nutrition are:

_____, _____, and _____.

7. The body mass index, a number based on a weight-to-height ratio, provides a quick reference to a person's nutritional status. A score of _____ is considered overweight, a score of _____ is considered obese, and a score greater than _____ is considered extremely obese.

8. Explain the concept of *negative nitrogen balance.*

_____

_____

9. Adolescent girls are particularly at risk for nutritional deficits in minerals, such as: _____,

_____, and _____.

Fill-In. *Correlate the following statements with the assessment most likely used to obtain the data. Write the word on the line provided.*

inspection
palpation
percussion
auscultation

1. Asymmetry of movement is associated with a central nervous system disorder. _____

2. Clubbing of the fingers is a diagnostic symptom of chronic pulmonary disorders. _____

3. Tenderness is present in the area of the thyroid isthmus. _____

4. Tactile fremitus is diagnostic of lung consolidation. _____

5. Tympanic or drumlike sounds are produced by pneumothorax. _____

6. The first heart sound is created by the simultaneous closure of the mitral and tricuspid valves. _____

7. A friction rub is present with pericarditis. _____

8. Nodules present with gout lie adjacent to the joint capsule. _____

Matching. *Match the body area listed in Column II with the descriptive sign of poor nutrition listed in Column I.*

Column I.	Column II
1._____ atrophic papillae	**a.** abdomen
2._____ brittle, dull, depigmented	**b.** eyes
3._____ cheilosis	**c.** hair
4._____ flaccid, underdeveloped	**d.** lips
5._____ fluorosis	**e.** muscles
6._____ xerophthalmia	**f.** skeleton
	g. teeth
	h. tongue

II. Critical Thinking Questions and Exercises

Clinical Situations

CASE STUDY: Calculating a Healthy Diet

Read the following case study. Fill in the blanks below.

Mrs. Allred is a 40-year-old, Hispanic woman, 5ft 5 in tall, with three children younger than 5 years of age. She had no known history of any physical illness before experiencing fatigue and irritability that she believed was the result of her parenting responsibilities. Mrs. Allred does not exercise regularly, eats snack foods while watching television with her children, and is too tired to prepare balanced meals for her family. She orders fast food or pizza for dinner at least three times a week.

Part I: *Estimate ideal body weight*

1. Calculate Mrs. Allred's frame size based on a wrist circumference of 16 cm.
   a. small frame
   b. medium frame
   c. large frame

2. Mrs. Allred's ideal body weight (IBW) is:_____ lb. Therefore, she needs to: _____ (gain/lose)

   approximately_____lb.

Part II: *Calculate a balanced diet for Mrs. Allred's ideal body weight, as determined in Part I. Use the Food Guide Pyramid (Figure 5–7, page 73) and Chart 5–3 (page 70) as a reference.*

1. Convert IBW in pounds to kilograms. _____

2. Determine basal energy needs (1 kcal/kg/hr): _____calories

3. Increase activity by 40% (moderate activity): _____calories

4. Divide calories into carbohydrates (50%) _____, fats (30%) _____, and

   proteins (20%) _____.

5. Estimate grams for each: carbohydrates _____, fats _____,

   proteins _____

6. Patient teaching guidelines:

   _____

   _____

UNIT 2
Biophysical and Psychosocial Concepts in Nursing Practice

6

Homeostasis, Stress, and Adaptation

I. Interpretation, Completion, and Comparison

Multiple Choice. *Read each question carefully. Circle your answer.*

1. Stress is a change state perceived as:
   a. challenging.
   b. damaging.
   c. threatening.
   d. having all of the above characteristics.

2. An individual's adaptation to stress is influenced by the stressor's:
   a. frequency and duration.
   b. number of occurrences and magnitude.
   c. sequencing (intermittent or enduring).
   d. combined characteristics as listed above.

3. An example of a functional, yet maladaptive, response of the body to a threat is:
   a. collateral circulation subsequent to diminished tissue perfusion.
   b. decreased cardiac output subsequent to cardiomegaly.
   c. increased pulmonary ventilation subsequent to increased levels of carbon dioxide.
   d. muscle atrophy subsequent to disuse.

4. Health promotion should be initiated before compensatory processes become maladaptive. Preventive nursing measures include all of the following *except:*
   a. demonstrating wound cleansing to a patient who has a necrotic leg ulcer resulting from vascular disease.
   b. showing a patient with a casted extremity how to perform isometric exercises.
   c. suggesting stress-reducing measures for a patient with a diagnosis of angina pectoris.
   d. teaching weight management to a patient who has a family history of obesity and a blood pressure reading of 125/90 mm Hg.

5. Maladaptive compensatory mechanisms result in disease processes in which cells may be:
   a. dead.
   b. diseased.
   c. injured.
   d. affected in all of the above ways.

6. Adaptation to a stressor is positively correlated with:
   a. previous coping mechanisms.
   b. the duration of the stressor.
   c. the severity of the stressor.
   d. all of the above.

7. During the initial stress response, primary appraisal refers to:
a. evaluating the effectiveness of several coping mechanisms.
b. organizing all available resources to deal with the stressor.
c. identifying support services needed for coping.
d. weighing the significance of the stressful event.

8. Helen, age 48, is diagnosed with pneumonia. She has been paralyzed from the chest down for 7 years. The nurse realizes that Helen needs additional support to cope with her infection because:
a. coping measures become less effective with advancing age.
b. the patient's available coping resources are already being used to manage the problems of immobility.
c. an acute infectious process requires more adaptive mechanisms than a chronic stressor does.
d. this additional physical stressor places unmanageable demands on the patient's internal and external resources.

9. Helen cooperates and willingly follows the treatment regimen. The nurse wonders how Helen can project such a positive outlook and cope with additional stress. Helen's ability to cope is probably due to all of the following *except*:
a. acceptance that "life is not fair" and that people have limited control over their health.
b. adoption of the problem-focused method of coping.
c. her ability to draw on past coping behaviors and apply them to new situations.
d. the support of family and friends who call and visit frequently

10. The neural and hormonal activities that respond to stress and maintain homeostasis are located in the:
a. cerebral cortex.
b. hypothalamus.
c. medulla oblongata.
d. pituitary gland.

11. Elizabeth is newly admitted to the medical unit. She has periodic episodes of shortness of breath and tightness in her throat. She is crying. To evaluate the impact of physiologic and psychological components on her illness, the nurse should:
a. perform a thorough physical examination and include subjective patient statements as well as objective laboratory data.
b. focus primary attention on the respiratory system, because this is the patient's chief complaint.
c. determine that the patient is not in acute distress, and then perform a complete physical examination and include data about the patient's lifestyle and social relationships.
d. attempt to discover the reasons behind the patient's anxieties, because stress can cause breathing difficulties.

12. During the nursing interview, a patient with shortness of breath reveals that she is in the process of getting a divorce. This information alerts the nurse to initially:
a. try to determine whether there is a psychological basis for the patient's physical symptoms.
b. restrict family members from visiting, because their presence may aggravate the patient's symptoms.
c. teach the patient specific breathing exercises that can be used to manage symptoms.
d. request that the physician recommend counseling services.

13. A patient is admitted to the emergency department for observation after a minor automobile accident. Based on an understanding of the sympathetic nervous system's response to stress, the nurse would expect to find all of the following during assessment *except*:
a. cold, clammy skin.
b. decreased heart rate.
c. rapid respirations.
d. skeletal muscle tension.

14. Physiologically, the sympathetic-adrenal-medullary response results in all of the following *except*:
a. decreased blood flow to the abdominal viscera.
b. decreased peripheral vasoconstriction.
c. increased myocardial contractility.
d. increased secretion of serum glucose.

15. The hypothalamic-pituitary response is a long-acting physiologic response to stress that involves:
    a. stimulation of the anterior pituitary to produce adrenocorticotropic hormone (ACTH).
    b. the production of cortisol from the adrenal cortex.
    c. protein catabolism and gluconeogenesis.
    d. all of the above mechanisms.

16. An example of a negative feedback process is increased:
    a. aldosterone secretion in burn trauma, resulting in excess sodium retention.
    b. cardiac output in hemorrhage, resulting in increased blood loss.
    c. secretion of antidiuretic hormone (ADH) in congestive heart failure, causing increased fluid retention.
    d. secretion of thyroid-stimulating factor (TSF), which stops when circulating thyroxin levels reach normal.

17. A patient experiences lower leg pain associated with lactic acid accumulation (an example of a local response involving a feedback loop). The nurse expects the pain to lessen when:
    a. aerobic metabolism is reinstated.
    b. anaerobic metabolism becomes the major pathway for energy release.
    c. muscle use and subsequent glucose catabolism increase.
    d. vasoconstriction diminishes blood flow, thereby slowing the removal of waste products.

18. A patient has a diagnosis of hypertrophy of the heart muscle (an example of cellular adaptation to injury). The nurse expects all of the following *except*:
    a. compromised cardiac output.
    b. muscle mass changes evident on radiologic examinations.
    c. cellular alteration compensatory to some stiumlus.
    d. decreased cell size, leading to more effective ventricular contractions.

19. Cell injury results when stressors interfere with the body's optimal balance by altering cellular ability to:
    a. grow and reproduce.
    b. synthesize enzymes.
    c. transform energy.
    d. do all of the above.

20. An adult patient's hemoglobin is 7g/dL. This should alert the nurse to assess for signs and symptoms associated with:
    a. hyperemia.
    b. hypertension.
    c. hypoglycemia.
    d. hypoxia.

21. A diabetic is admitted to the hospital with a blood sugar level of 320 mg/dL. The nurse decides to monitor fluid intake and output because:
    a. decreased blood osmolarity causes fluid to shift into the interstitial spaces, resulting in polydipsia.
    b. polydipsia occurs when glucose catabolism is accelerated, thereby increasing the body's need for fluids.
    c. polyuria results from osmotic diuresis, which is compensatory to hyperglycemia.
    d. the blood's hypotonicity will result in tissue fluid retention and weight gain.

22. Nursing care for a patient with a fever is based on all of the following body responses *except*:
    a. Diaphoresis, which is a compensatory mechanism that cools the body.
    b. Increased heart rate, which helps to meet increased metabolic demands.
    c. Increased nutrient catabolism, which influences the body's caloric needs.
    d. Vasodilation of surface blood vessels, which prevents excessive heat loss.

23. Anti-infective drugs are not useful against biologic agents known as:
    a. bacteria.
    b. fungi.
    c. mycoplasmas.
    d. viruses.

24. Viruses are infectious agents that:
    a. burst out of invaded cells to enter other cells.
    b. infect specific cells.
    c. replicate within invaded cells.
    d. do all of the above.

25. Genetic disorders arising from inherited traits include all of the following *except*:
a. hemophilia.
b. meningitis.
c. phenylketonuria.
d. sickle cell anemia.

26. A nurse who is caring for a patient with a localized response to a bee sting expects symptoms to include all of the following *except*:
a. blanching due to compensatory vasoconstriction.
b. hyperemia due to increased blood flow.
c. pain due to pressure on the nerve endings.
d. swelling due to increased vascular permeability.

27. While caring for a patient with an infected surgical incision, the nurse observes for signs of a systemic response. These include all of the following *except*:
a. leukopenia owing to increased white blood cell production.
b. a febrile state caused by the release of pyrogens.
c. anorexia, malaise, and weakness.
d. loss of appetitie and complaints of aching.

28. Research has shown that the single most important fator influencing an individual's health is:
a. health insurance coverage.
b. income.
c. level of education.
d. social relationships.

29. Nursing assessment to determine individual social support systems includes obtaining information about the person's:
a. belief that he or she belongs to a group that is mutually dependent and communicative.
b. concept of being cared for and loved.
c. impression of being esteemed and valued.
d. perception of all of the above.

30. Mrs. Talbot is scheduled for a breast biopsy in the morning. There is a history of breast malignancy in her family. While caring for her the evening before surgery, the most appropriate nursing action would be to:
a. administer a soothing back massage to promote relaxation and decrease stress.
b. make sure she eats all of her evening meal, because she will be NPO after midnight.
c. minimize the emotional impact of surgery by encouraging her to socialize with other patients.
d. sit with her and provide an opportunity for her to talk about her concerns.

Matching. *Match the primary category of stressors listed in Column II with its associated stressors listed in Column I.*

Column I

1._____ anxieties

2._____ genetic disorders

3._____ hypoxia

4._____ infectious agents

5._____ life changes

6._____ nutritional imbalance

7._____ social relationships

8._____ trauma

Column II

a. physiologic

b. psychosocial

Fill-In. *Read each statement carefully. Write your response in the space provided.*

1. Define a *maladaptive* response to a stressor. _____

2. Explain why *hyperpnea,* after intense exercise, is considered an adaptive response to a physiologic stressor.

_____

_____

3. Give an example of an *acute, time-limited* stressor versus a *chronic, enduring* stressor.

_____

4. Psychosocial stressors are classified as day-to-day occurrences (daily hassles), major events that affect large groups, and those infrequently occurring situations that directly affect a person. List two examples from your personal experiences that could be included under each classification.

a. Day-to-day occurrences   a. _____

                 _____

b. Major events that affect large groups of people b. _____

                 _____

c. Infrequently occurring major stressors   c. _____

5. Discuss the linkage between illness and critical life events.

_____

_____

_____

6. Discuss how internal cognitive processes and external resources are used by an individual to manage stress.

_____

_____

_____

7. Define stress according to Hans Selye:

_____

_____

II. Critical Thinking Questions and Exercises

Clinical Situations

Complete the flow chart. Fill in the physiologic reactions of the body that respond to sympathetic, nervous system stimulation, and provide the rationale for each reaction.

General body arousal	*Physiologic Reaction*	*Rationale*
↑ Norepinephrine =	↑_____	_____
	↑_____	↑_____
	↑_____	_____
	↑_____	↑_____
↓		
Effects on:		
Skeletal muscles	_____	↑_____
Pupils	_____	↑_____
Ventilation	_____	_____

Read the following case study. Fill in the blanks below.

CASE STUDY: Hypertensive Heart Disease

The body is capable of integrated responses to stress mediated by the sympathetic nervous system and the hypothalamic-pituitary-adrenocortical axis (see Fig. 6–2, p. 85 in the text). Use the clinical diagnosis, hypertensive heart disease, as an example of the body's response to stress.

Renin secretion is compensatory to decreased renal blood flow. Renin indirectly leads to sodium and water retention by stimulating the release of aldosterone. This mechanism initially results in increased cardiac output. For each compensatory mechanism shown, list nursing implications (assessment, nursing diagnoses/collaborative problems, planning, implementation, and evaluation) and give a rationale for each.

Selected Compensatory Mechanisms	*Nursing Implications*	*Rationale*
a. Renal blood flow is decreased as a result of hypertensive heart disease.	Assessment _____ _____ _____ Nursing Diagnoses _____ _____ Collaborative Problems _____ _____ Planning _____ Implementation _____ Evaluation	_____ _____ _____ _____ _____ _____ _____ _____ _____ _____ _____
b. Arteriole constriction occurs, resulting from renin secretion.		
c. Sodium and water retention occurs subsequent to aldosterone secretion.		
d. Increased cardiac output occurs as a result of increased extracellular fluid.		

Identifying Patterns

The sympathetic-adrenal-medullary response and the hypothalamic-pituitary response to stressors are adaptive and protective mechanisms that maintain homeostasis in the body.

Based on the information provided in the text, please complete the following flow chart.

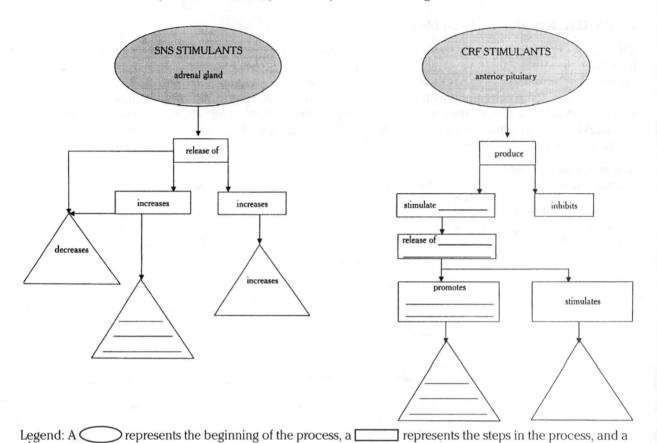

Legend: A ⬭ represents the beginning of the process, a ▭ represents the steps in the process, and a △ represents the physiologic end responses. Use pages 75–78 and Figure 6–1 as a guide.

7

Individual and Family Considerations Related to Illness

I. Interpretation, Completion, and Comparison

Multiple Choice. *Read each question carefully. Circle your answer.*

1. Compelling research has been established to show that the health of the immune system is correlated to the functioning of the:
   a. central nervous system.
   b. emotional moods and behavior.
   c. neuroendocrine responses.
   d. interconnections among all of the above.

2. To examine an individual's response to illness, a nurse should:
   a. analyze the way the patient thinks about stress, illness, and adaptive behavior.
   b. observe the patient's present behavior.
   c. obtain a description of the patient's previous coping mechanisms
   d. do all of the above.

3. A person's perception of illness as a stressor is primarily influenced by:
   a. finances.
   b. intelligence.
   c. occupational status.
   d. previous coping experiences.

4. The basic system disturbance believed to be responsible for the symptoms of posttraumatic stress disorder (PTSD) is in the:
   a. cardiopulmonary system.
   b. neurologic system.
   c. renal system.
   d. respiratory system.

5. The incidence of PTSD in high-risk groups is approximately:
   a. 10%–15%.
   b. 30%.
   c. 50%.
   d. 75% or greater.

6. In the United States, approximately _____ of clinically depressed individuals commit suicide.
   a. 5%
   b. 15%
   c. 25%
   d. 40%

7. Which of the following is *not* considered a risk for suicide?
   a. altered body image.
   b. family history.
   c. female gender.
   d. age 25–35 years.

8. It took Mr. A 3 months to admit that he was sick and in need of medical and nursing care and to accept his diagnosis of adenocarcinoma of the right kidney. An initial emotional response the nurse would expect to see associated with loss and grief is:
a. shame.
b. denial.
c. guilt and shame.
d. regression.

9. Nursing interventions to help a patient deal with denial include:
a. allowing the patient to use denial when it serves an immediate purpose and is not harmful.
b. challenging the patient's use of denial as a defense mechanism.
c. encouraging the use of denial as a satisfactory method of dealing with illness.
d. supporting the denial behavior, knowing that the patient needs this coping mechanism.

10. A communication breakdown will most probably occur if a nurse:
a. anticipates barriers to communication and works out solutions in advance.
b. clarifies facts about an illness with the patient during the patient's denial of that illness.
c. plans a teaching session for a time when the patient is free from pain.
d. presents a teaching program when the patient demonstrates a readiness to learn.

11. Mrs. Renton is hospitalized in the final states of metastatic carcinoma. She tells her physician that she will accept her prognosis if he can keep her alive until her grandchild is born in 3 months. Mrs. Renton is in that stage of dying identified by Kubler-Ross as:
a. isolation.
b. anger.
c. bargaining.
d. depression.

Fill-In. *Read each statement carefully. Write your response in the space provided.*

1. Write the most commonly accepted definition of a mental disorder.

_____

2. List the five major family functions described by Wright and Leahy (2000) that significantly influence an individual's response to illness.

a. _____   d. _____

b. _____   e. _____

c. _____

3. Record seven traits identified by Burr and associates (1994) that enhance coping of family members under stress.

a. _____   e. _____

b. _____   f. _____

c. _____   g. _____

d. _____

4. Identify five common emotional responses to post-traumatic stress disorder (PTSD).

a. _____   d. _____

b. _____   e. _____

c. _____

5. Three physiologic responses to PTSD are increased:_____, _____, and

_____ .

6. Document seven life events that are known to trigger symptoms of PTSD.

a. _____   e. _____

b. _____   f. _____

c. _____   g. _____

d. _____

7. List two common substance abuse problems.

a. _____

b. _____

Matching. *Match the classification of a complementary and alternative therapy listed in Column II with a specific type of holistic care listed in Column I.*

Column I

1._____ hypnosis

2._____ reiki

3._____ acupuncture

4._____ chiropracty

5._____ dietary plans

6._____ Ayuveda

7._____ therapeutic touch

8._____ homeopathic medicine

9._____ dance and music

10._____ Qi gong

Column II

a. alternative medical systems

b. biologically based systems

c. energy therapies

d. manipulative methods

e. mind-body interventions

II. Critical Thinking Questions and Exercises

Recognizing Contradictions

Rewrite each statement correctly. Underline the key concepts.

1. Since 1980, there has been a gradual decline in the number of individuals who seek holistic health care treatment.

2. The philosophical framework supporting holistic health care is emphasis on the spiritual domain of healing.

3. Clinical depression is a common response to health problems, especially for the young and the elderly.

4. The majority of people who commit suicide are depressed, isolated from friends, and have not sought personal or professional help.

5. A diagnosis of clinical depression requires repeated episodes of sadness over a 4-week period.

Clinical Situations

Read the following case studies. Circle the correct answer.

CASE STUDY: Hodgkin's Disease

Joan, a 29-year-old mother of two, works 20 hours a week as a secretary. She was diagnosed with Hodgkin's disease the week of her 29th birthday.

1. Joan's reaction to the diagnosis was to increase her working time to 40 hours per week and to increase her social activities. Joan's response is characteristic of the:
   a. first stage of illness.
   b. second stage of illness.
   c. third stage of illness.
   d. fourth stage of illness.

2. The most prominent emotion the nurse would expect Joan to experience at the time of her diagnosis is:
   a. acceptance.
   b. denial.
   c. depression.
   d. guilt.

3. Nursing intervention at the time of the diagnosis would *not* include:
   a. answering questions.
   b. listening to the patient ventilate.
   c. reinforcing reality.
   d. supporting denial.

CASE STUDY: Radical Mastectomy

Kathy, a 45-year-old, single executive with a major oil company, lives alone in a high-rise city apartment. She is recovering from a right radical mastectomy performed 3 days ago.

1. Kathy is firm about not bathing in the morning because her normal home routine involves a nightly relaxing tub bath. The nurse should:
   a. document in the plan of care that bathing is to take place near bedtime.
   b. explain the clinical routine to Kathy to help her understand the necessity for each patient to comply so that all patients will receive optimum care.
   c. gently remind Kathy that she is not in control in a hospital; the nurses decide when baths will be taken.
   d. give Kathy a choice of morning bath care or evening shower care, because staffing on the evening shift is not sufficient to meet her needs.

2. Kathy refuses to acknowledge that her breast was removed. She believes that her breast is intact under the dressings. The nurse should:
   a. call the physician to change the dressings so that Kathy can see the incision.
   b. recognize that Kathy is experiencing denial, a normal stage of the grieving process.
   c. reinforce Kathy's belief for several days, until her body can adjust to the stress of surgery.
   d. remind Kathy that she needs to accept her diagnosis so that she can begin rehabilitation exercises.

3. Kathy screams at her nurse because the nurse is 10 minutes late administering Kathy's pain medication. The nurse is aware that anger:
   a. is a maladaptive response to a stressful situation.
   b. is an anticipated reaction to a change in body appearance.
   c. should be reinforced to help reality orientation.
   d. should be repressed so that Kathy can gain control of her surroundings.

4. To help Kathy adjust to her altered body image, the nurse should:
   a. offer acceptance.
   b. reinforce Kathy's concept of self-worth.
   c. understand Kathy's emotional responses to her illness and her surgery.
   d. all of the above.

8

Perspectives in Transcultural Nursing

I. Interpretation, Completion, and Comparison

Multiple Choice. Read each question carefully. Circle your answer.

1. Choose the minority group in the United States that is not federally recognized as a minority:
   a. Asian/Pacific Islanders.
   b. Hispanic Americans.
   c. Native Americans.
   d. Islamics.

2. The most common non-English language spoken in the United States is:
   a. German.
   b. French.
   c. Italian.
   d. Spanish.

3. Madeline Leininger's theory of transcultural nursing supports providing care that:
   a. allows for restructuring.
   b. can be accommodated.
   c. is congruent.
   d. reflects all of the above characteristics.

4. Personal space is a culturally defined phenomenon. In comparing cultures, individuals who require the *most* personal space between themselves and others would be from:
   a. Japan.
   b. Latin America.
   c. the Middle East.
   d. the United States.

5. Choose the culture that does *not* consider eye contact to be impolite when speaking with another:
   a. American.
   b. Arabian.
   c. Indo-Chinese.
   d. Native American.

6. The cultural group in which staring at the floor during conversation is considered behavior conveying respect is the:
   a. Asian.
   b. Appalachian.
   c. Indo-Chinese.
   d. Native American.

7. The cultural group that has a wide frame of reference for attitudes about time is the:
   a. Hispanic.
   b. Arabian.
   c. Native American.
   d. Asian.

8. The nurse would expect that a woman from the _____ culture would want only a female physician to examine her.
   a. Arabian.
   b. Asian.
   c. Japanese.
   d. Latin American.

9. Choose the religious group that shuns the use of caffeine-containing beverages:
   a. Hindu.
   b. Jewish.
   c. Mormon.
   d. Seventh Day Adventist.

10. The yin-yang theory of harmony and illness is rooted in the _____ paradigm of health and illness.
    a. biomedical.
    b. holistic.
    c. religious.
    d. scientific.

Fill In. Read each statement carefully. Write your response in the space provided.

1. The founder of transcultural nursing is: _____

2. Name the four basic characteristics of culture.

   _____, _____,

   _____, and _____

3. Three elements used to identify diversity are: _____, _____, and

   _____.

4. Give at least five examples of groupings that can be used to identity subcultures.

   _____, _____, _____,

   _____, and _____

5. List four strategies that individuals tend to use when communication has broken down.

   _____, _____,

   _____, and _____

6. Name four religious groups that routinely incorporate fasting into the religious practice.

   _____, _____,

   _____, and _____

7. Explain the concept of yin-yang.

   _____

   _____

II. Critical Thinking Questions and Exercises

Discussion and Analysis

1. Explain the goal of Madeleine Leininger's comprehensive theory, "Culture Care Diversity and Universality."

   _____

   _____

2. Explain the concepts of *culture care accommodation* and *culture care restructuring,* according to Leininger.

   _____

   _____

3. Distinguish between the terms *acculturation* and *cultural imposition*.

   _____

   _____

9

Genetics Perspectives in Nursing

1. Interpretation, Completion, and Comparison

Multiple Choice. *Read each question carefully. Circle your answer.*

1. The study of gene mapping and function is known as:
   a. genetics.
   b. genomics.
   c. meiosis.
   d. mitosis.

2. Chromosomes are located within the nucleus of a cell. The human body has _____ chromosomes.
   a. 23.
   b. 46.
   c. 69.
   d. 92.

3. *Trisomy* refers to a condition in which cellular division results in an extra chromosome. An example of trisomy is:
   a. Down's syndrome.
   b. sickle cell anemia.
   c. Tay-Sachs disease.
   d. Turner's syndrome.

4. Stephanie has learned that her ovarian cancer syndrome is an autosomal dominant inherited condition. Stephanie knows that her daughter has a _____ chance of inheriting the gene mutation for this disease.
   a. 10%–15%
   b. 25%
   c. 50%
   d. 60%–80%

5. An example of an autosomal recessive inherited condition is:
   a. cystic fibrosis.
   b. hereditary breast cancer.
   c. Huntington's disease.
   d. familial hypercholesterolemia.

6. Katie has just been told that she has the *BRCA1* hereditary breast cancer gene mutation. At age 32, she knows that her risk of developing cancer by the age of 65 years is:
   a. 25%.
   b. 50%.
   c. 80%.
   d. 100%.

7. Kurt and Kathy are carriers for thalassemia. They are thinking about starting a family. A nurse tells them that they have a _____ risk of having a child who will inherit the gene.
   a. 25%.
   b. 50%.
   c. 75%.
   d. 100%.

8. An example of an X-linked, recessive inherited condition, which a mother (carrier) has a 50% chance of passing onto her son, is:

a. cystic fibrosis.

b. hemophilia.

c. phenylketonuria.

d. Tay-Sachs disease.

9. A multifactorial genetic condition that tends to cluster in families is:

a. galactosemia.

b. Duchenne muscular dystrophy.

c. neurofibromatosis.

d. neural tube defects.

10. When assessing patient information as part of genetic counseling, the nurse knows that Tay-Sachs disease is most common among:

a. Ashkenazi Jews.

b. Italian Americans.

c. American Indians.

d. African Americans.

Fill-In. *Read each statement. Write your response in the space provided.*

1. The term *genomic medicine* refers to:

_____

2. The nurse uses a framework for integrating genetics into nursing practice when he or she:

a. _____

b. _____

c. _____

d. _____

3. The term *penetrance* refers to: _____

4. Name the common chromosomal condition that occurs with greater frequency in pregnancies of women who are 35 years of age or older: _____.

5. The frequency of chromosomal abnormalities in newborns is: _____.

6. Define the term *pharmacogenetics:*

_____

7. The most common adult-onset condition in Causasian populations is: _____.

8. List five nursing activities in genetics-related nursing practice:

a. _____

b. _____

c. _____

d. _____

e. _____

Matching. _Match the age of adult onset in Column II with the specific disorder listed in Column I._

Column I

1. _____ spinocerebellar ataxia, type 2

2. _____ Huntingdon's disease

3. _____ early-onset familial Alzheimer's disease

4. _____ hereditary hemochromatosis

5. _____ spinocerebellar ataxia, type 3

6. _____ polycystic kidney disease

7. _____ familial hypercholesterolemia

8. _____ amotrophic lateral sclerosis (ALS)

Column II

a. mean age of 30 years

b. 30–40 years

c. 35–44 years

d. 40–60 years

e. 60–65 years

f. 50–70 years

10

Chronic Illness

I. Interpretation, Completion, and Comparison

Multiple Choice. Read each question carefully. Circle your answer.

1. A medical condition is considered *chronic* when long-term management is required for a *minimum* of:
   a. 8 weeks.
   b. 3 months.
   c. 16 weeks.
   d. 6 months.

2. It is estimated that the number of people afflicted with chronic conditions will _____ by the year 2030.
   a. decrease by 25%
   b. double
   c. increase by 50%
   d. triple

3. It is projected that the direct medical costs for those with chronic illness, over the next 10 years, will:
   a. decrease by 5%.
   b. grow about 1% per year.
   c. increase by 20%.
   d. remain the same.

4. As chronic conditions increase over the next 20 years, it is expected that the percentage of individuals with limitations of a major activity will approach:
   a. 30%.
   b. 40%.
   c. 50%.
   d. 75%.

5. The most disabling chronic condition in the United States is projected to be:
   a. extremity paralysis.
   b. mental retardation.
   c. multiple sclerosis.
   d. respiratory cancers.

6. Identify the chronic illness that is increasing rapidly and is directly related to an unhealthy lifestyle.
   a. diabetes mellitus
   b. breast cancer
   c. emphysema
   d. colorectal cancer

7. A major health-promoting behavior that can significantly improve the quality of life for those with a chronic condition is:
   a. diet.
   b. exercise.
   c. hydration.
   d. rest.

8. A person who is at risk for developing a chronic condition because of genetic factors is said to be in the _____ phase of the Trajectory Model.
   a. pretrajectory
   b. trajectory
   c. unstable
   d. acute

9. Chronic illness can be monitored using the Trajectory Model. The phase in which a nursing diagnosis can help in care planning is known as:
   a. pretrajectory.
   b. trajectory.
   c. crisis.
   d. downward course.

10. Remission after an exacerbation represents the Trajectory Model phase known as:
    a. acute.
    c. comeback.
    b. crisis.
    d. downward course.

Fill-In. Read each statement carefully. Write your response in the space provided.

1. List four factors believed to significantly increase the occurrence of chronic conditions in the United States.

   _____, _____,

   _____, and _____

2. List three characteristics common to all forms of chronic illness: _____,
   _____, and _____.

3. The two most frequent interferences with activities of daily living (ADL) related to chronic illness are:

   _____ and _____.

4. The occurrence of most chronic conditions can be traced to three activities that can be modified to prevent the severity of the condition. The activities are: _____, _____,

   and _____.

5. List six common management problems related to chronic conditions.

   a. _____   d. _____

   b. _____   e. _____

   c. _____   f. _____

6. Define the concept of the Trajectory Model as it relates to chronic illness.

   _____

   _____

II. Critical Thinking Questions and Exercises

Examining Associations

Listed below are some characteristics of chronic illness. For each characteristic, write a description of its implications that can be affected by nursing care.

1. Managing chronic illness involves more than managing medical problems.

   _____

2. Chronic conditions are associated with different phases over a course of time.

   _____

3. Managing chronic conditions requires adherence to a therapeutic regimen.

   _____

4. Chronic illness affects the whole family.

5. Management is a collaborative process.

6. Chronic conditions mean living with uncertainty.

Clinical Applications

CASE STUDY: Use of the Trajectory Model

The focus of care for patients with chronic illness is determined by their phase of illness (refer to Chart 10–1). Each phase can be correlated to a step in the nursing process. For each step below, discuss the role of nursing, which includes assessment, diagnosis, planning, implementation, and evaluation. Use as an example a 32-year-old mother of one who works full-time as a teacher and has just been diagnosed with rheumatoid arthritis.

Step 1: Identify the Trajectory Phase
Step 2: Establish goals
Step 3: Establish a plan to meet the identified goals
Step 4: Identify factors that facilitate or hinder the attainment of goals.
Step 5: Implement interventions

11

Principles and Practices of Rehabilitation

I. Interpretation, Completion, and Comparison

Multiple Choice. Read each question carefully. Circle your answer.

1. Rehabilitation, an integral part of nursing, should begin:
   a. after the patient feels comfortable in the clinical setting.
   b. after the physician has prescribed rehabilitative goals.
   c. when an exercise program has been initiated.
   d. with initial patient contact.

2. In the United States, approximately _____ of Americans have some form of disability.
   a. 10%
   b. 20%
   c. 40%
   d. 60%

3. The normal first emotional reactions to a disability are:
   a. anger and hostility.
   b. confusion and denial.
   c. depression and regression.
   d. grief and mourning.

4. The key member of the rehabilitation team is the:
   a. nurse.
   b. patient.
   c. physical therapist.
   d. physician.

5. The occurrence of spinal cord and traumatic brain injuries is directly associated with substance abuse, alcohol, and the use of illegal drugs. The percentage of patients who are under the influence at the time of injury is as high as:
   a. 50%.
   b. 75%.
   c. 80%.
   d. 95%.

6. The PULSES profile uses six components to evaluate self-care independence. The assessment of bladder control would be documented under:
   a. "E," excretory function.
   b. "L," lower system functions.
   c. "P," physical condition.
   d. "S," sensory functions.

7. The *least* common position used in positioning a patient in bed to prevent musculoskeletal complications is:
   a. prone.
   b. semi-Fowler's.
   c. side-lying.
   d. supine

8. A nurse who wants to help a patient assume the side-lying position would:
a. align the lower extremities in a neutral position.
b. extend the legs with a firm support under the popliteal area.
c. place the uppermost hip slightly forward in a position of slight abduction.
d. position the trunk so that hip flexion is minimized.

9. A quick method used to measure for crutches is to use the patient's height and:
a. add 6 inches.
b. add 12 inches.
c. subtract 8 inches.
d. subtract 16 inches.

10. A pressure ulcer is associated with the presence of:
a. dehydration and skin dryness.
b. excessive skin moisture.
c. inflammation and infection.
d. small nutrient vessel compression.

11. Initial skin redness in a patient susceptible to pressure sores should be documented as tissue:
a. anoxia.
b. eschar.
c. hyperemia.
d. ischemia.

12. A patient at potential risk for a pressure ulcer is assessed by the nurse. A laboratory study the nurse should examine is:
a. serum albumin.
b. serum glucose.
c. prothrombin time.
d. sedimentation rate.

13. A diet recommended for hypoproteinemia that "spares" protein is one high in:
a. carbohydrates.
b. fats.
c. minerals.
d. vitamins.

14. Wound healing depends on collagen formation, which depends on vitamin:
a. A.
b. C.
c. D.
d. K.

15. A rehabilitation program for an elderly patient with a hip fracture must focus on the:
a. impact of multiple system pathology on recovery.
b. influence of mental status changes on health improvement.
c. periodic physiologic evaluation of bone repair.
d. value of all of the above factors.

16. Insufficient cerebral circulation can result from the use of the tilt table and can be identified by:
a. diaphoresis.
b. nausea.
c. tachycardia.
d. all of the above.

17. Weight bearing on long bones is essential for preventing:
a. calcium loss.
b. potassium loss.
c. protein loss.
d. sodium loss.

18. To initiate a schedule of bladder training, the nurse should:
a. encourage the patient to wait 30 minutes after drinking a measured amount of fluid before attempting to void.
b. give up to 2500 mL of fluid daily.
c. teach bladder massage to increase intra-abdominal pressure.
d. do all of the above.

19. Successful bowel training depends on:
a. a daily defecation time that is within 15 minutes of the same time every day.
b. an adequate intake of fiber-containing foods.
c. fluid intake between 2 and 4 L/day.
d. all of the above.

20. Sexual problems faced by the disabled include:
a. impaired self-image.
b. lack of opportunities to form friendships.
c. limited access to information about sexuality.
d. all of the above.

Fill-In. *Read each statement carefully. Write your response in the space provided.*

1. The American with Disabilities Act went into effect in July 1992. This act requires employers to provide access to facilitate employment of a person with a disability. The two phrases that mandate compliance are: _____ and _____.

2. Define the term *contracture* as it relates to impaired physical mobility.

   _____

3. List three complications commonly associated with prolonged or impaired physical immobility: _____, _____, and _____.

4. Two common musculoskeletal complications for patients who are in bed for prolonged periods are:

   _____ and _____.

5. Four factors that contribute to footdrop are: _____, _____,

   _____, and _____.

6. A joint should be moved through its range of motion _____ times, at least once a day.

7. For crutch-walking, the sequence for the four-point gait begins with the _____ crutch and ends with the _____ foot.

8. Examples of orthotic devices include:

   _____

9. Life-threatening complications of pressure sores include:

   _____

10. Eschar covering an ulcer should be removed surgically because eschar:

    _____

Matching. *Match the explanations of range-of-motion techniques listed in Column II with their associated terms in Column I.*

Column I	Column II
1.____ adduction	a. bending of the foot toward the leg
2.____ dorsiflexion	b. increasing the angle of a joint
3.____ extension	c. movement away from the midline of the body
4.____ inversion	d. movement that turns the sole of the foot inward
5.____ pronation	e. movement toward the midline of the body
6.____ abduction	f. rotating the forearm so that the palm is down

II. Critical Thinking Questions, Exercises, and Issues

Discussion and Analysis

1. A 65-year-old woman is recovering from surgery to repair a compound fracture of the femur. She will be discharged to home in 24 hours. One nursing diagnosis is Self-care deficit, bathing and dressing. After assessing her limitations in performing activities of daily living (ADL), the nurse designs a plan of care. Refer to Chart 11–2 on page 164 to outline specific nursing activities related to teaching ADL.

2. A patient has been diagnosed with impaired physical mobility due to a lower leg deformity. After assessment, the nurse selects a nursing diagnosis that can be used to design a plan of care. List several possible nursing diagnoses.

Clinical Situations

View Figure 11–4, page 176 of the text, and answer the following clinically focused questions regarding impaired skin integrity.

1. Define the term *pressure ulcer.*

_____

2. The initial sign of pressure is _____ caused by _____.

3. The two most susceptible surfaces for pressure ulcer formation are the _____ and the

_____.

4. The least favorable position to use to shift body weight would be:
   a. prone.
   b. recumbent.
   c. semi-Fowler's.
   d. side-lying.

5. The patient should be repositioned:
   a. every 30 minutes.
   b. hourly.
   c. every 3 to 4 hours.
   d. once per shift.

6. Based on the _____ law, explain why a gel-type flotation pad and an air-fluidized bed reduce pressure:

_____

7. Explain why the shearing force is increased when the head of the bed is raised, even if only by a few centimeters.

_____

Read the following case studies. Circle the correct answers.

CASE STUDY: Traumatic Amputation Psychosocial Perspective

Oliver, a 42-year-old mechanical engineer, works at a major paper mill. While he was doing routine maintenance work, his foot slipped, and he fell against an industrial paper cutter. He suffered a traumatic amputation of his left hand.

1. The nurse expects Oliver's initial emotional reaction on admission to the emergency department to be one of:
   a. adjustment and acceptance.
   b. anger and regression.
   c. denial and confusion.
   d. grief and depression.

2. If Oliver begins to mourn for his missing body part, the nurse should:
   a. emphasize all the abilities he has with his remaining hand.
   b. encourage him to cheer up.
   c. listen as he talks about his loss.
   d. remind him of his limited abilities, to reinforce reality.

3. The nurse notices that Oliver blames his loss on his family, because he has rationalized that he had to work in a dangerous area to generate sufficient income to support his seven children and his dependent parents. A nursing care plan for Oliver should include:
   a. advising him about budgeting his income to minimize the stress associated with financial worries.
   b. allowing him to project his emotions.
   c. demonstrating self-assistive devices that will help him meet his activities of daily living.
   d. encouraging him to have a positive attitude toward his disability to facilitate his recovery.

4. After several weeks, Oliver seems to be adjusting to his disability. Behaviors consistent with this period include:
   a. acceptance of his limitations.
   b. interest in obtaining information about his disability.
   c. redirecting his energies toward coping.
   d. all of the above.

CASE STUDY: Buck's Extension Traction

Patricia is 67 years old and has limited mobility as a result of a right hip fracture. She is in Buck's extension traction awaiting surgery.

1. During morning care, the nurse suggests that Patricia attempt isometric exercises of her legs. This suggestion is based on the nurse's goal of:
   a. encouraging normal muscle function.
   b. maintaining muscle strength while immobilizing the joints.
   c. providing resistance to increase muscle strength.
   d. retaining as much joint range of motion as possible.

2. The nursing goals associated with therapeutic isometric exercises include all of the following *except:*
   a. enhanced joint mobility.
   b. improved patient well-being.
   c. increased strength of the musculature that controls the joints.
   d. prevention of venous stasis.

3. To assist Patricia with isometric exercises of her lower extremities, the nurse should teach her to:
   a. contract or tighten her thigh and calf muscles without moving her knees and hip joints, hold for several seconds, and then "let go."
   b. slowly move her legs through limited range of motion while the nurse stabilizes the proximal joint and supports the distal part.
   c. move her legs through their full range of motion while the nurse supports each distal part.
   d. put each leg through full range of motion while the nurse offers slight resistance to the movement.

CASE STUDY: Assisted Ambulation: Crutches

Rita, a 17-year-old college student, is in a full leg cast because of a compound fracture of the left femur. Rita is to be discharged from the hospital in several days. She lives with her parents in a split-level house.

1. The exercises that the nurse would recommend to strengthen Rita's upper extremity muscles are:
   a. isometric exercises of the biceps.
   b. push-ups performed in a sitting position.
   c. gluteal setting.
   d. quadriceps setting.

2. Rita is 5 feet, 5 inches tall. Her crutches should measure:
   a. 45 inches.
   b. 49 inches.
   c. 54 inches.
   d. 59 inches.

3. Before teaching a crutch gait, the nurse directs Rita to assume the tripod position. In this basic crutch stance, the crutches are placed in front and to the side of Rita's toes, at an approximate distance of:
   a. 4–6 inches.
   b. 6–8 inches.
   c. 8–10 inches.
   d. 10–12 inches.

4. Because Rita is not allowed to bear weight on her casted leg, she should be taught the:
   a. two-point gait.
   b. three-point gait.
   c. four-point gait.
   d. swing-through gait.

12

Health Care of the Older Adult

I. Interpretation, Completion, and Comparison

Multiple Choice. Read each question carefully. Circle your answer.

1. The study of old age is referred to as:
   a. ageism.
   b. geriatrics.
   c. gerontonics.
   d. gerontology.

2. Psychological adjustment to aging is believed to be related to the successful completion of:
   a. aging.
   b. developmental tasks.
   c. physical adjustment.
   d. societal position.

3. Nursing interventions to help older people deal with psychological aging include:
   a. attentive listening.
   b. discussing their personal plans for the future.
   c. focusing their attention on the present.
   d. all of the above.

4. All of the following statements are true concerning Erikson's task of ego integrity *except:*
   a. one accepts one's lifestyle as it is.
   b. one feels dissatisfied with life.
   c. one is still in control of one's life.
   d. one has made the best choices for particular situations.

5. Choose the sociologic theory that suggests that adjustment to old age depends on the person's ability to continue life patterns throughout his or her lifetime.
   a. Activity
   b. Continuity
   c. Disengagement
   d. Adaptation

6. The process most sensitive to deterioration with aging seems to be:
   a. creativity.
   b. judgment.
   c. intelligence.
   d. short-term memory.

7. The leading cause of death in the aged is a disorder or dysfunction of the _____ system.
   a. cardiovascular
   b. genitourinary
   c. integumentary
   d. reproductive

8. The primary cause of hospitalization among the elderly is:
   a. congestive heart failure.
   b. emphysema.
   c. chronic renal failure.
   d. cancer of the lung.

9. The cardiac condition most frequently seen among the aged is:
  a. aortic stenosis.
  b. coronary artery disease.
  c. mitral valve prolapse.
  d. ventricular tachycardia.

10. Respiratory changes associated with aging include all of the following *except:*
  a. decreased residual volume.
  b. changes in the anteroposterior diameter of the chest.
  c. loss of elastic tissue surrounding the alveoli.
  d. reduced vital capacity.

11. All of the following statements concerning genitourinary system changes in the older adult are true *except*:
  a. The renal filtration rate decreases.
  b. The acid–base balance is restored more slowly.
  c. Bladder capacity increases with advanced age.
  d. Urinary frequency, urgency, and incontinence are common problems.

12. Dietary intake should emphasize fruits, vegetables and fish. The daily intake of carbohydrates should be about:
  a. 20%–25%.
  b. 40%–45%.
  c. 55%–60%.
  d. 70%–75%.

13. Bone changes associated with aging frequently result from a loss of:
  a. calcium.
  b. magnesium.
  c. vitamin A.
  d. vitamin C.

14. Nervous system changes associated with aging include all of the following *except:*
  a. a decrease in brain weight subsequent to the destruction of brain cells.
  b. an increase in blood flow to the brain to compensate for the gradual loss of brain cells.
  c. atrophy of the convolutions of the brain surface.
  d. widening and deepening of the spaces between the convolutions of the brain.

15. Nursing measures to deal with sensory changes in the aged include:
  a. increasing room lighting without increasing glare.
  b. speaking louder than normal.
  c. suggesting appetite stimulants before meals.
  d. all of the above actions.

16. The most common affective or mood disorder of old age is:
  a. Alzheimer's disease.
  b. delirium.
  c. depression.
  d. multi-infarct dementia.

17. The most common and preventable source of mortality and morbidity in older adults is:
  a. dehydration.
  b. emphysema.
  c. falls.
  d. melenoma.

18. Drug dosages must be reduced in the elderly because:
  a. cardiac output is significantly reduced.
  b. the number of mucosal cells in the gastrointestinal tract is reduced.
  c. drug biotransformation takes longer in older persons.
  d. all of the above are true.

19. The medications that remain in the body longer in the elderly because of increased body fat are:
  a. anticoagulants.
  b. barbiturates.
  c. digitalis glycosides.
  d. diuretics.

20. The seventh leading cause of death in older persons is:
  a. accidents and injuries.
  b. drug toxicity.
  c. elder abuse.
  d. malnutrition.

21. The major source of public funding that provides nursing home care for the poor elderly is:
  a. Medicaid.
  b. Medicare.

Fill-In. *Read each statement carefully. Write your response in the space provided.*

1. In approximately _____ years, there will be a higher percentage (_____%) of people older than 65 years of age than of those younger than 18 years of age (_____%).

2. A 75-year old woman today can expect to live to be about _____ years of age

3. The major cause of disability in those older than 65 years of age is _____.

4. The leading cause of death in those older than 65 years of age is _____, followed by _____ and _____.

5. The elderly's use of Medicare funding for hospitalization is about _____%.

6. The ability to acquire new information and learn new skills significantly decreases after the age of _____ years.

7. The dementias in older adults are characterized by a decrease in the following intellectual skills: _____, _____, _____, and _____.

8. List the five most common infections in the elderly.

   a. _____   d. _____

   b. _____   e. _____

   c. _____

II. Critical Thinking Questions and Exercises

Interpreting Data

Refer to Figure 12–1 to answer the following questions.

1. In the decade between the years 2000 and 2010, the percentage of people older than 65 years of age will increase by _____%.

2. In the decade between 2010 and 2020, the percentage increase in people older than 65 years will be _____%, more than _____ that of the prior 10 years (2000–2010).

3. Will the percentage of people older than 65 years of age continue to increase from 2020 to 2030 at a slower, equal, or greater rate? _____. The percentage increase for the decade is projected to be _____%.

4. The number of persons older than 65 years of age increased at an equal rate of growth (_____%) over the two time spans of _____ and _____.

5. By the year 2030, approximately _____ million individuals will be older than 65 years of age.

Recognizing Contradictions

Rewrite each statement correctly. Underline the key concepts.

1. Bones are composed of postmiotic cells that diminish and cause bone density.

2. Osteoporosis, accelerated by the loss of estrogen, can be reversed with a high-calcium diet.

3. If the symptoms of delirium go untreated, they will eventually decrease, and the person will regain his or her previous level of consciousness.

4. Older persons should "take it easy" and avoid vigorous activity.

5. Baseline body temperature is usually 1°F higher than normal in an older person because dehydration is common.

Clinical Situations

Read the following case studies. Circle the correct answer.

CASE STUDY: Loneliness

Suzanne is an 80-year-old retired schoolteacher. She was recently widowed and lives alone. She in financially secure but socially isolated, because she has outlived most of her friends. Her children are self-sufficient and are very busy with their own lives.

1. Psychological threats that Suzanne may experience include:
   a. a deterioration of self-concept.
   b. a loss of self-esteem.
   c. extensive grief over frequently occurring losses.
   d. all of the above.

2. Suzanne is concerned about the dryness of her skin. Suggestions for skin care include:
   a. applying ointment to the skin several times a day.
   b. avoiding overexposure to the sun.
   c. patting the skin dry instead of rubbing it with a towel.
   d. all of the above measures.

3. Suzanne notices that food does not taste the same as before. She needs to be aware that this sensory change is most probably related to:
   a. a decrease in the number of taste buds.
   b. a loss of appetite associated with a decreased sense of smell.
   c. altered enzyme secretions.
   d. diminished gastric secretions.

4. An analysis of Suzanne's diet shows that it does not contain adequate protein. Her daily protein intake, for a body weight of 134 lb, should be about:
   a. 30 g.
   b. 40 g.
   c. 50 g.
   d. 60 g.

5. Most accidents among older people involve falls within the home. Preventive nursing measures include advising Suzanne to:
   a. avoid climbing and bending.
   b. keep personal items stored at a level between her hips and her eyes.
   c. make certain that all her shoes fit securely.
   d. do all of the above.

CASE STUDY: Alzheimer's Disease

Thomas, a 75-year-old retired bricklayer, lives at home with Anne, his 65-year-old wife, who is healthy and active. Lately Anne has noticed that Thomas is negative, hostile, and suspicious of her. He gets lost in his own home, and his conversations have been accompanied by forgetfulness. Recently, Thomas' physician has indicated a probable diagnosis of Alzheimer's disease.

1. Choose the statement that is false concerning Alzheimer's disease.
   a. It is found only in old persons.
   b. The disease process is irreversible.
   c. The probable cause is neuropathologic and biochemical.
   d. The cells that are affected by the disease are the ones that use acetylcholine.

2. The nurse should suggest that Anne deal with Thomas' behavior by:
   a. reasoning with him.
   b. providing reality orientation.
   c. providing a calm and predictable environment.
   d. not structuring activities for him.

3. An important point to communicate to Anne is that:
   a. there are no realistic goals appropriate for Thomas.
   b. lists and written instructions will only tend to confuse Thomas.
   c. Thomas should be restrained when agitated.
   d. maintaining personal dignity and autonomy is still an important part of Thomas' life.

4. Caregivers of patients with Alzheimer's disease should be aware that:
   a. Alzheimer's support groups exist.
   b. Alzheimer's disease does not eliminate the need for intimacy.
   c. socializing with old friends may be comforting.
   d. all of the above are appropriate.

CASE STUDY: Dehydration

Vera, an 89-year-old widow, was transferred from a nursing home to a hospital with a diagnosis of dehydration. Vera needs to be in bed because of her generalized weakness. She is occasionally confused and disoriented.

1. From knowledge of temperature regulation in the elderly, the nurse should:
   a. make sure that the environmental temperature is adequate.
   b. palpate Vera's skin periodically to assess for warmth.
   c. place extra blankets at Vera's bedside in case she becomes cold, especially in the evening.
   d. do all of the above.

2. The nurse initiates a 2-hour turning schedule for Vera, based on the knowledge that the underlying cause of all decubiti is:
   a. altered skin turgor.
   b. nutritional deficiency.
   c. pressure.
   d. vasoconstriction.

3. Vera has been incontinent of urine since admission. Nursing interventions include all of the following *except:*
   a. initiating a bladder training program.
   b. offering fluids frequently to maintain a minimum daily intake of 2 to 3 L.
   c. providing means for limited daily exercises and ambulation.
   d. securing a physician's order for urethral catheterization.

4. The nurse suggests that Vera sit in a rocking chair for 20 minutes, four times a day. This suggestion is based on the knowledge that rocking:
   a. discourages hypostatic pulmonary congestion.
   b. increases pulmonary ventilation.
   c. improves venous return through contraction of the calf muscles.
   d. does all of the above.

UNIT 3

Concepts and Challenges in Patient Management

13

Pain Management

I. Interpretation, Completion, and Comparison

Multiple Choice. Read each question carefully. Circle your answer.

1. Although the criterion is arbitrary, acute pain can be classified as chronic when it has persisted for:
   a. 1–2 months.
   b. 3 months.
   c. 3–5 months.
   d. longer than 6 months.

2. Acute pain may be described as having the following characteristic.
   a. It does not usually respond well to treatment.
   b. It is associated with a specific injury.
   c. It serves no useful purpose.
   d. It responds well to placebos.

3. A physiologic response not usually associated with acute pain is:
   a. decreased cardiac output.
   b. altered insulin response.
   c. increased metabolic rate.
   d. decreased production of cortisol.

4. Chronic pain may be described as:
   a. attributable to a specific cause.
   b. prolonged in duration.
   c. rapidly occurring and subsiding with treatment.
   d. separate from any central or peripheral pathology.

5. An example of chronic benign pain is:
   a. a migraine headache.
   b. an exacerbation of rheumatoid arthritis.
   c. low back pain.
   d. sickle cell crisis.

6. A chemical substance thought to inhibit the transmission of pain is:
   a. acetylcholine.
   b. bradykinin.
   c. enkephalin.
   d. histamine.

7. All of the following statements about endorphins are true *except*:
   a. Their release inhibits the transmission of painful impulses.
   b. They represent the same mechanism of pain relief as non-narcotic analgesics.
   c. They are endogenous neurotransmitters structurally similar to opioids.
   d. They are found in heavy concentrations in the central nervous system.

8. The nurse assessing for pain should:
   a. believe a patient when he or she states that pain is present.
   b. doubt that pain exists when no physical origin can be identified.
   c. realize that patients frequently imagine and state that they have pain without actually feeling painful sensations.
   d. do all of the above.

9. When a nurse asks a patient to describe the quality of his or her pain, the nurse expects the patient to use a descriptive term such as:
   a. burning.
   b. chronic.
   c. intermittent.
   d. severe.

10. A physiologic indicator of acute pain is:
   a. diaphoresis.
   b. bradycardia.
   c. hypotension.
   d. lowered respiratory rate.

11. A nursing measure to manage anxiety during the anticipation of pain should include:
   a. focusing the patient's attention on another problem.
   b. teaching about the nature of the impending pain and associated relief measures.
   c. using an anxiety-reducing technique, such as desensitization.
   d. any or all of the above.

12. A nursing plan of care for pain management should include:
   a. altering factors that influence the pain sensation.
   b. determining responses to the patient's behavior toward pain.
   c. selecting goals for nursing intervention.
   d. all of the above.

13. The nurse's major area of assessment for a patient receiving patient-controlled analgesia (PCA) is assessment of the _____ system.
   a. cardiovascular
   b. integumentary
   c. neurologic
   d. respiratory

14. Pain in the elderly requires careful assessment, because older people:
   a. are expected to experience chronic pain.
   b. have a decreased pain threshold.
   c. experience reduced sensory perception.
   d. have increased sensory perception.

15. Administration of analgesics to the elderly requires careful patient assessment, because older people:
   a. metabolize drugs more rapidly.
   b. have increased hepatic, renal, and gastrointestinal function.
   c. are more sensitive to drugs.
   d. have lower ratios of body fat and muscle mass.

16. A preventive approach to pain relief with nonsteroidal anti-inflammatory drugs (NSAIDs) means that the medication is given:
   a. before the pain becomes severe.
   b. before the pain is experienced.
   c. when pain is at its peak.
   d. when the level of pain tolerance has been exceeded.

17. The advantage of using intraspinal infusion to deliver analgesics is:
   a. reduced side effects of systemic analgesia.
   b. reduced effects on pulse, respirations, and blood pressure.
   c. reduced need for frequent injections.
   d. all of the above.

18. The drug of choice for epidural administration of analgesia is:
   a. codeine.
   b. Demerol.
   c. Dilaudid.
   d. morphine.

19. The most worrisome adverse effect of epidural opioids is:
   a. asystole.
   b. hypertension.
   c. bradypnea.
   d. tachycardia.

20. Cutaneous stimulation is helpful in reducing painful sensations, because it:
   a. provides distraction from the pain source and decreases awareness.
   b. releases endorphins.
   c. stimulates large-diameter nerve fibers and reduces the intensity of pain.
   d. accomplishes all of the above.

Fill-In. *Read each statement carefully. Write your response in the space provided.*

1. Name three categories used to describe pain: _____, _____, and _____.

2. Pain transmission to and from the brain involves nerve mechanisms and structures known as:

   _____ and _____.

3. List five algogenic substances that are released into the tissues and affect the sensitivity of nociceptors:

   _____, _____, _____, _____, and _____.

4. List eight common physiologic responses to pain: _____, _____, _____,

   _____, _____, _____, _____, and _____.

5. Name the three general categories of analgesic agents that are used in some combination form to achieve

   balanced anesthesia: _____, _____ and _____.

6. The two most common types of electrical stimulation are: _____ and _____.

Complete the following crossword puzzle using terminology associated with pain management.

Down

1. Pain receptors in the skin.

2. Nonsteroidal agents that decrease inflammation and increase the effects of analgesics.

3. A type of analgesia that is controlled by the patient using a special pump.

4. A drug is prescribed on an "as needed" basis for pain management.

5. The only commercially available transdermal opioid medication.

6. Significantly increases a person's response to pain.

Across

1. Chemicals known to inhibit the transmission or perception of pain.

2. This substance, released in response to a painful stimuli, causes vasodilation.

3. An inactive substance given in place of pain medication.

4. Medication administration directly into the subarachnoid space and cerebrospinal fluid.

5. A type of cutaneous stimulation that decreases pain transmission through the descending pain pathway.

6. Transcutaneous stimulation of nonpain receptors in the same area of an injury.

7. Term used to describe a pain's rhythm.

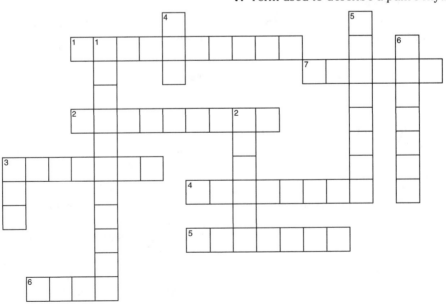

II. Critical Thinking Questions and Exercises

Discussion and Analysis

1. Explain what characteristics need to be present for pain to be classified as *chronic*.
2. Describe the classic *Gate Control Theory* of pain as described by Melzack and Well in 1965.
3. Explain how the technique of *distraction* works to relieve acute and chronic pain.

Clinical Situations

Read the following case study. Circle the correct answer.

CASE STUDY: Pain Experience

Courtney is a young, healthy adult who slipped off the stairs going down to the basement and struck her forehead on the cement flooring. Courtney did not lose consciousness but did sustain a mild concussion and a hematoma that was 5 cm in width and protruded outward about 6 cm. She experienced immediate acute pain at the site of injury plus a pounding headache.

1. An immediate assessment of the localized pain, based on the patient's description, is that it should be:
   a. brief in duration.
   b. mild in intensity.
   c. persistent after healing has occurred.
   d. recurrent for 3 to 4 months.

2. During the assessment process, the nurse attempts to determine Courtney's physiologic and behavioral responses to her pain experience. The nurse is aware that a patient can be in pain yet appear to be "pain free." A behavioral response indicative of acute pain is:
   a. an expressionless face.
   b. clear verbalization of details.
   c. muscle tension.
   d. physical inactivity.

3. The nurse uses distraction to help Courtney cope with her pain experience. A suggested activity is:
   a. promoting relaxation.
   b. playing music or using a videotape.
   c. using cutaneous stimulation.
   d. any or all of the above.

4. After treatment, Courtney is discharged to home while still in pain. The nurse should:
   a. clarify that Courtney knows what type of pain signals a problem.
   b. remind Courtney that acute pain may persist for several days.
   c. review methods of pain management.
   d. do all of the above.

14

Fluids and Electrolytes: Balance and Distribution

I. Interpretation, Completion, and Comparison

Multiple Choice. Read each question carefully. Circle your answer.

1. The average daily urinary output in an adult is:
   a. 0.5 L.
   b. 1.0 L.
   c. 1.5 L.
   d. 2.5 L.

2. A febrile patient's fluid output is in excess of normal because of diaphoresis. The nurse should plan fluid replacement based on the knowledge that insensible losses in an *afebrile* person are normally not greater than:
   a. 300 mL/24 hr.
   b. 600 mL/24 hr.
   c. 900 mL/24 hr.
   d. 1200 mL/24 hr.

3. A patient's serum sodium is within the normal range. The nurse estimates that the serum osmolality should be:
   a. less than 136 mOsm/kg.
   b. 280 to 295 mOsm/kg.
   c. greater than 408 mOsm/kg.
   d. 350 to 544 mOsm/kg.

4. The nurse expects that a decrease in serum osmolality would occur with:
   a. diabetes insipidus.
   b. hyperglycemia
   c. renal failure.
   d. uremia.

5. One of the best indicators of renal function is:
   a. blood urea nitrogen.
   b. serum creatintine.
   c. specific gravity.
   d. urine osmolality.

6. A patient is hemorrhaging from multiple trauma sites. The nurse expects that compensatory mechanisms associated with hypovolemia would cause all of the following symptoms *except:*
   a. hypertension.
   b. oliguria.
   c. tachycardia.
   d. tachypnea.

7. A nurse is directed to administer a hypotonic intravenous solution. Looking at the following labeled solutions, she should choose:
a. 0.45% sodium chloride.
b. 0.90% sodium chloride.
c. 5% dextrose in water.
d. 5% dextrose in normal saline solution.

8. An isotonic solution that contains electrolytes similar to the concentration used in plasma is:
a. 5% dextrose in water.
b. lactated Ringer's solution.
c. 3% NaCl solution.
d. 5% NaCl solution.

9. Nursing intervention for a patient with a diagnosis of hyponatremia includes all of the following *except:*
a. assessing for symptoms of nausea and malaise.
b. encouraging the intake of low-sodium liquids, such as coffee or tea.
c. monitoring neurologic status.
d. restricting tap water intake.

10. A patient with abnormal sodium losses is receiving a house diet. To provide 1600 mg of sodium daily, the nurse could supplement the patient's diet with:
a. one beef cube and 8 oz of tomato juice.
b. four beef cubes and 8 oz of tomato juice.
c. one beef cube and 16 oz of tomato juice.
d. one beef cube and 12 oz of tomato juice.

11. To return a patient with hyponatremia to normal sodium levels, it is safer to restrict fluid intake than to administer sodium:
a. in patients who are unconscious.
b. to prevent fluid overload.
c. to prevent dehydration.
d. in patients who show neurologic symptoms.

12. Hypernatremia is associated with a:
a. serum osmolality of 245 mOsm/kg.
b. serum sodium of 150 mEq/L.
c. urine specific gravity lower than 1.003.
d. combination of all of the above.

13. One of the dangers of treating hypernatremia is:
a. red blood cell crenation.
b. red blood cell hydrolysis.
c. cerebral edema.
d. renal shutdown.

14. A semiconscious patient presents with restlessness and weakness. He has a dry, swollen tongue. His body temperature is 99.3°F, and his urine specific gravity is 1.020. Choose the most likely serum sodium (Na$^+$) value for this patient.
a. 110 mEq/L
b. 140 mEq/L
c. 155 mEq/L
d. 165 mEq/L

15. A patient is admitted who has had severe vomiting for 24 hours. She states that she is exhausted and weak. The results of an admitting electrocardiogram(ECG) show flat T waves and ST-segment depression. Choose the most likely potassium (K$^+$) value for this patient.
a. 4.0 mEq/L
b. 8.0 mEq/L
c. 2.0 mEq/L
d. 2.6 mEq/L

16. The ECG change that is specific to hypokalemia is:
a. a depressed ST segment.
b. a flat T wave.
c. an elevated U wave.
d. an inverted T wave.

17. To supplement a diet with foods high in potassium, the nurse should recommend the addition of:
a. fruits such as bananas and apricots.
b. green leafy vegetables.
c. milk and yogurt.
d. nuts and legumes.

18. If a patient has severe hyperkalemia, it is possible to administer calcium gluconate intravenously to:
a. immediately lower the potassium (K$^+$) level by active transport.
b. antagonize the action of K$^+$ on the heart.
c. prevent transient renal failure (TRF).
d. accomplish all of the above.

19. Cardiac effects of hyperkalemia are usually present when the serum potassium level reaches:
a. 5 mEq/L.
b. 6 mEq/L.
c. 7 mEq/L.
d. 8 mEq/L.

20. A patient complains of tingling in his fingers. He has positive Trousseau's and Chvostek's signs. He says that he feels depressed. Choose the most likely serum calcium (Ca^{++}) value for this patient.
   a. 11 mg/dL
   b. 9 mg/dL
   c. 7 mg/dL
   d. 5 mg/dL

21. Management of hypocalcemia includes all of the following actions *except* administration of:
   a. fluid to dilute the calcium levels.
   b. the diuretic furosemide (Lasix), without saline, to increase calcium excretion through the kidneys.
   c. inorganic phosphate salts.
   d. intravenous phosphate therapy.

22. A patient is admitted with a diagnosis of renal failure. He also mentions that he has had stomach distress and has ingested numerous antacid tablets over the past 2 days. His blood pressure is 110/70 mm Hg, his face is flushed, and he is experiencing generalized weakness. Choose the most likely magnesium (Mg^{++}) value for this patient.
   a. 11 mEq/L
   b. 5 mEq/L
   c. 2 mEq/L
   d. 1 mEq/L

23. Management of the foregoing patient should include:
   a. a regular diet with extra fruits and green vegetables.
   b. potassium-sparing diuretics.
   c. discontinuance of any oral magnesium salts.
   d. all of the above measures.

24. The most common buffer system in the body is the:
   a. plasma protein buffer system.
   b. hemoglobin buffer system.
   c. phosphate buffer system.
   d. bicarbonate–carbonic acid buffer system.

25. The kidneys regulate acid–base balance by all of the following mechanisms *except:*
   a. excreting hydrogen ions (H^+).
   b. reabsorbing or excreting HCO_3^- into the blood.
   c. reabsorbing carbon dioxide into the blood.
   d. retaining hydrogen ions (H^+).

26. The lungs regulate acid–base balance by all of the following mechanisms *except:*
   a. excreting HCO_3^- into the blood.
   b. slowing ventilation.
   c. controlling carbon dioxide levels.
   d. increasing ventilation.

27. Choose the condition that exhibits blood values with a low pH and a low plasma bicarbonate concentration.
   a. Respiratory acidosis
   b. Respiratory alkalosis
   c. Metabolic acidosis
   d. Metabolic alkalosis

28. The nursing assessment for a patient with metabolic alkalosis includes evaluation of laboratory data for all of the following *except:*
   a. hypocalcemia.
   b. hypoglycemia.
   c. hypokalemia.
   d. hypoxemia.

29. Choose the condition that exhibits blood values with a low pH and a high PCO_2.
   a. Respiratory acidosis
   b. Respiratory alkalosis
   c. Metabolic acidosis
   d. Metabolic alkalosis

30. A normal oxygen saturation value for arterial blood is:
   a. 90%.
   b. 92%.
   c. 93%.
   d. 95%.

Fill-In. *Read each statement carefully. Write your response in the space provided.*

1. The major positively charged ion in intracellular fluid is _____; the major positively charged ion in extracellular fluid is _____.

2. Define *colloidal osmotic pressure.*

_____

_____

3. The major organ that carefully regulates serum potassium balance is the _____.

4. Calcium levels are primarily regulated by_____.

5. The normal blood pH is _____.

6. The upper and lower blood pH levels that are incompatible with life are _____ and

_____.

7. Indicate which of the following factors contribute to hyponatremia by writing "LOW" in the space provided, and indicate which contribute to hypernatremia by writing "HIGH" in the space provided.
   a. _____ vomiting
   b. _____ diarrhea
   c. _____ watery diarrhea
   d. _____ inability to quench thirst
   e. _____ burns over a large surface area
   f. _____ diuretics
   g. _____ heat stroke
   h. _____ adrenal insufficiency
   i. _____ syndrome of inappropriate antidiuretic hormone
   j. _____ status post therapeutic abortion
   k. _____ diabetes insipidus with water restriction
   l. _____ excessive parenteral administration of dextrose and water solution

8. Indicate which of the following factors contribute to hypokalemia by writing "LOW' in the space provided, and indicate which contribute to hyperkalemia by writing "HIGH" in the space provided.
   a. _____ alkalosis
   b. _____ too tight a tourniquet when collecting a blood sample
   c. _____ vomiting
   d. _____ gastric suction
   e. _____ leukocytosis
   f. _____ anorexia nervosa
   g. _____ hyperaldosteronism
   h. _____ furosemide (Lasix) administration
   i. _____ steroid administration
   j. _____ renal failure
   k. _____ penicillin administration
   l. _____ adrenal steroid deficiency

9. Indicate which of the following factors contribute to hypocalcemia by writing "LOW" in the space provided, and indicate which contribute to hypercalcemia by writing "HIGH" in the space provided.
   a. _____ hyperparathyroidism
   b. _____ massive administration of citrated blood
   c. _____ malignant tumors
   d. _____ immobilization because of multiple fractures
   e. _____ pancreatitis
   f. _____ thiazide diuretics
   g. _____ renal failure
   h. _____ aminoglycoside administration

10. Indicate which of the following factors contribute to hypomagnesemia by writing "LOW" in the space provided, and indicate which contribute to hypermagnesemia by writing "HIGH" in the space provided.
   a. _____ alcohol abuse
   b. _____ renal failure
   c. _____ diarrhea
   d. _____ gentamicin administration
   e. _____ untreated ketoacidosis

11. Indicate which of the following factors contribute to hypophosphatemia by writing "LOW" in the space provided, and indicate which contribute to hyperphosphatemia by writing "HIGH" in the space provided.

a. _____ hyperparathyroidism
b. _____ renal failure
c. _____ major thermal burns
d. _____ alcohol withdrawal
e. _____ neoplastic disease chemotherapy

12. For each of the following factors, indicate the probable cause by writing "M-ACID" for metabolic acidosis, "M-ALKA" for metabolic alkalosis, "R-ACID" for respiratory acidosis, or "R-ALKA" for respiratory alkalosis.

a. _____ sedative overdose
b. _____ lactic acidosis
c. _____ ketoacidosis
d. _____ severe pneumonia
e. _____ hypoxemia
f. _____ acute pulmonary edema
g. _____ diarrhea
h. _____ vomiting
i. _____ hypokalemia
j. _____ gram-negative bacterial infection

13. Explain why the administration of a 3% to 5% sodium chloride solution requires intense monitoring.

_____

14. List several symptoms associated with air embolism, a complication of intravenous therapy.

_____

15. The major complication of intravenous therapy is: _____.

II. Critical Thinking Questions and Exercises

Discussion and Analysis.

Read the following statements and answer the questions.

1. Explain why decreased urine output, despite adequate fluid intake, is an early indicator of a third space fluid shift.

2. Explain the important role of two opposing forces, *hydrostatic pressure* and *osmotic pressure*, in maintaining fluid movement through blood vessels.

3. Determine the normal daily urine output of an adult. Calculate the usual per hour output for adults with the following weights: 110 lb, 132 lb, and 176 lb.

Examining Associations.

Examine the relationships between the following and answer each question.

1. The regulation of body fluid compartments depends on many factors. Examine the association between *osmosis, diffusion*, and *filtration* and give an example of each.

2. Explain the interdependence of renin, angiotensin, and the aldosterone system on the fluid regulation cycle.

3. Correlate the associations between these three columns. First, match the statement about body fluid listed in Column III with its body fluid space listed in Column II. Then match the fluid space in Column II with an associated fact in Column I. Write the associated Roman numeral and small letter in the space provided.

Column I	Column II	Column III
1. _____ third space fluid shift	a. _____ intracellular space	I. comprises the cerebrospinal and pericardial fluids
2. _____the smallest compartment of the extracellular fluid space	b. _____ extracellular fluid compartment	II. is equal to about 8 L in an adult
3. _____ space where plasma is contained	c. _____ intravascular space	III. signs include hypotension, edema, and tachycardia
4. _____ comprises the intravascular, interstitial, and transcellular fluid	d. _____ transcellular space	IV. found mostly in skeletal muscle mass
5. _____ comprises about 60% of body fluid	e. _____ interstitial space	V. comprises about one third of body fluid
6. _____ comprises fluid surrounding cell	f. _____ intravascular fluid volume deficit	VI. comprises 50% of blood volume

Clinical Situations

Read the following case studies. Circle the correct answer.

CASE STUDY: Extracellular Fluid Volume Deficit

Harriet, 30 years old, has been admitted to the burn treatment center with full-thickness burns over 30% of her upper body. Her diagnosis is consistent with extracellular fluid volume deficit (FVD).

1. The major indicator of extracellular FVD can be identified by assessing for:
   a. a full and bounding pulse.
   b. a drop in postural blood pressure.
   c. an elevated temperature.
   d. pitting edema of the lower extremities.

2. Manifestations of extracellular FVD include all of the following *except:*
   a. collapsed neck veins.
   b. decreased serum albumin.
   c. elevated hematocrit.
   d. weight loss.

3. A nursing plan of care for Harriet should include assessing blood pressure with the patient in the supine and upright positions. A diagnostic reading that should be recorded and reported is:
   a. supine, 140/90; sitting, 120/80; standing, 110/70 mm Hg.
   b. supine, 140/90; sitting, 130/90; standing, 130/90 mm Hg.
   c. supine, 140/90; sitting, 140/85; standing, 135/85 mm Hg.
   d. supine, 140/90; sitting, 140/90; standing, 130/90 mm Hg.

4. Nursing intervention for Harriet includes all of the following *except:*
   a. monitoring urinary output to assess kidney perfusion.
   b. placing the patient in the Trendelenburg position to maximize cerebral blood flow.
   c. positioning the patient flat in bed with legs elevated to maintain adequate circulating volume.
   d. teaching leg exercises to promote venous return and prevent postural hypotension when the patient stands.

CASE STUDY: Congestive Heart Failure

George, 88 years old, is suffering from congestive heart failure. He was admitted to the hospital with a diagnosis of extracellular fluid volume excess. He was frightened, slightly confused, and dyspneic on exertion.

1. During the assessment process, the nurse expects to identify the following *except:*
   a. a full pulse.
   b. decreased central venous pressure.
   c. edema.
   d. neck vein distention.

2. A manifestation of extracellular volume excess is:
   a. altered serum osmolality.
   b. hyponatremia.
   c. increased hematocrit when volume excess develops quickly.
   d. rapid weight gain.

3. A nursing plan of care for George should include:
   a. auscultating for abnormal breath sounds.
   b. inspecting for leg edema.
   c. weighing the patient daily.
   d. all of the above.

4. Nursing intervention for George should include all of the following *except:*
   a. administering diuretics, as prescribed, to help remove excess fluid.
   b. assisting the patient to a recumbent position to minimize his breathing effort.
   c. inspecting for sacral edema to note the degree of fluid retention.
   d. teaching dietary restriction of sodium to help decrease water retention.

CASE STUDY: Diabetes Mellitus

Isaac, 63 years old, was admitted to the hospital with a diagnosis of diabetes mellitus. On his admission, the nurse observed rapid respirations, confusion, and signs of dehydration.

1. Isaac's arterial blood gas values are pH, 7.27; HCO_3, 20 mEq/L; PaO_2, 33 mm Hg. These values are consistent with a diagnosis of compensated:
   a. metabolic acidosis.
   b. metabolic alkalosis.
   c. respiratory acidosis.
   d. respiratory alkalosis.

2. A manifestation *not* associated with altered acid–base balance is:
   a. bradycardia.
   b. hypertension.
   c. lethargy.
   d. hypokalemia.

3. In terms of cellular buffering response, the nurse should expect the major electrolyte disturbance to be:
   a. hyperkalemia.
   b. hypernatremia.
   c. hypocalcemia.
   d. hypokalemia.

4. The nurse should anticipate that the physician will attempt to reverse this acid–base imbalance by prescribing intravenous administration of:
   a. potassium chloride.
   b. potassium iodide.
   c. sodium bicarbonate.
   d. sodium chloride.

15

Shock and Multisystem Failure

I. Interpretation, Completion, and Comparison

Multiple Choice. Read each question carefully. Circle your answer.

1. Calculate a patient's mean arterial pressure (MAP) when the blood pressure is 110/70 mm Hg.
   a. 65   c. 83
   b. 73   d. 91

2. Baroreceptors are a primary mechanism of blood pressure regulation which results from the initial stimulation of _____ receptors.
   a. chemical   c. neural
   b. hormonal   d. pressure

3. The stage of shock characterized by a normal blood pressure is the _____ stage.
   a. initial   c. progressive
   b. compensatory   d. irreversible

4. The nurse assesses a patient in compensatory shock whose lungs have decompensated. The nurse would *not* expect to find the following symptoms:
   a. a heart rate greater than 100 bpm   c. lethargy and mental confusion
   b. crackles   d. respirations fewer than 15/min

5. Oliguria occurs in the progressive stage of shock because the kidneys decompensate. To assess for this condition, the nurse should look for the following signs or symptoms:
   a. congestive heart failure   c. increased blood urea nitrogen and serum
   b. decreased capillary permeability and localized   creatinine
      edema   d. systolic blood pressure greater than 120 mm Hg

6. Hematologic system changes in progressive shock would *not* be characterized by:
   a. generalized hypoxemia.   c. metabolic acidosis.
   b. hypertension.   d. sluggish blood flow.

7. Depleted adenosine triphosphate (ATP) stores and multiple organ failure are characteristic of the _____ stage of shock.
   a. initial   c. progressive
   b. compensatory   d. irreversible

8. Patients receiving fluid replacement should frequently be monitored for:
   a. adequate urinary output.
   b. changes in mental status.
   c. vital sign stability.
   d. all of the above.

9. The most commonly used colloidal solution to treat hypovolemic shock is:
   a. blood products.
   b. 5% albumin.
   c. 6% dextran.
   d. 6% hetastarch.

10. Vasoactive agents are effective in treating shock because of their ability to:
    a. decrease blood pressure.
    b. decrease stroke volume.
    c. increase cardiac output.
    d. increase cardiac preload.

11. A common vasoactive agent used to improve cardiac contractility is:
    a. dopamine.
    b. epinephrine.
    c. nitroprusside.
    d. phenylephrine.

12. Hypovolemic shock occurs when intravascular volume decreases by:
    a. 5%–10%.
    b. 15%–25%.
    c. 30%–50%.
    d. more than 60%.

13. The primary goal in treating cardiogenic shock is to:
    a. improve the heart's pumping mechanism.
    b. limit further myocardial damage.
    c. preserve the healthy myocardium.
    d. treat the oxygenation needs of the heart muscle.

14. The drug of choice for cardiac pain relief is intravenous:
    a. codeine.
    b. Demerol.
    c. Dilaudid.
    d. morphine.

15. Sympathomimetic drugs increase cardiac output by all of the following measures *except*:
    a. decreasing preload and afterload.
    b. increasing myocardial contractility.
    c. tachycardia.
    d. vasoconstriction.

16. The vasoactive effects of dopamine are diminished when high doses are given, because vasoconstriction increases cardiac workload. Doses are titrated for therapeutic range. A nontherapeutic drug dose for a 154-lb (70-kg) man would be:
    a. 210 mg/min.
    b. 350 mg/min.
    c. 490 mg/min.
    d. 630 mg/min.

17. The negative effect of intravenous nitroglycerin (Tridil) for shock management is:
    a. reduced preload.
    b. reduced afterload.
    c. increased cardiac output.
    d. increased blood pressure.

18. Intra-aortic balloon counterpulsation (IABC) is a mechanical, assistive device used as a temporary means of improving the heart's pumping ability. IABC is primarily meant to:
    a. decrease cardiac work.
    b. decrease stroke volume.
    c. increase preload.
    d. maintain current coronary circulation.

19. The primary etiology of distributive shock is:
    a. arterial and venous dilatation.
    b. compromised cardiac contractility.
    c. decreased blood volume.
    d. obstructed blood flow.

20. The sequence of multiple-organ dysfunction syndrome (MODS) usually begins in the:
    a. heart.
    b. kidneys.
    c. liver.
    d. lungs.

21. A 40% mortality rate can be found with early stage MODS that is associated with:
    a. autocatabolism.
    b. a hypermetabolic phase.
    c. septic shock.
    d. all of the above.

Read the definitions of the terms related to shock and multisystem failure. Find each term in the scramblegram and circle it. Terms may be written in any direction.

Definitions of Terms

1. A syndrome of inadequate blood flow to body tissues.
2. Nutrients, chemically broken down within the cell, are stored in this form.
3. Substance is responsible for the conversion of angiotensin I.
4. Hormone, secreted by the pituitary gland, that causes the kidneys to retain fluid.
5. Insufficient oxygenation of the blood.
6. The degree of stretch of cardiac muscle before its contraction.
7. Urinary output less than 30 mL/hr.
8. A colloid that rapidly expands plasma volume.
9. A popular vasoactive agent that improves cardiac contractility.
10. The most common type of distributive shock.
11. A central line used to monitor venous pressure.
12. The most common side effect of fluid replacement in shock.
13. These solutions are used to expand intravascular volume in shock.
14. Multiple organ failure usually begins in this organ.
15. A vasodilator used to reduce the heart's demand for oxygen in conditions of shock.

D	A	O	L	E	R	P	B	D	F	H	R
B	L	C	F	I	L	U	M	P	R	E	T
C	B	A	J	A	R	L	D	G	N	H	G
Y	U	D	K	S	E	M	J	I	L	F	K
L	M	G	W	F	B	O	N	E	D	N	O
M	I	S	P	T	G	N	S	G	N	U	L
A	N	D	T	C	R	A	R	M	I	H	I
I	V	I	A	D	H	Y	I	R	P	D	G
M	L	O	R	O	C	Y	P	J	R	K	U
E	A	L	T	P	X	E	L	S	I	O	R
X	C	L	B	A	I	D	M	N	D	M	I
O	S	O	K	M	W	E	S	O	E	P	A
P	V	C	O	I	L	M	A	H	K	I	F
Y	R	A	Q	N	F	A	N	T	O	C	P
H	T	R	C	E	S	E	P	T	I	C	J
C	K	G	P	N	W	T	U	C	M	B	K
F	H	J	M	E	S	B	M	E	D	I	A
H	A	D	G	K	O	R	H	L	O	B	F

Match the type of shock listed in Column II with its associated cause listed in Column I. An answer may be used more than once.

Column I

1._____ valvular damage

2._____ peritonitis

3._____ burns

4._____ bee sting allergy

5._____ immunosuppression

6._____ spinal cord injury

7._____ dysrhythmias

8._____ vomiting

9._____ pulmonary embolism

10._____ penicillin sensitivity

Column II

a. hypovolemic, owing to an internal fluid shift

b. hypovolemic, owing to an external fluid loss

c. cardiogenic

d. distributive of a neurogenic nature

e. distributive of an anaphylactic nature

f. distributive of a septic nature

g. noncoronary cardiogenic shock

II. Critical Thinking Questions and Exercises

Examining Associations

Chart the physiologic sequence of events in hypovolemic shock.

Flow Chart: Hypovolemic Shock

↓ _____ from hemorrhage or severe dehydration

results in

↓ _____ and ↓ _____

which causes

↓ _____ and ↓ _____

which leads to

↓ _____ and _____

Clinical Situations:

Read the following case studies. Fill in the blanks or circle the correct answer.

CASE STUDY: Hypovolemic Shock

Mr. Mazda is a 57-year-old, 154-lb (70-kg) patient, who was received on the nursing unit from the recovery room after having a hemicolectomy for colon cancer. On initial assessment, Mr. Mazda was alert, yet anxious; his skin was cool, pale, and moist; and his abdominal dressings were saturated with bright red blood. Urinary output was 100 mL over 4 hours. The patient was receiving 1000 mL of lactated Ringer's solution. Vital signs were blood pressure, 80/60 mm Hg; heart rate, 126 bpm; and respirations 40/minute (baseline vital signs were 130/70, 84, and 22, respectively). The nurse assessed that the patient was experiencing hypovolemic shock.

1. The nurse understands that hypovolemic shock will occur with an intravascular volume reduction of 15% to 25%. Therefore, the nurse determines that Mr. Mazda, who weighs 70 kg, has probably lost:
   a. 200 mL of blood.
   b. 500 mL of blood.
   c. 750 mL of blood.
   d. 1000 mL of blood.

2. The nurse knows to monitor vital signs every 5 to 15 minutes and to be concerned about the patient's pulse pressure of

   _____

3. The nurse knows that the progressive pattern of changes in vital signs is more important than the exact readings. A _____ in pulse rate, followed by a _____ in blood pressure, is indicative of shock.

4. The nurse understands that a systolic reading of 80 mm Hg is serious, because a systolic reading lower than _____ mm Hg in a normotensive person indicates well-advanced shock.

5. Urinary output will be measured hourly. An output less than _____ mL/hr is indicative of decreased glomerular filtration.

6. Nursing interventions include notifying the physician, reinforcing the abdominal dressings, and treating the patient for shock by administering fluids ordered, such as:

   a. _____

   b. _____

   c. _____

   d. _____

CASE STUDY: Septic Shock

Mr. Dressler, a 43-year-old Caucasian, was admitted to the medical-surgical unit on the third postoperative day after a vertical bonded gastroplasty for morbid obesity. He had initially transferred to the intensive care unit from the recovery room. Mr. Dressler had a normal postoperative recovery period until his first afternoon on the unit. The RN went into his room to assess 4:00 pm vital signs and noted that his temperature was 102°F, he was shaking with chills, his skin was warm and dry, yet his extremities were cool to the touch. The nurse, assessing that Mr. Dressler was probably experiencing septicemia, immediately notified the physician.

Answer the following questions based on your knowledge of septicemia and shock.

1. Septic shock is most commonly caused by gram-negative organisms. Give an example of a common gram-negative bacteria: _____.

2. The nurse knows that the mortality rate associated with septic shock is between _____% and _____%.

3. The nurse expects that the physician will request body fluid specimens for culture and sensitivity tests. The nurse prepares to collect specimens of: _____, _____, _____, and _____.

4. Four modalities of treatment are essential to manage the septic shock: _____, _____, _____, and _____.

5. The two most common and serious side effects of fluid replacement are: _____ and _____.

6. A central venous pressure line (CVP) helps monitor fluid replacement. A normal CVP value is _____.

16

Oncology: Nursing Management in Cancer Care

I. Interpretation, Completion, and Comparison

Multiple Choice. Read each question carefully. Circle your answer.

1. As a cause of death in the United States, cancer ranks:
   a. first.
   b. second.
   c. third.
   d. fourth.

2. Cancer mortality in the United States is highest among:
   a. African Americans.
   b. American Indians.
   c. Caucasians.
   d. Hispanics.

3. The etiology of cancer can be associated with specific agents or factors such as:
   a. dietary and genetic factors.
   b. hormonal and chemical agents.
   c. viruses.
   d. all of the above.

4. David, age 67 years, is admitted for diagnostic studies to rule out cancer. He is white, has been employed as a landscaper for 40 years, and has a 36-year history of smoking one pack of cigarettes a day. David has three risk factors associated with the development of cancer. Choose the *least* significant risk factor among the following:
   a. age
   b. sex
   c. occupation
   d. race

5. Cancer cells can affect the immune system by:
   a. stimulating the release of T lymphocytes into the circulation.
   b. suppressing the patient's natural defenses.
   c. mobilizing macrophages.
   d. all of the above.

6. To reduce nitrate intake because of possible carcinogenic action, the nurse suggests that a patient decrease his or her intake of:
   a. eggs and milk.
   b. fish and poultry.
   c. ham and bacon.
   d. green, leafy vegetables.

7. An endoscopic procedure can be used to remove an entire piece of suspicious tissue growth. The diagnostic biopsy method used for this procedure is known as:
   a. excisional biopsy.
   b. incisional biopsy.
   c. needle biopsy.
   d. staging.

8. A patient is admitted for an excisional biopsy of a breast lesion. The nurse should do all of the following *except*:
   a. clarify information provided by the physician.
   b. provide aseptic care to the incision postoperatively.
   c. provide time for the patient to discuss her concerns.
   d. counsel the patient about the possibility of losing her breast.

9. Surgery done to remove lesions that are likely to develop into cancer is known as:
   a. diagnostic.
   b. palliative.
   c. prophylactic.
   d. reconstructive.

10. An example of palliative surgery is a:
    a. colectomy.
    b. cordotomy.
    c. mastectomy.
    d. nephrectomy.

11. The *incorrect* rationale for the effectiveness of radiation therapy is its ability to:
    a. cause cell death.
    b. break the strands of the DNA helix.
    c. disrupt mitosis by slowing dividing cells.
    d. interrupt cellular growth when a nonsurgical approach is needed.

12. Radiation therapy for the treatment of cancer is administered over several weeks to:
    a. allow time for the patient to cope with the treatment.
    b. allow time for the repair of healthy tissue.
    c. decrease the incidence of leukopenia and thrombocytopenia.
    d. accomplish all of the above.

13. A patient with uterine cancer is being treated with internal radiation therapy. A primary nursing responsibility is to:
    a. explain to the patient that she will continue to emit radiation for approximately 1 week after the implant is removed.
    b. maintain as much distance as possible from the patient while in the room.
    c. alert family members that they should restrict their visiting to 5 minutes at any one time.
    d. wear a lead apron when providing direct patient care.

14. A major disadvantage of chemotherapy is that it:
    a. attacks cancer cells during their vulnerable phase.
    b. functions against disseminated disease.
    c. is systemic.
    d. targets normal body cells as well as cancer cells.

15. When a patient takes vincristine, a plant alkaloid, the nurse should assess for symptoms of toxicity affecting the:
    a. gastrointestinal system.
    b. nervous system.
    c. pulmonary system.
    d. urinary system.

16. Initial nursing action for extravasation of a chemotherapeutic agent includes all of the following *except*:
    a. applying warm compresses to the phlebitic area.
    b. immediately discontinuing the infusion.
    c. injecting an antidote, if required.
    d. placing ice over the site of infiltration.

17. Realizing that chemotherapy can result in renal damage, the nurse should:
    a. encourage fluid intake to dilute the urine.
    b. take measures to acidify the urine and thus prevent uric acid crystallization.
    c. withhold medication when the blood urea nitrogen level exceeds 20 mg/dL.
    d. limit fluids to 1000 mL daily to prevent accumulation of the drugs' end products after cell lysis.

18. Allopurinol may be prescribed for a patient who is receiving chemotherapy to:
   a. stimulate the immune system against the tumor cells.
   b. treat drug-related anemia.
   c. prevent alopecia.
   d. lower serum and urine uric acid levels.

19. The use of hyperthermia as a treatment modality for cancer may cause:
   a. fatigue, nausea, and vomiting.
   b. hypotension, skin burn, and tissue damage.
   c. thrombophlebitis, diarrhea, and peripheral neuropathies.
   d. all of the above side effects.

20. Bacille Calmétte-Guerin (BCG) is a biologic response modifier that is a standard form of treatment for cancer of the:
   a. bladder.
   b. breast.
   c. lungs.
   d. skin.

21. The nurse should assess a cancer patient's nutritional status by:
   a. weighing the patient daily.
   b. monitoring daily calorie intake.
   c. observing for proper wound healing.
   d. doing all of the above.

22. The most frequently occurring gram-positive cause of infection in cancer patients is:
   a. *Candida albicans.*
   b. *Escherichia coli.*
   c. *Pseudomonas aeruginosa.*
   d. *Staphylococcus.*

23. The most common cause of bleeding in cancer patients is:
   a. anemia.
   b. coagulation disorders.
   c. hypoxemia.
   d. thrombocyotpenia.

Fill-In. Write the definition for each of the following words.

1. anaplasia _____

2. alopecia _____

3. carcinogenesis _____

4. cytokines _____

5. metastasis _____

6. nadir _____

7. vesicant _____

8. xerostomia _____

Fill-In. Read each statement carefully. Write your response in the space provided.

1. List in order of frequency the three leading causes of cancer deaths in the United States.

Men	*Women*
a. _____	a. _____
b. _____	b. _____
c. _____	c. _____

2. Distinguish between the terms *invasion* and *metastasis* as they relate to the spread of cancerous cells.
   Invasion: _____
   Metastasis: _____

3. List two significant tumor-specific antigens present in cancer cells that help with diagnosis and treatment:
   _____ and _____.

4. At least _____% of all cancers are thought to be related to the environment around us.

5. Three cruciferous vegetables that appear to reduce cancer risk are _____, _____, and _____.

6. Describe what is meant by primary and secondary prevention of cancer, and provide an example of how nurses can participate in both types of prevention.

Definition

Primary: _____

Secondary: _____

Example

Primary: _____

Secondary: _____

7. Distinguish among the three goals of cancer treatment.

Cure: _____

Control: _____

Palliation: _____

8. Toxicity occurs with radiation therapy. For each heading in Column I, list several examples of side effects in Column II.

Column I

1. Skin

2. Oral mucosal membrane

3. Stomach or colon

4. Bone marrow-producing sites

Column II

a. _____

b. _____

c. _____

a. _____

b. _____

c. _____

d. _____

a. _____

b. _____

c. _____

d. _____

a. _____

b. _____

c. _____

9. Describe the modes of action in the following classifications of chemotherapeutic agents.

Cell cycle–specific: _____

Cell cycle–nonspecific: _____

10. List five signs that indicate that an extravasation of an infusion of a cancer chemotherapeutic agent has occurred.

a. _____

b. _____

c. _____

d. _____

e. _____

11. Describe the role of hyperthermia in the treatment of cancer.

_____

12. Describe the role of interferons in the treatment of cancer.

_____

Matching. Match the type of neoplasm in Column II with its associated description listed in Column I.

Column 1

1.____ Cells bear little resemblance to the normal cells of the tissue from which they arose.

2.____ Rate of growth is usually slow.

3.____ Tumor tissue is encapsulated.

4.____ Tumor spreads by way of blood and lymph channels to other areas of the body.

5.____ Growth tends to recur when removed.

Column 2

a. benign

b. malignant

Matching. Match the drug category listed in Column II with an associated antineoplastic agent listed in Column I. An answer may be used more than once.

Column I

1.____ vincristine

2.____ 5-fluorouracil

3.____ cisplatin

4.____ estrogens

5.____ thiotepa

6.____ lomustine

7.____ mitomycin

8.____ amsacrine

9.____ pentostatin

10.____ paclitaxel (Taxol)

Column II

a. alkylating agent

b. nitrosourea

c. antimetabolite

d. antitumor antibiotic

e. plant alkaloid/natural product

f. hormonal agent

II. Critical Thinking Questions and Exercises

Examining Associations

Read each analogy. Fill in the space provided with the best response.

1. Primary cancer prevention: preventing or reducing the risk of cancer :: Secondary prevention: _____.

2. Staging of tumor cells: tumor size and existence of metastasis :: Grading: _____.

3. Allogenic bone marrow transplant: an unrelated donor :: Syngenic bone marrow transplant: _____.

4. Stomatitis: oral tissue inflammation :: Alopecia: _____.

5. Anorexia: loss of appetite :: Cachexia: _____.

Clinical Situations

Read the following case studies. Fill in the space or circle the correct answer.

CASE STUDY: Cancer of the Breast

Kim is a 45-year-old mother of four who, after a needle aspiration biopsy, is diagnosed as having a malignant breast tumor, stage III. She was scheduled for a modified radical mastectomy. On assessment, her breast tissue had a dimpling or "orange-peel" appearance. Nursing diagnoses included (a) fear and ineffective coping related to the diagnosis and (b) disturbance in self-concept related to the nature of the surgery.

1. Realizing that Kim's mother died of breast cancer, the nurse correlates the cause of Kim's diagnosis to:
   a. environmental factors.
   b. genetics.
   c. dietary factors.
   d. chemical agents.

2. To assist Kim in adapting to the loss of her breast, the nurse should assess Kim's:
   a. attitude toward her body image.
   b. feelings of self-esteem.
   c. social and sexual values.
   d. attitudes and values regarding all of the above.

3. Kim's husband refuses to participate in any discussion about his wife's diagnosis. The nurse realizes that he is using the defense mechanism of:
   a. denial.
   b. depression.
   c. rationalization.
   d. repression.

4. Postoperatively, Kim experiences severe incisional pain. The nurse realizes that Kim's perception of pain is possibly influenced by:
   a. tissue manipulation during surgery.
   b. apprehension regarding the prognosis of her condition.
   c. anger stemming from her change in body image.
   d. all of the above.

Kim is scheduled to begin radiation therapy, followed by chemotherapy with 5-fluorouracil.

5. Realizing the side effects of radiation therapy, the nurse should prepare Kim for all of the following *except*:
   a. her lungs may possibly produce more mucus.
   b. the skin at the treatment area may become red and inflamed.
   c. she may tire more easily and require additional rest periods.
   d. alopecia will occur as a result of the quickly growing hair follicles.

6. The nurse should teach Kim what she can do to protect her skin between radiation treatments. Measures include all of the following *except*:
   a. handle the area gently.
   b. avoid irritation with soap and water.
   c. use a heat lamp once a day directed to the radiation site to promote tissue repair.
   d. wear loose-fitting clothing.

After radiation therapy, Kim begins a regimen of chemotherapy with 5-fluorouracil. Three weeks after treatment begins, Kim develops a fever, sore throat, and cold symptoms.

7. The nurse knows that Kim's symptoms could be due to all of the following *except*:
   a. hypercalcemia.
   b. bone marrow depression.
   c. altered nutrition.
   d. leukopenia.

8. Nursing assessment during Kim's chemotherapy includes observing for:
   a. evidence of stomatitis.
   b. renal and hepatic abnormalities.
   c. symptoms of infection owing to granulocytopenia.
   d. all of the above.

9. Kim is diagnosed as having thrombocytopenia. The nurse should assess for all of the following *except*:
   a. hematuria.
   b. fever.
   c. hematemesis.
   d. ecchymosis.

CASE STUDY: Cancer of the Lung

Mr. Donato is a 48-year-old accountant who has been a one-pack-a-day smoker for 23 years. He has had a persistent cough for 1 year that is hacking and nonproductive and has had repeated unresolved upper respiratory tract infections. He went to see his physician because he was fatigued, had been anorexic, and had lost 12 pounds over the last 3 months. Diagnostic evaluation led to the diagnosis of a localized tumor with no evidence of metastatic spread. Mr. Donato is scheduled for a lobectomy in 3 days.

1. Because infection is the leading cause of mortality in the oncology population, the nurse preoperatively notes the significance of a(n):
   a. basophil count of 1.3%.
   b. eosinophil count of 4.5%.
   c. lymphocyte count of 23%.
   d. neutrophil count of 20%.

2. The nurse is concerned that the patient's nutritional status is compromised based on his recent weight loss. Impaired nutritional status contributes to: _____, _____,

   _____, _____ and _____.

3. List five factors that the nurse would assess to determine the patient's experience with pain, in order to develop a plan of care for pain management: _____, _____,

   _____, _____ and _____.

4. The nurse knows that a diagnosis of cancer is accompanied by grieving. Usually the first reaction in the grieving process is:
   a. bargaining.
   b. acceptance.
   c. denial.
   d. depression.

5. List four activities the nurse can do to support the patient and family during the grieving process:

   _____, _____, _____ and _____.

6. The nurse knows that postopertive care needs to be directed toward the prevention of

   _____, the leading cause of death in cancer patients.

7. Two major gram-negative bacilli that cause infection in an immunosuppressed patient are:

   _____ and _____.

8. The nurse will also assess for the postoperative complication of septic shock, which is associated with all of the following *except*:
   a. dysrhythmias.
   b. hypertension.
   c. metabolic acidosis.
   d. oliguria.

17

End-of-Life Care

I. Interpretation, Completion, and Comparison

Multiple Choice. *Read each question carefully. Circle your answer.*

1. The major causes of death in this century are diseases that are _____ in nature.
   a. communicable
   b. degenerative
   c. genetic
   d. infectious

2. A common, initial patient response to the seriousness of a terminal illness is:
   a. acceptance.
   b. anger.
   c. denial.
   d. bargaining.

3. Patients enrolled in hospice care are terminally ill with a life expectancy of:
   a. 3 months.
   b. 6 months.
   c. 6–9 months.
   d. about 1 year.

4. Hospice care is utilized by about _____ of eligible patients.
   a. 15%
   b. 30%
   c. 50%
   d. 75%

5. When a person authorizes another to make medical decisions on his or her behalf, the person has written:
   a. an advance directive.
   b. a living will.
   c. a standard addendum to a will.
   d. a proxy directive.

6. A dying patient wants to talk to the nurse about his fears. The patient states, " I know I'm dying, aren't I"? An appropriate nursing response would be:
   a. "This must be very difficult for you."
   b. "Tell me more about what's on your mind."
   c. "I'm so sorry. I know just how you feel."
   d. "You know you're dying?"

7. One of the most common and feared responses to terminal illness is:
   a. anorexia.
   b. cachexia.
   c. dyspnea.
   d. pain.

8. The anorexia-cachexia syndrome that is common toward the end of life is characterized by:
   a. anemia.
   b. alterations in carbohydrate metabolism.
   c. endocrine dysfunction.
   d. all of the above, plus altered fat and altered protein metabolism.

Fill-In. Read each statement carefully. Write your response in the space provided.

1. Dr. _____ spearheaded a movement to increase an awareness of the dying process among health care practitioners.

2. Distinguish between the terms *assisted suicide* and *physician-assisted suicide*.

3. The first state to legalize physician-assisted suicide was _____ in the year _____.

4. Name the primary distinction between *palliative care* and *hospice care*:

   _____

5. Define the term *hospice care*. _____

6. List four medications that are commonly used to stimulate appetite in anorexic patients:

   _____, _____, _____, and _____.

II. Critical Thinking Questions and Exercises

Discussion and Analysis

1. How a person and his or her family cope with the dying process is influenced by many cultural, psychological, and socioeconomic factors. Analyze the role of the nurse in assessing values, preferences, and practices for a patient influenced by the Western culture of autonomy over care decisions and for a patient influenced by an Eastern culture of interdependence with care decisions.

2. Consider a recent clinical experience involving a dying patient. Draft an outline of nursing interventions that were or could have been used to support the patient's ability to maintain "hope" within the context of realism for the patient.

3. Review Dr. Kubler-Ross' five stages of dying and discuss nursing implications for each stage. Use some recent clinical examples if possible.

UNIT 4
Perioperative Concepts and Nursing Management

18

Preoperative Nursing Management

I. Interpretation, Comparison, and Completion

Multiple Choice. Read each question carefully. Circle your answer.

1. An example of a surgical procedure classified as urgent is:
   a. an appendectomy.
   b. an exploratory laparotomy.
   c. a repair of multiple stab wounds.
   d. a face lift.

2. A mammoplasty would be classified as surgery that is:
   a. elective.
   b. optional.
   c. required.
   d. reconstructive.

3. An informed consent is required for:
   a. closed reduction of a fracture.
   b. insertion of an intravenous catheter.
   c. irrigation of the external ear canal.
   d. urethral catheterization.

4. Protein replacement for nutritional balance can be accomplished with a diet that:
   a. is high in carbohydrates.
   b. is high in protein.
   c. is low in fats.
   d. includes all of the above.

5. A significant mortality rate exists for those alcoholics who experience "delirium tremens" postoperatively. When caring for the alcoholic, the nurse should assess for symptoms of alcoholic withdrawal:
   a. within the first 12 hours.
   b. about 24 hours postoperatively.
   c. on the second or third day.
   d. 4 days after surgery.

6. It is recommended that those who smoke cigarettes should stop smoking at least _____ before surgery.
   a. 2 months
   b. 3 months
   c. 2 weeks
   d. 3 weeks

7. Because liver disease is associated with a high surgical mortality rate, the nurse knows to alert the physician for:
   a. a blood ammonia concentration of 180 mg/dL.
   b. a lactate dehydrogenase concentration of 300 units.
   c. a serum albumin concentration of 5.0 g/dL.
   d. a serum globulin concentration of 2.8 g/dL.

8. Surgery would be contraindicated for a renal patient with:
   a. a blood urea nitrogen level of 42 mg/dL.
   b. a creatine kinase level of 120 U/L.
   c. a serum creatinine level of 0.9 mg/dL.
   d. a urine creatinine level of 1.2 mg/dL.

9. The chief life-threatening hazard for surgical patients with uncontrolled diabetes is:

   a. dehydration.

   b. hypertension.

   c. hypoglycemia.

   d. glucosuria.

10. The goal for the diabetic patient undergoing surgery is to maintain a blood glucose level of:

   a. 140–200 mg/dL.

   b. 200–240 mg/dL.

   c. 250–300 mg/dL.

   d. 300–350 mg/dL.

11. A nursing history of prior drug therapy is based on the particular concern that:

   a. phenothiazines may increase the hypotensive action of anesthetics.

   b. thiazide diuretics may cause excessive respiratory depression during anesthesia.

   c. tranquilizers may cause anxiety and even seizures if withdrawn suddenly.

   d. all of the above potential complications could occur.

12. The potential effects of medication therapy must be evaluated before surgery. A drug classification that may cause electrolyte imbalance is:

   a. corticosteroids.

   b. diuretics.

   c. phenothiazines.

   d. insulin.

13. Assessment of a gerontologic patient reveals bilateral dimmed vision. This information alerts the nurse to plan for:

   a. a safe environment.

   b. restrictions of the patient's unassisted mobility activities.

   c. probable cataract extractions.

   d. referral to an ophthalmologist.

14. Hazards of surgery for the geriatric patient are directly related to the:

   a. number of coexisting health problems.

   b. type of surgical procedure.

   c. severity of the surgery.

   d. all of the above.

15. Obesity is positively correlated with surgical complications of:

   a. the cardiovascular system.

   b. the gastrointestinal system.

   c. the pulmonary system.

   d. all of the systems listed.

16. The nursing goal of encouraging postoperative body movement is to:

   a. contribute to optimal respiratory function.

   b. improve circulation.

   c. prevent venous stasis.

   d. promote all of the above activities.

17. Food and water are usually withheld beginning at midnight of the surgical day. However, if necessary, water may be given up to:

   a. 8 hours before surgery.

   b. 6 hours before surgery.

   c. 4 hours before surgery.

   d. 2 hours before surgery.

18. The primary goal in withholding food before surgery is to prevent:

   a. aspiration.

   b. distention.

   c. infection.

   d. obstruction.

19. Expected patient outcomes for relief of anxiety related to a surgical procedure include all of the following *except*:

   a. understands the nature of the surgery and voluntarily signs an informed consent.

   b. verbalizes an understanding of the preanesthetic medication.

   c. requests a visit with a member of the clergy.

   d. questions the anesthesiologist about anesthesia-related concerns.

20. Choose a statement that indicates that a patient is knowledgeable about his or her impending surgery. The patient:

   a. participates willingly in the preoperative preparation.

   b. discusses stress factors that are making him or her depressed.

   c. expresses concern about postoperative pain.

   d. verbalizes his or her fears to family.

21. Hidden fears may be indicated when a patient:
   a. avoids communication.
   b. repeatedly asks questions that have previously been answered
   c. talks incessantly.
   d. does all of the above.

22. Choose the appropriate response to the statement, "I'm so nervous about my surgery."
   a. "Relax. Your recovery period will be shorter if you're less nervous."
   b. "Stop worrying. It only makes you more nervous."
   c. "You needn't worry. Your doctor has done this surgery many times before."
   d. "You seem nervous about your surgery."

23. The purpose of preoperative skin preparation is to:
   a. reduce the number of microorganisms.
   b. remove all resident bacteria.
   c. render the skin sterile.
   d. accomplish all of the above.

24. The least desirable method of hair removal is use of:
   a. electric clippers.
   b. a depilatory cream in nonsensitive patients.
   c. a razor with an extruded blade.
   d. scissors for long hair (more than 3 mm).

25. Purposes of preanesthetic medication include all of the following *except*:
   a. facilitation of anesthesia induction.
   b. lowering of the dose of the anesthetic agent used.
   c. potentiation of the effects of anesthesia.
   d. reduction of preoperative pain.

Fill-In. Read each statement carefully. Write your response in the space provided.

1. The term used to describe the period of time that constitutes the surgical experience is:_____.

2. The intraoperative phase begins when the patient _____ and ends when _____.

3. Informed consent for a surgical procedure is necessary when a procedure meets the following four conditions: _____, _____, _____ and _____.

4. List three significant nutritional concerns for the elderly surgical patient: _____, _____ and _____.

5. Name three primary goals necessary to promote postopertive mobility: _____, _____, and _____.

6. Explain why food is withheld before surgery. _____

II. Critical Thinking Questions and Exercises

Identifying Patterns

For each drug classification below, list the potential effects of prior drug therapy on a patient's surgical course.

Drug Classification	*Potential Effects of Drug Therapy*
Anticoagulants	_____
Diuretics	_____
Phenothiazines	_____
Tranquilizers	_____

Antidepressants   _____

Insulin   _____

Antibiotics   _____

For each essential preoperative nursing intervention listed in Column I, write an appropriate nursing goal under Column II.

Column I: Nursing Activity	*Column II: Nursing Goals*
Restriction of nutrition and fluids	_____
Intestinal preparation	_____
Preoperative skin preparation (cleansing)	_____
Urinary catheterization	_____
Administration of preoperative medications	_____
Transportation of patient to presurgical suite	_____

Recognizing Contradictions

Rewrite each statement correctly. Underline the key concepts.

1. The majority of surgical procedures performed today require overnight hospitalization, because "high-tech" interventions require intense postoperative monitoring.

2. The intraoperative phase of perioperative nursing ends when surgery is completed.

3. Cosmetic surgery is a type of elective surgery.

4. Vitamin K is an essential vitamin requirement for surgery, because it is needed for collagen synthesis.

5. Corticosteroids should always be given up to the day before surgery, so that the immune system can fight off postoperative infection.

Clinical Applications

Look at the figure below. List the five preoperative teaching points you would mention to instruct a patient how to cough correctly.

1. _____

2. _____

3. _____

4. _____

5. _____

19

Intraoperative Nursing Management

I. Interpretation, Completion, and Comparison

Multiple Choice. Read each question carefully. Circle your answer.

1. The circulating nurse's responsibilities, in contrast to the scrub nurse's responsibilities, include:
   a. assisting the surgeon.
   b. monitoring aseptic practices.
   c. setting up the sterile tables.
   d. all of the above functions.

2. Preoperatively, an anesthesiologist is responsible for:
   a. assessing pulmonary status.
   b. inquiring about preexisting pulmonary infections.
   c. knowing the patient's history of smoking.
   d. all of the above.

3. The anesthesiologist classifies a person's physical status for anesthesia before surgery. A nurse should know that a preoperative classification of II refers to patients with:
   a. mild systemic disease.
   b. no systemic abnormality.
   c. severe systemic disease.
   d. an incapacitating systemic disease.

4. A nurse knows that perioperative risks increase with age because:
   a. ciliary action decreases, reducing the cough reflex.
   b. fatty tissue increases, prolonging the effects of anesthesia.
   c. liver size decreases, reducing the metabolism of anesthetics.
   d. all of the above biologic changes exist.

5. A general anesthetic can be administered:
   a. by inhalation.
   b. intravenously.
   c. rectally.
   d. by all of these methods.

6. The nurse should know that, postoperatively, a general anesthetic is primarily eliminated by:
   a. the kidneys.
   b. the lungs.
   c. the skin.
   d. all of these routes.

7. An example of a stable and safe nondepolarizing muscle relaxant is:
   a. Anectine (succinylcholine chloride).
   b. Norcuron (vercuronium bromide).
   c. Pavulon (pancuronium bromide).
   d. Syncurine (decamethonium).

8. Postoperative nursing assessment for a patient who has received a depolarizing neuromuscular blocking agent includes careful monitoring of the:
  a. cardiovascular system.
  b. endocrine system.
  c. gastrointestinal system.
  d. genitourinary system.

9. A factor involved in post–spinal anesthesia headaches is the:
  a. degree of patient hydration.
  b. leakage of spinal fluid from the subarachnoid space.
  c. size of the spinal needle used.
  d. combination of the above mechanisms.

10. Epinephrine is often used in combination with a local infiltration anesthetic, because it:
  a. causes vasoconstriction.
  b. prevents rapid absorption of the anesthetic drug.
  c. prolongs the local action of the anesthetic agent.
  d. does all of the above.

11. A local infiltration anesthetic can last for up to:
  a. 1 hour.
  b. 3 hours.
  c. 5 hours.
  d. 7 hours.

12. Recent research has indicated that inadvertent hypothermia in gerontologic patients can be effectively and inexpensively prevented by:
  a. placing the patient on a hyperthermia blanket.
  b. maintaining environmental temperature at 37°C.
  c. covering the top of the patient's head with an ordinary plastic shower cap during anesthesia.
  d. frequent massage of the extremities with warmed skin lotion.

13. The nurse caring for a patient who is at risk for malignant hyperthermia subsequent to general anesthesia would assess for the most frequent early sign of:
  a. hypertension.
  b. muscle rigidity ("tetany-like" movements).
  c. oliguria.
  d. tachycardia.

14. If an operating room nurse is to assist a patient to the Trendelenburg position, she would place him:
  a. flat on his back with his arms next to his sides.
  b. on his back with his head lowered so that the plane of his body meets the horizontal on an angle.
  c. on his back with his legs and thighs flexed at right angles.
  d. on his side with his uppermost leg adducted and flexed at the knee.

Fill-In. *Read each statement carefully. Write your response in the space provided.*

1. Anesthesia dosage is reduced with age, because _____.

2. List four responsibilities of a Registered Nurse First Assistant (RNFA): _____,
_____, _____, and _____.

3. The type of anesthesia most likely to be used for a patient undergoing a colonoscopy is _____,
and the most frequently used agents are _____ and _____.

4. The anesthetic most commonly used for general anesthesia by intravenous injection
is _____, which can cause _____ as a serious, toxic side effect.

5. Spinal anesthesia is a conduction nerve block that occurs when a local anesthetic is injected into
_____.

6. The conduction block anesthesia commonly used in labor is the _____.

7. What nursing assessment indicates that a patient has recovered from the effects of spinal anesthesia?
_____

8. List six potential intraoperative complications:

a. _____   d. _____

b. _____   e. _____

c. _____   f. _____

9. The mortality rate of malignant hypothermia currently exceeds _____.

II. Critical Thinking Questions and Exercises

Discussion and Analysis

1. Explain why the elderly are at a higher risk of complications from anesthesia because of biologic changes that occur in later life.

2. Describe the role of the perioperative nurse.

Recognizing Contradictions

Rewrite each statement correctly. Underline the key concepts.

1. Older patients need more anesthetic agent to produce anesthesia, because they eliminate anesthetic agents more quickly.

2. A scrub nurse controls the environment, coordinates the activities of other personnel, and monitors the patient.

3. If there is any doubt about the sterility of an area, it is considered sterile.

4. A draped table is considered sterile from the top to the edge of the drapes.

5. Only the circulating nurse can extend an arm over the sterile area to deliver sterile supplies.

Clinical Situations

Read the following case studies. Circle the correct answer.

CASE STUDY: General Anesthesia

Anne, age 34, is in excellent health and is scheduled for open reduction of a fractured femur. The general anesthetic drugs to be used include enflurane and nitrous oxide.

1. The nurse knows that the advantages of enflurane (Ethrane) include all of the following *except*:
  a. fast recovery.   c. potent analgesia.
  b. low incidence of respiratory depression.   d. rapid induction.

2. The major disadvantage of nitrous oxide is its ability to cause:
  a. hypertension.   c. liver damage.
  b. hypoxia.   d. nausea and vomiting.

3. The major postoperative nursing assessment after administration of Ethrane is observation for:
  a. anuria.   c. respiratory depression.
  b. laryngospasm.   d. tachycardia.

CASE STUDY: Intravenous Anesthesia

Brian is scheduled to have a wisdom tooth extracted. The anesthetic agent of choice is thiopental sodium (Pentothal).

1. The nurse anticipates that the route of administration will be:
   a. by inhalation.
   b. by mask.
   c. intramuscular.
   d. intravenous.

2. The nurse is aware that after anesthetic administration, Brian will be unconscious in:
   a. 30 seconds.
   b. 60 seconds.
   c. 2 minutes.
   d. 3 minutes.

3. The chief danger with thiopental sodium is its:
   a. β-adrenergic blocking action.
   b. depressant action on the respiratory system.
   c. nephrotoxicity.
   d. rapid onset and prolonged duration.

20

Postoperative Nursing Management

I. Interpretation, Completion, and Comparison

Multiple Choice. Read each question carefully. Circle your answer.

1. The primary nursing goal in the immediate postoperative period is maintenance of pulmonary function and prevention of:
   a. laryngospasm.
   b. hyperventilation.
   c. hypoxemia and hypercapnia.
   d. pulmonary edema and embolism.

2. Unless contraindicated, any unconscious patient should be positioned:
   a. flat on his or her back, without elevation of the head, to facilitate frequent turning and minimize pulmonary complications.
   b. in semi-Fowler's position, to promote respiratory function and reduce the incidence of orthostatic hypotension when the patient can eventually stand.
   c. in Fowler's position, which most closely simulates a sitting position, thus facilitating respiratory as well as gastrointestinal functioning.
   d. on his or her side with a pillow at the patient's back and his or her chin extended, to minimize the dangers of aspiration.

3. A major postoperative nursing responsibility is assessing for cardiovascular function by monitoring:
   a. arterial blood gases.
   b. central venous pressure.
   c. vital signs.
   d. all of the above.

4. In the immediate postoperative period, a nurse should immediately report:
   a. a systolic blood pressure lower than 90 mm Hg.
   b. a temperature reading between 97°F and 98°F.
   c. respirations between 20 and 25 per minute.
   d. all of the above assessments.

5. Patients remain in the recovery room or postanesthesia care unit (PACU) until they are fully recovered from anesthesia. This is evidenced by:
   a. a patient airway.
   b. a reasonable degree of consciousness.
   c. a stable blood pressure.
   d. indication that all of the above have have occurred.

6. When a PACU room scoring guide is used, a patient can be transferred out of the recovery room with a minimum score of:
   a. 5.
   b. 6.
   c. 7.
   d. 8.

7. With the PACU room scoring guide, a nurse would give a patient an admission cardiovascular score of 2 if the patient's systolic arterial pressure is ____ of his or her preanesthetic level.
   a. 80%
   b. 75%–60%
   c. 60%–50%
   d. less than 50%

8. When vomiting occurs postoperatively, the most important nursing intervention is to:
   a. measure the amount of vomitus to estimate fluid loss, in order to accurately monitor fluid balance.
   b. offer tepid water and juices to replace lost fluids and electrolytes.
   c. support the wound area so that unnecessary strain will not disrupt the integrity of the incision.
   d. turn the patient's head to prevent aspiration of vomitus into the lungs.

9. Postoperatively, the nurse monitors urinary function. An abnormal outcome that should be reported to the physician is a 2-hour output that is:
   a. less than 30 mL.
   b. between 75 and 100 mL.
   c. between 100 and 200 mL.
   d. greater than 200 mL.

10. Most surgical patients are encouraged to be out of bed:
   a. within 6 to 8 hours after surgery.
   b. between 10 and 12 hours after surgery.
   c. as soon as it is indicated.
   d. on the second postoperative day.

11. The most common postoperative respiratory complication in elderly patients is:
   a. pleurisy.
   b. pneumonia.
   c. hypoxemia.
   d. pulmonary edema.

12. The proliferative stage of wound healing is characterized by:
   a. deposition of a fibrinoplatelet clot.
   b. histamine release and increased capillary permeability.
   c. fibroblast stimulation of collagen synthesis.
   d. scar formation.

13. A nurse wants to document the presence of granulation tissue in a healing wound. She describes the tissue as:
   a. necrotic and hard.
   b. pale yet able to blanch with digital pressure.
   c. pink to red and soft, noting that it bleeds easily.
   d. white with long, thin areas of scar tissue.

14. A physician's admitting note lists a wound as healing by second intention. The nurse expects to see:
   a. a deep, open wound that was previously sutured.
   b. a sutured incision with a little tissue reaction.
   c. a wound with a deep, wide scar that was previously resutured.
   d. a wound in which the edges were not approximated.

15. A wound that has hemorrhaged carries an increased risk of infection, because:
   a. reduced amounts of oxygen and nutrients are available.
   b. the tissue becomes less resilient.
   c. retrograde bacterial contamination may occur.
   d. dead space and dead cells provide a culture medium.

16. Postoperative abdominal distention seems to be directly related to:
   a. a temporary loss of peristalsis and gas accumulation in the intestines.
   b. beginning food intake in the immediate postoperative period.
   c. improper body positioning during the recovery period.
   d. the type of anesthetic administered.

17. A nursing measure for evisceration is to:
   a. apply an abdominal binder snugly so that the intestines can be slowly pushed back into the abdominal cavity.
   b. approximate the wound edges with adhesive tape so that the intestines can be gently pushed back into the abdomen.
   c. carefully push the exposed intestines back into the abdominal cavity.
   d. cover the protruding coils of intestines with sterile dressings moistened with sterile saline solution.

18. The characteristic sign of a paralytic ileus is:
   a. abdominal tightness.
   b. abdominal distention.
   c. absence of peristalsis.
   d. increased abdominal girth.

19. The most common postoperative nosocomial infections occur in the incisional area in:
   a. 5% to 15% of surgical patients.
   b. 15% to 25% of surgical patients.
   c. 25% to 50% of surgical patients.
   d. approximately 67% of surgical patients.

20. One of the major dangers associated with deep venous thrombosis is:
   a. pulmonary embolism.
   b. immobility because of calf pain.
   c. marked tenderness over the anteromedial surface of the thigh.
   d. swelling of the entire leg owing to edema.

21. Nursing measures to prevent thrombophlebitis include:
   a. assisting the patient with leg exercises.
   b. encouraging early ambulation.
   c. avoiding placement of pillows or blanket rolls under the patient's knees.
   d. all of the above.

22. One of the most effective nursing procedures for reducing nosocomial infections is:
   a. administration of prophylactic antibiotics.
   b. aseptic wound care.
   c. control of upper respiratory tract infections.
   d. proper hand-washing techniques.

23. The nurse recognizes that a clean-contaminated wound has a relative probability of infection of:
   a. 1% to 3%.
   b. 7% to 16%.
   c. 3% to 7%.
   d. more than 16%.

Fill-In. *Read each statement carefully. Write your response in the space provided.*

1. List five areas of concern for a recovery room PACU nurse who has just received a patient from the operating room.
   a. _____
   b. _____
   c. _____
   d. _____
   e. _____

2. The primary nursing priorities during immediate postoperative assessment are evaluation of:

_____

_____

3. Explain the differences among the three classifications of hemorrhage.

Primary:

_____

_____

Intermediary:

_____

_____

Secondary:

_____

_____

4. The most serious and most frequent postoperative complications involve the _____ system.

5. Several psychological factors that can influence a patient's pain experience are: _____

_____

_____

_____

6. Explain patient-controlled analgesia (PCA). _____

_____

_____

7. Explain why the postoperative complications of atelectasis and hypostatic pneumonia are reduced as a result of early ambulation. _____

_____

_____

8. Name three criteria that must be met before a postoperative patient can be given fluids:

   a. _____

   b. _____

   c. _____

9. The return of peristalsis in the postoperative period can be determined by the presence of:

_____ and _____, both of which are assessed by the nurse.

II. Critical Thinking Questions and Exercises

Discussion and Analysis

1. Describe expected nursing interventions to treat hypopharyngeal obstruction.

2. Discuss at least 5 of 12 major nursing diagnoses for the postoperative patient.

3. Describe three postoperative conditions that put a patient at risk for common respiratory complications.

Applying Concepts

Read the case study. Fill in the spaces provided.

CASE STUDY: Postoperative Pain

Mr. Flynn's pain medication was frequently delayed because his staff nurses were busy with other patients. As a nursing supervisor, you stressed the necessity of preventing or managing postoperative pain, knowing that there is a positive correlation between pain experience and the frequency of complications. Support your argument by filling in these blank spaces.

Pain stimulates _____, which increases _____ and

_____.

Noxious impulses stimulate _____, which increases _____ and

_____.

Hypothalmic stress responses increase _____ and _____,

   which can lead to _____ and _____.

Bendetti (1992) found that _____ can be _____ times more

   frequent and _____ can be _____ times greater with
   adequate postoperative control.

Clinical Situations

Read the following case studies. Circle the correct answer.

CASE STUDY: Hypovolemic Shock

Mario is admitted to the emergency department with a diagnosis of hypovolemic shock secondary to a 30% blood volume loss resulting from a motorcycle accident.

1. A primary nursing objective is to:
   a. administer vasopressors.
   b. ensure a patent airway.
   c. minimize energy expenditure.
   d. provide external warmth.

2. With a diagnosis of hypovolemic shock, the nurse expects to assess all of the following *except*:
   a. a decreased and concentrated urinary output.
   b. an elevated central venous pressure reading.
   c. hypotension with a small pulse pressure.
   d. tachycardia and a thready pulse.

3. The nurse takes blood pressure readings every 5 minutes. She knows that shock is well advanced when the systolic reading drops below:
   a. 90 mm Hg.
   b. 100 mm Hg.
   c. 110 mm Hg.
   d. 120 mm Hg.

4. A urinary catheter is inserted to measure hourly output. The nurse knows that inadequate volume replacement is reflected by an output of less than:
   a. 30 mL/hr.
   b. 50 mL/hr.
   c. 80 mL/hr.
   d. 100 mL/hr.

5. The physician prescribes crystalloid solution to be administered to restore blood volume. The nurse knows that a crystalloid solution is:
   a. a blood transfusion.
   b. lactated Ringer's solution.
   c. plasma or a plasma substitute.
   d. serum albumin.

CASE STUDY: Hypopharyngeal Obstruction

Daena is unconscious when she is transferred to the recovery room. She has experienced prolonged anesthesia, and all her muscles are relaxed.

1. During the initial assessment, the nurse diagnosed hypopharyngeal obstruction. This difficulty is signaled by:
   a. choking.
   b. cyanosis.
   c. irregular respirations.
   d. all of the above.

2. To treat hypopharyngeal obstruction, the nurse would:
   a. flex the neck and pull the lower jaw down toward the chest.
   b. hyperextend the neck and push forward on the angle of the lower jaw.
   c. raise the head and open the mouth as far as possible.
   d. rotate the head to either side and unclench the teeth.

3. The nurse knows that the most accurate way to determine whether Daena is breathing is to:
   a. auscultate for breath sounds.
   b. inspect for diaphragmatic movement.
   c. palpate for thoracic changes.
   d. place her palm over Daena's nose and mouth.

4. The anesthesiologist chose to leave a plastic airway in Daena's mouth. The nurse knows that an airway should not be removed:
   a. without a physician's order.
   b. until the patient's secretions have been aspirated.
   c. until signs indicate that reflexes are returning.
   d. until arterial blood gas measurements indicate adequate PO_2 levels.

CASE STUDY: Wound Healing

Elizabeth is returned from the recovery room to a patient care area after a routine cholecystectomy.

1. The nurse expects that the inflammatory phase of wound healing should last for about:
   a. 1 day.
   b. 3 days.
   c. 5 days.
   d. 4 days.

2. When both sides of the wound approximate within 24 to 48 hours, the healing is said to be by ____ intention.
   a. first
   b. second
   c. third
   d. spontaneous

3. Those clinical manifestations associated with the inflammatory phase of wound healing that the nurse would expect to see postoperatively are:
   a. pain.
   b. redness.
   c. warmth.
   d. all of the above.

4. Nursing measures to promote adequate tissue oxygenation during the inflammatory phase of wound healing include:
   a. applying warm compresses to the incision every 4 hours for 2 to 3 days to stimulate vasodilation.
   b. encouraging coughing and deep breathing to enhance pulmonary and cardiovascular functions.
   c. helping Elizabeth stay in bed for 4 to 6 days to prevent unnecessary strain on the suture line.
   d. leaving soiled dressings in place to prevent airborne microorganisms from entering the wound and setting up a localized infection.

Clinical Situation: Phlebothrombosis

View Figure 20–8, page 456, and answer the following clinically focused questions.

1. Look at (A) and explain what the nurse is doing.

   _____

   _____

2. Describe how the nurse would assess for a positive Homans' sign:

   _____

   _____

3. Describe what phlebothrombosis is:

   _____

   _____

4. Look at (B), and explain why a tape measure is around the calf muscle.

   _____

   _____

UNIT 5
Gas Exchange and Respiratory Function

21

Assessment of Respiratory Function

I. Interpretation, Completion, and Comparison

Multiple Choice. Read each question carefully. Circle your answer.

1. The purpose of the cilia is to:
   a. produce mucus.
   b. phagocytize bacteria.
   c. contract smooth muscle.
   d. move the mucous back to the larynx.

2. A patient with sinus congestion points to the area on the inside of the eye as a point of pain. The nurse knows that the patient is referring to the _____ sinus.
   a. frontal
   b. ethmoidal
   c. maxillary
   d. sphenoidal

3. The lungs are enclosed in a serous membrane called the:
   a. diaphragm.
   b. mediastinum.
   c. pleura.
   d. xiphoid process.

4. The left lung, in contrast to the right lung, has:
   a. one less lobe.
   b. one more lobe.
   c. the same number of lobes.
   d. two more lobes.

5. The divisions of the lung lobe proceed in the following order, beginning at the main stem bronchi:
   a. lobar bronchi, bronchioles, segmented bronchi, subsequent bronchi.
   b. segmented bronchi, subsegmented bronchi, lobar bronchi, bronchioles.
   c. lobar bronchi, segmented bronchi, subsegmented bronchi, bronchioles.
   d. subsegmented bronchi, lobar bronchi, bronchioles, segmented bronchi.

6. Choose the initial part of the respiratory tract that is not considered part of the gas-exchange airways.
   a. Bronchioles
   b. Respiratory bronchioles
   c. Alveolar duct
   d. Alveolar sacs

7. Choose the alveolar cells that secrete surfactant.
   a. Type I cells
   b. Type II cells
   c. Type III cells
   d. Type I and type II cells

8. Gas exchange between the lungs and blood and between the blood and tissues is called:
   a. active transport.
   b. respiration.
   c. ventilation.
   d. cellular respiration.

9. The exchange of oxygen and carbon dioxide from the alveoli into the blood occurs by:
a. active transport.
b. diffusion.
c. osmosis.
d. pinocytosis.

10. Airflow into the lungs during inspiration depends on all of the following *except*:
a. contraction of the muscles of respiration.
b. enlargement of the thoracic cavity.
c. lowered intrathoracic pressure.
d. relaxation of the diaphragm.

11. The pulmonary circulation is considered a:
a. high-pressure, high-resistance system.
b. low-pressure, low-resistance system.
c. high-pressure, low-resistance system.
d. low-pressure, high-resistance system.

12. The maximum volume of air that can be inhaled after a normal inhalation is known as:
a. inhalation reserve volume.
b. expiratory reserve volume.
c. tidal volume.
d. residual volume.

13. Tidal volume, which may not significantly change with disease, has a normal value of approximately:
a. 300 mL.
b. 500 mL.
c. 800 mL.
d. 1000 mL.

14. Uneven perfusion of the lung is primarily due to:
a. pulmonary artery pressure.
b. gravity.
c. alveolar pressure.
d. all of the above.

15. A nurse caring for a patient with a pulmonary embolism understands that a high ventilation–perfusion ratio may exist. This means that:
a. perfusion exceeds ventilation.
b. there is an absence of perfusion and ventilation.
c. ventilation exceeds perfusion.
d. ventilation matches perfusion.

16. A nurse understands that a safe but low level of oxygen saturation provides for adequate tissue saturation but allows no reserve for situations that threaten ventilation. A safe but low oxygen saturation level is:
a. 40 mm Hg.
b. 75 mm Hg.
c. 80 mm Hg.
d. 95 mm Hg.

17. When taking a respiratory history, the nurse should assess:
a. the previous history of lung disease in the patient or family.
b. occupational and environmental influences.
c. smoking and exposure to allergies.
d. all of the above.

18. Bacterial pneumonia can be indicated by the presence of all of the following except:
a. green, purulent sputum.
b. thick, yellow sputum.
c. thin, mucoid sputum.
d. rusty sputum.

19. Nursing assessment for a patient with chest pain includes:
a. determining whether there is a relationship between the pain and the patient's posture.
b. evaluating the effect of the phases of respiration on the pain.
c. looking for factors that precipitate the pain.
d. all of the above.

20. Chest pain described as knifelike on inspiration would most likely be diagnostic of:
a. bacterial pneumonia.
b. bronchogenic carcinoma.
c. lung infarction.
d. pleurisy.

21. Hemoptysis, a symptom of cardiopulmonary disorders, is characterized by all of the following *except*:
a. a coffeeground appearance.
b. an alkaline pH.
c. a sudden onset.
d. bright red bleeding mixed with sputum.

22. A patient exhibits cyanosis when _____ g/dL of hemoglobin is unoxygenated.
a. 0.77
b. 2.3
c. 15.0
d. 5.0

23. The nurse inspects the thorax of a patient with advanced emphysema. The nurse expects chest configuration change consistent with a deformity known as:
   a. barrel chest.
   c. kyphoscoliosis.
   b. funnel chest.
   d. pigeon chest.

24. Breath sounds that originate in the smaller bronchi and bronchioles and are high-pitched, sibilant, and musical are called:
   a. wheezes.
   c. rales.
   b. rhonchi.
   d. crackles.

25. The arterial blood gas measurement that best reflects the adequacy of alveolar ventilation is the:
   a. PaO_2.
   c. pH.
   b. $PaCO_2$.
   d. SaO_2.

26. Nursing directions to a patient from whom a sputum specimen is to be obtained should include all of the following *except* directing the patient to:
   a. initially clear his or her nose and throat.
   c. take a few deep breaths before coughing.
   b. spit surface mucus and saliva into a sterile specimen container.
   d. use diaphragmatic contractions to aid in the expulsion of sputum.

27. A physician wants a study of diaphragmatic motion because of suspected pathology. The physician would most likely order a:
   a. barium swallow.
   c. fluoroscopy.
   b. bronchogram.
   d. tomogram.

28. Nursing instructions for a patient who is scheduled for a perfusion lung scan should include informing the patient that:
   a. a mask will be placed over his or her nose and mouth during the test.
   c. the imaging time will amount to 20 to 40 minutes.
   d. all of the above will occur.
   b. he or she will be expected to lie under the camera.

29. The nurse should advise the prebronchoscope patient that he or she will:
   a. have his or her nose sprayed with a topical anesthetic.
   c. receive preoperative medication.
   d. experience all of the above.
   b. be required to fast before the procedure.

Fill-In. *Read each statement carefully. Write your response in the space provided.*

1. Explain the difference between ventilation and respiration.

   _____

2. Explain the function of the epiglottis.

   _____

3. Explain this statement: A patient with atelectasis and pulmonary fibrosis has decreased lung compliance.

   _____

4. Name two centers in the brain that are responsible for the neurologic control of ventilation:

   _____ and _____

5. The alveoli begin to lose elasticity at about age _____ years, resulting in decreased gas diffusion.

6. Explain the breathing pattern characterized as Cheyne-Stokes respirations.

   _____

II. Critical Thinking Questions and Exercises

Clinical Situations

Read the following case studies. Circle the correct answer.

CASE STUDY: Bronchoscopy

Mr. Kecklin is scheduled for a bronchoscopy for the diagnostic purpose of locating a pathologic process.

1. Because a bronchoscopy was ordered, the nurse knows that the suspected lesion was not in the:
   a. bronchus.
   b. larynx.
   c. pharynx.
   d. trachea.

2. Nursing measures before the bronchoscopy include:
   a. obtaining an informed consent.
   b. supplying information about the procedure.
   c. withholding food and fluids for 6 hours before the test.
   d. all of the above.

3. The nurse is aware that possible complications of bronchoscopy include all of the following *except*:
   a. aspiration.
   b. gastric perforation.
   c. infection.
   d. pneumothorax.

4. After the bronchoscopy, Mr. Kecklin must be observed for:
   a. dyspnea.
   b. hemoptysis.
   c. tachycardia.
   d. all of the above.

5. After the bronchoscopy, Mr. Kecklin:
   a. can be given ice chips and fluids after he demonstrates that he can perform the gag reflex.
   b. should immediately be given a house diet to alleviate the hunger resulting from the required fast.
   c. should initially be given iced ginger ale to prevent vomiting and possible aspiration of stomach contents.
   d. will need to remain NPO for 6 hours to prevent pharyngeal irritation.

CASE STUDY: Thoracentesis

Mrs. Lomar is admitted to the clinical area for a thoracentesis. The physician wants to remove excess air from the pleural cavity.

1. Nursing responsibilities before the thoracentesis should include:
   a. informing Mrs. Lomar about pressure sensations that will be experienced during the procedure.
   b. making sure that chest roentgenograms ordered in advance have been completed.
   c. seeing that the consent form has been explained and signed.
   d. all of the above.

2. For the thoracentesis, the patient is assisted to any of the following positions *except*:
   a. lying on the unaffected side with the bed elevated 30 to 40 degrees.
   b. lying prone with the head of the bed lowered 15 to 30 degrees.
   c. sitting on the edge of the bed with her feet supported and her arms and head on a padded overbed table.
   d. straddling a chair with her arms and head resting on the back of the chair.

3. Nursing intervention includes exposing the entire chest even though the thoracentesis site is normally in the midclavicular line between the:
   a. first and second intercostal spaces.
   b. second and third intercostal spaces.
   c. third and fourth intercostal spaces.
   d. fourth and fifth intercostal spaces.

4. Nursing observations after the thoracentesis include assessment for:

a. blood-tinged mucus.

b. signs of hypoxemia.

c. tachycardia.

d. all of the above.

5. A chest x-ray film is usually ordered after the thoracentesis to rule out:

a. pleurisy.

b. pneumonia.

c. pneumothorax.

d. pulmonary edema.

Interpreting Data

Review the figure below and explain in your own words what the oxygen-hemoglobin curve depicts. Also explain expected changes with clinical conditions (see pages 470–471 of the text).

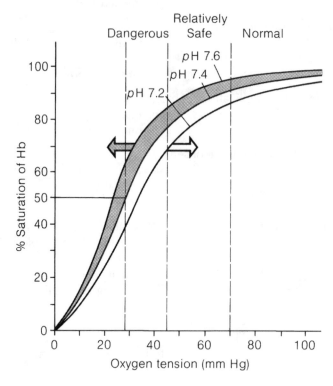

Oxyhemoglobin dissociation curve.

The oxyhemoglobin dissociation curve is marked to show three oxygen levels:

1. normal levels (PaO_2 greater than 70 mm Hg),

2. relatively safe levels (PaO_2 45 to 70 mm Hg), and

3. dangerous levels (PaO_2 lower than 40 mm Hg). The normal (middle) curve shows that 75% saturation occurs at a PaO_2 of 40 mm Hg. If the curve shifts to the right, the same saturation (75%) occurs at the higher PaO_2 of 57 mm Hg. If the curve shifts to the left, 75% saturation occurs at a PaO_2 of 25 mm Hg.

Explain the concepts supporting the basis for the oxygen–hemoglobin dissociation curve in your own words. Interpret the relevance of the data depicted in the figure.

_____

_____

_____

_____

22

Management of Patients With Upper Respiratory Tract Disorders

I. Interpretation, Completion, and Comparison

Multiple Choice. *Read each question carefully. Circle your answer.*

1. Nursing measures associated with the uncomplicated common cold include all of the following *except*:
   a. administering prescribed antibiotics to decrease the severity of the viral infection.
   b. informing the patient about the symptoms of secondary infection, the major complication of a cold.
   c. suggesting adequate fluid intake and rest.
   d. teaching people that the virus is contagious for 2 days before symptoms appear and during the first part of the symptomatic phase.

2. Health teaching for viral rhinitis includes advising the patient to:
   a. blow his or her nose gently to prevent spread of the infection.
   b. blow through both nostrils to equalize the pressure.
   c. rest, to promote overall comfort.
   d. do all of the above.

3. The herpes virus, which remains latent in cells of the lips or nose, usually subsides spontaneously in:
   a. 5 days.
   b. 1 week.
   c. 10–14 days.
   d. 3–4 weeks.

4. Acyclovir, an antiviral agent, is recommended for:
   a. herpes simplex infection.
   b. rhinitis.
   c. sinusitus.
   d. bronchitis.

5. About 60% of cases of acute sinusitis are caused by bacterial organisms. A second-line antibiotic used is:
   a. Augmentin
   b. Amoxil
   c. erythromycin.
   d. septra.

6. Nursing suggestions for a patient with acute or chronic sinusitis include:
   a. adequate fluid intake.
   b. increased humidity.
   c. local heat applications to promote drainage.
   d. all of the above.

7. Acute pharyngitis of a bacterial nature is most commonly caused by:
   a. group A, beta-hemolytic streptococci.
   b. gram-negative *Klebsiella*.
   c. *Pseudomonas*.
   d. *Staphylococcus aureus*.

8. A complication of acute pharyngitis is:
   a. mastoiditis.
   b. otitis media.
   c. peritonsillar abscess.
   d. all of the above.

9. Nursing management for a patient with acute pharyngitis includes:
   a. applying an ice collar for symptomatic relief of a severe sore throat.
   b. encouraging bed rest during the febrile stage of the illness.
   c. suggesting a liquid or soft diet during the acute stage of the disease.
   d. all of the above measures.

10. The most common organism associated with tonsillitis and adenoiditis is:
    a. group A, beta-hemolytic streptococcus.
    b. gram-negative *Klebsiella*.
    c. *Psuedomonas*.
    d. *Staphylococcus aureus*.

11. Potential complications of enlarged adenoids include all of the following *except*:
    a. bronchitis.
    b. nasal obstruction.
    c. allergies.
    d. acute otitis media.

12. To assess for an upper respiratory tract infection, the nurse should palpate:
    a. the frontal and maxillary sinuses.
    b. the trachea.
    c. the neck lymph nodes.
    d. all of the above areas.

13. To assess for an upper respiratory tract infection, the nurse should inspect:
    a. the nasal mucosa.
    b. the frontal sinuses.
    c. the tracheal mucosa.
    d. all of the above.

14. Airway clearance in a patient with an upper airway infection is facilitated by all of the following *except*:
    a. decreasing systemic hydration.
    b. humidifying inspired room air.
    c. positional drainage of the affected area.
    d. administering prescribed vasoconstrictive medications.

15. Nursing intervention for a patient with a fractured nose includes all of the following *except*:
    a. applying cold compresses to decrease swelling and control bleeding.
    b. assessing respirations to detect any interference with breathing.
    c. observing for any clear fluid drainage from either nostril.
    d. packing each nostril with a cotton pledget to minimize bleeding and help maintain the shape of the nose during fracture setting.

16. Surgical reduction of nasal fractures is usually performed _____ after the fracture.
    a. within 24 hours
    b. 7–10 days
    c. 2–3 weeks
    d. 2 months

17. The glottis is also known as the:
    a. larynx.
    b. cricoid cartilage.
    c. "Adam's apple."
    d. opening between the vocal chords.

18. To correctly perform the Heimlich maneuver, a person should forcefully apply pressure against the victim's:
    a. abdomen.
    b. diaphragm.
    c. lungs.
    d. trachea.

19. An early sign of cancer of the larynx in the glottic area (66% of cases) is:
    a. affected voice sounds.
    b. burning of the throat when hot liquids are ingested.
    c. enlarged cervical nodes.
    d. dysphagia.

20. Assessment of a patient admitted for laryngeal carcinoma includes:

    a. palpation of the frontal and maxillary sinuses to detect infection or inflammation.

    b. palpation of the neck for swelling.

    c. inspection of the nasal mucosa for polyps.

    d. all of the above techniques.

21. A patient with a total laryngectomy would no longer have:

    a. natural vocalization.

    b. protection of the lower airway from foreign particles.

    c. a normal effective cough.

    d. all of the above mechanisms.

22. Patient education for a laryngectomy includes:

    a. advising that large amounts of mucus can be coughed up through the stoma.

    b. cautioning about preventing water from entering the stoma.

    c. telling the patient to expect a diminished sense of taste and smell.

    d. doing all of the above.

Fill-In. *Read each statement carefully. Write your response in the space provided.*

1. Explain how rhinitis can lead to sinusitis.

_____

2. Name three bacterial organisms that account for more than 60% of all cases of acute sinusitis:

_____, _____ and _____.

3. The most common cause of laryngitis is _____, with symptoms including _____,

_____ and _____.

4. List five potential complications of an upper airway infection: _____, _____,

_____, _____, and _____.

5. Explain the clinical manifestations that are used to diagnose obstructive sleep apnea:

_____

II. Critical Thinking Questions and Exercises

Clinical Situations

Read the following case studies. Fill in the blanks or circle the correct answer.

CASE STUDY: Tonsillectomy and Adenoidectomy

Isabel, a 14-year-old girl, has just undergone a tonsillectomy and adenoidectomy. The staff nurse assists her with transport from the recovery area to her room.

1. Based on knowledge about tonsillar disease, the nurse knows that Isabel must have experienced symptoms that required surgical intervention. Clinical manifestations may have included:

    a. hypertrophy of the tonsils.

    b. repeated attacks of otitis media.

    c. suspected hearing loss secondary to otitis media.

    d. all of the above.

2. The nurse assesses Isabel's postoperative vital signs and checks for the most significant postoperative complication of:

    a. epiglottis.

    b. eustachian tube perforation.

    c. hemorrhage.

    d. oropharyngeal edema.

3. The nurse maintains Isabel in the recommended postoperative position of:

    a. prone with her head on a pillow and turned to the side.

    b. reverse Trendelenburg with the neck extended.

    c. semi-Fowler's with the neck flexed.

    d. supine with her neck hyperextended and supported with a pillow.

4. Isabel is to be discharged the same day of her tonsillectomy. The nurse makes sure that her family knows to:

    a. encourage her to eat a house diet to build up her resistance to infection.

    b. offer her only clear liquids for 3 days, to prevent pharyngeal irritation.

    c. offer her soft foods for several days to minimize local discomfort and supply her with necessary nutrients.

    d. supplement her diet with orange and lemon juices because of the need for vitamin C to heal tissues.

CASE STUDY: Epistaxis

Gilberta, a 14-year-old high school student, is sent with her mother to the emergency department of a local hospital for uncontrolled epistaxis.

1. Describe what the school nurse should tell Gilberta to manage the bleeding site while being transported to the hospital.

_____

_____

2. Initial nursing measures in the emergency room that can be used to stop the nasal bleeding include:

    a. compressing the soft outer portion of the nose against the midline septum continuously for 5 to 10 minutes.

    b. keeping Gilberta in the upright position with her head tilted forward to prevent swallowing and aspiration of blood.

    c. telling Gilberta to breathe through her mouth and to refrain from talking.

    d. all of the above.

3. The nurse expects that emergency medical treatment may include insertion of a cotton pledget moistened with:

    a. an adrenergic blocking agent.

    b. aqueous epinephrine.

    c. protamine sulfate.

    d. vitamin K.

4. The nurse is aware that nasal packing used to control bleeding can be left in place:

    a. no longer than 2 hours.

    b. an average of 12 hours.

    c. an average of 24 hours.

    d. anywhere from 2 to 6 days.

CASE STUDY: Laryngectomy

Jerome, a 52-year-old widower, is admitted for a laryngectomy owing to a malignant tumor.

1. Before developing a care plan, the nurse needs to know whether Jerome's voice will be preserved. The surgical procedure that would not damage the voice box is a:

    a. partial laryngectomy.

    b. supraglottic laryngectomy.

    c. thyrotomy.

    d. total laryngectomy.

2. Jerome is scheduled for a total laryngectomy. Preoperative education includes:

    a. informing him that there are ways he will be able to carry on a conversation without his voice.

    b. making sure that he knows he will require a permanent tracheal stoma.

    c. reminding him that he will not be able to sing, whistle, or laugh.

    d. all of the above.

3. Postoperative nutrition is usually maintained by way of a nasogastric catheter. The nurse needs to tell Jerome that oral feedings usually begin after:

    a. 24 hours.

    b. 2–3 days.

    c. 5–6 days.

    d. 1 week.

4. Postoperative nursing measures to promote respiratory effectiveness include:

a. assisting with turning and early ambulation.

b. positioning Jerome in semi- to high Fowler's position.

c. reminding him to cough and take frequent deep breaths.

d. all of the above.

5. Jerome needs to know that the laryngectomy tube will be removed when:

a. esophageal speech has been perfected.

b. he requests that it be removed.

c. oral feedings are initiated.

d. the stoma is well healed.

23

Management of Patients With Chest and Lower Respiratory Tract Disorders

I. Interpretation, Comprehension, and Comparison

Multiple Choice. *Read each question carefully. Circle your answer*

1. Nursing management for a person diagnosed as having acute tracheobronchitis includes:
   a. increasing fluid intake to remove secretions.
   b. encouraging the patient to remain in bed.
   c. using cool-vapor therapy to relieve laryngeal and tracheal irritation.
   d. all of the above.

2. The nurse knows that a sputum culture is necessary to identify the causative organism for acute tracheobronchitis. If the culture identifies a fungal agent, the nurse knows it would most likely be:
   a. *Aspergillius.*
   b. *Haemophilus.*
   c. *Mycoplasma pneumoniae.*
   d. *Streptococcus pneumoniae.*

3. In the United States, the most common cause of death from infectious diseases is:
   a. atelectasis.
   b. pulmonary embolus.
   c. pneumonia.
   d. traceobronchitis.

4. *Streptococcus pneumoniae* is the most common organism responsible for _____ pneumonia.
   a. hospital-acquired
   b. immunocompromised
   c. aspiration-specific
   d. community-acquired

5. Characteristics of the *Mycobacterium tuberculosis* include all of the following *except*:
   a. it can be transmitted only by droplet nuclei.
   b. it is acid-fast.
   c. it is able to lie dormant within the body for years.
   d. it survives in anaerobic conditions.

6. It is estimated that *Mycobacterium tuberculosis* infects about _____ of the world's population.
   a. 10%
   b. 25%
   c. 35%
   d. 50%

7. For the tubercle bacillus to multiply and initiate a tissue reaction in the lungs, it must be deposited in:
   a. the alveoli.
   b. the bronchi.
   c. the trachea.
   d. all of the above.

8. A Mantoux skin test is considered not significant if the size of the induration is:
    a. 3–4 mm.
    b. 5–6 mm.
    c. 7–8 mm.
    d. >9 mm.

9. Prophylactic INH drug treatment is necessary for about _____ months.
    a. 3
    b. 3–5
    c. 6–12
    d. 13–18

10. Diagnostic confirmation of a lung abscess is made by:
    a. chest radiograph.
    b. bronchoscopy.
    c. sputum culture.
    d. evaluating all of the above studies.

11. The most diagnostic clinical symptom of pleurisy is:
    a. dullness or flatness on percussion over areas of collected fluid.
    b. dyspnea and coughing.
    c. fever and chills.
    d. stabbing pain during respiratory movement.

12. A pleural effusion results when fluid accumulation in the pleural space is greater than:
    a. 5 mL.
    b. 10 mL.
    c. 15 mL.
    d. 20 mL.

13. Auscultation can be used to diagnose the presence of pulmonary edema when the following adventitious breath sounds are present:
    a. crackles in the posterior bases.
    b. low-pitched rhonchi during expiration.
    c. pleural friction rub.
    d. sibilant wheezes.

14. Acute respiratory failure (ARF) occurs when oxygen tension (PaO_2) falls below _____ mm Hg (hypoxemia) and carbon dioxide tension ($PaCO_2$) rises to greater than _____ mm Hg (hypercapnia).
    a. 50   b. 60   c. 75   d. 80

15. The pathophysiology of ARF is directly related to:
    a. decreased respiratory drive.
    b. chest wall abnormalities.
    c. dysfunction of lung parenchyma.
    d. all of the above mechanisms.

16. Neuromuscular blockers are given to patients who are on ventilators in ARF to accomplish all of the following *except*:
    a. maintain positive end-expiratory pressure (PEEP).
    b. maintain better ventilation.
    c. increase the respiratory rate.
    d. keep the patient from fighting the ventilator.

17. A key characteristic feature of adult respiratory distress syndrome (ARDS) is:
    a. arterial hypoxemia.
    b. diminished alveolar dilation.
    c. tachypnea.
    d. increased PaO_2.

18. A 154-lb, 60-year-old woman is being treated for ARDS. The nurse knows that the minimum daily caloric requirement to meet normal requirements is:
    a. 1200–1800 cal.
    b. 1800–2200 cal.
    c. 2000–2400 cal.
    d. 2500–3000 cal.

19. A nurse knows to assess a patient with pulmonary hypertension for the primary symptoms of:
    a. ascites.
    b. dyspnea.
    c. hypertension.
    d. syncope.

20. Clinical manifestations directly related to cor pulmonale include all of the following *except*:
    a. dyspnea and cough.
    b. diminished peripheral pulses.
    c. distended neck veins.
    d. edema of the feet and legs.

21. The nurse assesses a patient for a possible pulmonary embolism. The nurse looks for _____, the most frequent sign.
    a. cough
    b. hemoptysis
    c. syncope
    d. tachypnea

22. Anticoagulation with heparin attempts to maintain the partial thromboplastin time (PTT) at times _____ normal.
a. 0.5–1.0
b. 1.5–2.5
c. 2.5–3.0
d. >3.0

23. Nursing measures to assist in the prevention of pulmonary embolism in a hospitalized patient include all of the following *except*:
a. a liberal fluid intake.
b. assisting the patient to do leg elevations above the level of the heart.
c. encouraging the patient to dangle his or her legs over the side of the bed for 30 minutes, four times a day.
d. the use of elastic stockings, especially when decreased mobility would promote venous stasis.

24. To assess for a positive Homan sign, the nurse should:
a. dorsiflex the foot while the leg is elevated to check for calf pain.
b. elevate the patient's legs for 20 minutes and then lower them slowly while checking for areas of inadequate blood return.
c. extend the leg, plantar flex the foot, and check for the patency of the dorsalis pedis pulse.
d. lower the patient's legs and massage the calf muscles to note any areas of tenderness.

25. As a cause of death among men in the United States, lung cancer ranks:
a. first.
b. second.
c. third.
d. fourth.

26. More than 85% of all lung cancers are primarily caused by:
a. cigarette smoking.
b. fibrosis.
c. inhalation of environmental carcinogens.
d. tuberculosis.

27. The most prevalent lung carcinoma that is peripherally located and frequently metastasizes is:
a. adenocarcinoma.
b. broncheoalveolar.
c. large cell.
d. squamous cell.

28. The most frequent symptom of lung cancer is:
a. copious sputum production.
b. coughing.
c. dyspnea.
d. severe pain.

29. The nurse is aware that the most common surgical procedure for a small, apparently curable tumor of the lung is a:
a. lobectomy.
b. pneumonectomy.
c. segmentectomy.
d. wedge resection.

30. Paradoxical chest movement is associated with the following chest disorder:
a. pneumothorax.
b. flail chest.
c. ARDS.
d. tension pneumothorax.

31. An initial characteristic symptom of a simple pneumothorax is:
a. ARDS.
b. severe respiratory distress.
c. sudden onset of chest pain.
e. tachypnea and hypoxemia.

Fill-In. *Complete the following questions related to the condition of atelectasis, a pulmonary disorder that can lead to life-threatening acute respiratory failure.*

Atelectasis, which refers to closure or collapse of alveoli, may be chronic or acute in nature.

1. Relate the etiology of atelectasis to 10 possible causes:
a. _____
b. _____
c. _____
d. _____
e. _____
f. _____
g. _____
h. _____
i. _____
j. _____

2. Explain 10 pathogenic mechanisms associated with atelectasis:

a. _____

b. _____

c. _____

d. _____

e. _____

f. _____

g. _____

h. _____

i. _____

j. _____

3. Describe why the alveoli shrinks in size because of reduced alveolar ventilation.

_____

4. Name eight possible clinical manifestations of atelectasis.

a. _____ e. _____

b. _____ f. _____

c. _____ g. _____

d. _____ h. _____

5. Identify eight nursing measures that can be used to prevent atelectasis.

a. _____ e. _____

b. _____ f. _____

c. _____ g. _____

d. _____ h. _____

6. The diagnosis of hospital-acquired pneumonia is usually associated with the presence of one of three

conditions:_____, _____ and

_____.

7. List three severe complications of pneumonia: _____, _____,

and _____.

8. Explain the meaning of the term *superinfection*.

_____

9. According to the World Health Organization(WHO), the leading cause of death among human immunodeficiency virus (HIV)–positive people is:

_____.

10. List four respiratory system mechanisms that can lead to acute respiratory failure (ARF):

_____ _____

_____ _____

II. Critical Thinking Questions and Exercises

Examining Associations

1. Diagram the sequence of pathophysiologic events that lead to pneumonia.

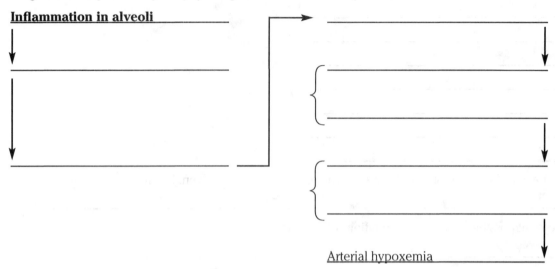

2. Diagram the sequence of pathophysiologic events that lead to ARDS.

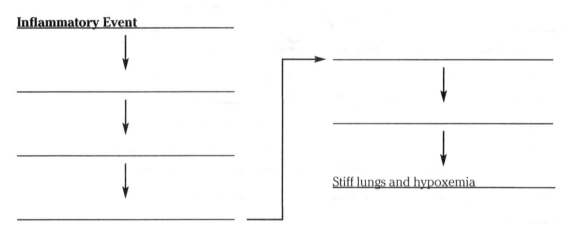

Clinical Situations

Read the following case studies. Circle the correct answer.

CASE STUDY: Community-Acquired Pneumonia

Theresa, a 20-year-old college student, lives in a small dormitory with 30 other students. Four weeks into the Spring semester, she was diagnosed as having bacterial pneumonia and was admitted to the hospital.

1. The nurse is informed that Theresa has the strain of bacteria most frequently found in community-acquired pneumonia. The nurse suspects that the infecting agent is:
   a. *Haemophilus influenzae*   c. *Pseudomonas aeruginosa*
   c. *Klebsiella*   d. *Streptococcus pneumoniae*

2. All of the following are manifestations of bacterial pneumonia *except*:

    a. fever.

    b. bradycardia.

    c. stabbing or pleuritic chest pain.

    d. tachypnea.

3. The nurse expects that Theresa will be medicated with the usual antibiotic of choice, which is:

    a. cephalosporin.

    b. clindamycin.

    c. erythromycin.

    d. penicillin G.

4. The nurse is aware that Theresa may develop arterial hypoxemia, because:

    a. bronchospasm causes alveolar collapse, which decreases the surface area necessary for perfusion.

    b. mucosal edema occludes the alveoli, thereby producing a drop in alveolar oxygen.

    c. venous blood is shunted from the right to the left side of the heart.

    d. all of the above are true.

5. Theresa is expected to respond to antibiotic therapy:

    a. within 6 hours.

    b. between 1 and 2 days.

    c. by the fourth day.

    d. after 7 days.

6. Nursing management includes assessment for complications such as:

    a. atelectasis.

    b. hypotension and shock.

    c. pleural effusion.

    d. all of the above.

CASE STUDY: Tuberculosis

Mr. Carrera, a 67-year-old retired baker and pastry chef, is admitted to the clinical area for confirmation of suspected tuberculosis. He is anorexic and fatigued and suffers from "indigestion." His temperature is slightly elevated every afternoon.

1. Mr. Carrera's Mantoux tuberculin test yields an induration area of 10 mm. This result is interpreted as indicating that:

    a. active disease is present.

    b. he has been exposed to *M. tuberculosis* or has been vaccinated with BCG.

    c. preventive treatment should be initiated.

    d. the reaction is doubtful and should be repeated.

2. After Mr. Carrera has undergone a series of additional tests, the diagnosis is confirmed by:

    a. a chest radiograph.

    b. acid-fast bacilli in a sputum smear.

    c. a positive multiple-puncture skin test.

    d. repeated Mantoux tests that yield indurations of 10 mm or greater.

3. Mr. Carrera is started on a multiple-drug regimen. Nursing management includes observing for ototoxicity and nephrotoxicity when _____ is used.

    a. ethambutol

    b. isoniazid

    c. rifampin

    d. streptomycin

4. Mr. Carrera needs to know that the initial intensive treatment is usually given daily for:

    a. 2 weeks.

    b. 2–4 weeks.

    c. 2 months.

    d. 4–6 months.

5. Mr. Carrera is informed that he will no longer be considered infectious after:

    a. repeat Mantoux tests are negative.

    b. serial chest radiographs show improvement.

    c. two consecutive sputum specimens are negative.

    d. all of the above parameters are met.

CASE STUDY: Acute Respiratory Distress Syndrome

Anne, 71 years of age and single, is admitted to the unit with a diagnosis of ARDS. She was receiving treatment at home for viral pneumonia and had appeared to be improving until yesterday.

1. During assessment, the nurse notes symptoms positively correlated with ARDS, including:

    a. dysrhythmias and hypotension.

    b. contraction of the accessory muscles of respiration.

    c. tachypnea and tachycardia.

    d. all of the above.

2. The nurse also observes symptoms of cerebral hypoxia, including:
   a. drowsiness.
   b. confusion.
   c. irritability.
   d. all of the above.

3. The nurse observes that Anne is receiving oxygen by way of a nasal cannula at 6 L/min. The nurse knows that Anne's FIO_2 is:
   a. 24%.   b. 34%.   c. 44%.   d. 54%.

4. Indications for ventilator support for ARDS include all of the following *except*:
   a. O_2 saturation greater than 90%.
   b. PaO_2 greater than 60%.
   c. respiratory rate greater than 35 bpm.
   d. vital capacity equal to 60 mL/kg of body weight.

5. It is decided that Anne needs a ventilator to help her breathe. Her physician prescribes PEEP. When PEEP is used, all of the following occur *except*:
   a. improved arterial oxygenation.
   b. improved ventilation-perfusion.
   c. increased alveolar dilation.
   d. increased functional residual capacity.

CASE STUDY: Pulmonary Embolism

Sandy, a 37-year-old recovering from multiple fractures sustained in a car accident, was admitted to the intensive care unit for treatment of a pulmonary embolism. Before admission, she was short of breath after walking up a flight of stairs.

1. On the basis of Sandy's medical history, the nurse suspects that a predisposing condition may have been:
   a. hypercoagulability.
   b. postoperative immobility.
   c. venous stasis.
   d. all of the above factors.

2. As part of her assessment information, the nurse knows that the majority of pulmonary emboli originate in the:
   a. deep leg veins.
   b. lung tissue.
   c. pelvic area.
   d. right atrium of the heart.

3. The most common symptom of pulmonary embolism is:
   a. chest pain.
   b. dyspnea.
   c. fever.
   d. hemoptysis.

4. Based on Sandy's diagnosis, the nurse knows to look for a decrease in:
   a. alveolar dead space.
   b. cardiac output.
   c. pulmonary arterial pressure.
   d. right ventricular work load of the heart.

5. A primary nursing problem for Sandy would be:
   a. atelectasis.
   b. bradycardia.
   c. dyspnea.
   d. hypertension.

6. The nurse knows that Sandy's diagnosis was probably confirmed by:
   a. a bronchogram.
   b. a chest roentgenogram.
   c. an electrocardiogram.
   d. a lung scan.

24

Management of Patients With Chronic Obstructive Pulmonary Disease

I. Interpretation, Completion, and Comparison

Multiple Choice. *Read each question carefully. Circle your answer.*

1. As a cause of death in the United States, chronic obstructive pulmonary disease (COPD) ranks:
   a. second.
   b. third.
   c. fourth.
   d. fifth.

2. The current new definition of COPD leaves only one disorder under its classification. That is:
   a. asthma.
   b. bronchiectasis.
   c. cystic fibrosis.
   d. emphysema.

3. The underlying pathophysiology of COPD is:
   a. inflamed airways that obstruct airflow.
   b. mucus secretions that block airways.
   c. overinflated alveoli that impair gas exchange.
   d. characterized by variations of all of the above.

4. The abnormal inflammatory response in the lungs occurs primarily in the:
   a. airways.
   b. parenchyma.
   c. pulmonary vasculature.
   d. areas identified in all of the above.

5. Two diseases common to the etiology of COPD are:
   a. asthma and atelectasis.
   b. bronchitis and emphysema.
   c. pneumonia and pleurisy.
   d. tuberculosis and pleural effusions.

6. For a patient with chronic bronchitis, the nurse expects to see the major clinical symptoms of:
   a. chest pain during respiration.
   b. dyspnea and a productive cough.
   c. fever, chills, and diaphoresis.
   d. tachypnea and tachycardia.

7. The major cause of emphysema is:
   a. air pollution.
   b. allergens.
   c. infectious agents.
   d. smoking.

8. The pathophysiology of emphysema is directly related to airway obstruction. The end result of deterioration is:
   a. diminished alveolar surface area.
   b. hypercapnia resulting from decreased carbon dioxide elimination.
   c. hypoxemia secondary to impaired oxygen diffusion.
   d. respiratory acidosis due to airway obstruction.

9. The primary presenting symptom of emphysema is:
a. chronic cough.
b. dyspnea.
c. tachypnea.
d. wheezing.

10. Bronchodilators are prescribed in emphysema primarily because they:
a. improve gas exchange.
b. interfere with mucosal edema.
c. improve airflow.
d. reverse bronchospasm.

11. A nurse notes that the FEV_1/FVC ratio is less than 70% for a patient with COPD. The nurse documents that the patient is in stage:
a. 0.
b. I.
c. II.
d. III.

12. Nursing assessment of a patient with bronchospasm associated with COPD would include assessment for:
a. compromised gas exchange.
b. decreased airflow.
c. wheezes.
d. all of the above.

13. A commonly prescribed methylxanthine used as a bronchodilator is:
a. Albuteral.
b. Levalbuteral.
c. Theophylline.
d. Terbutaline.

14. The nurse should be alert for a complication of bronchiectasis that results from a combination of retained secretions and obstruction. This complication is known as:
a. atelectasis.
b. emphysema.
c. pleurisy.
d. pneumonia.

15. Histamine, a mediator that supports the inflammatory process in asthma is secreted by:
a. eosinophils.
b. lymphocytes.
c. mast cells.
d. neutrophils.

16. Obstruction of the airway in the patient with asthma is caused by all of the following *except*:
a. thick mucus.
b. swelling of bronchial membranes.
c. destruction of the alveolar wall.
d. contraction of muscles surrounding the bronchi.

17. The major symptom of asthma is:
a. cough.
b. dyspnea.
c. wheezing.
d. all of the above.

18. A commonly prescribed mast cell stabilizer used for asthma is:
a. Albuteral.
b. Budesonide.
c. Cromolyn sodium.
d. Theophylline.

19. The nurse understands that a patient with status asthmaticus will likely initially evidence symptoms of:
a. metabolic acidosis.
b. metabolic alkalosis.
c. respiratory acidosis.
d. respiratory alkalosis.

20. A definitive diagnosis of cystic fibrosis is based on the following diagnostic test:
a. bronchoscopy.
b. computed tomography scan of lungs.
c. pulmonary function tests.
d. sweat chloride test.

Fill-In. Read each statement carefully. Write your response in the space provided.

1. Chronic airway inflammation in COPD results in: _____.

2. Define the term *emphysema* _____.

3. The most important risk factor for COPD is: _____.

4. A genetic risk factor for COPD is: _____.

5. The three *primary symptoms* associated with COPD are: _____, _____,

and _____.

6. The *single most effective* intervention to prevent COPD or slow its progression is:_____.

7. Primary causes for an acute exacerbation of emphysema are:_____ and

   _____.

8. In COPD, increasing the oxygen flow to a high rate may suppress the respiratory drive, because

   _____.

9. The strongest predisposing factor for asthma is: _____.

10. Complications of asthma may include: _____, _____,

    _____ and _____.

II. Critical Thinking Questions and Exercises

Identifying Patterns

Chart the sequence of events that illustrate the pathophysiology of chronic bronchitis.

Smoke and environmental pollutants irritate the airways

⬇

_____

_____

Reduced ciliary function ⬅

_____

_____

➡ *Bronchial wall thickening*

_____

_____

Adjacent alveoli may become damaged and fibrosed ⬅

➡ _____

⬇

_____

Respiratory infections (viral, bacterial and mycoplasmal)

Chart the sequence of events that illustrate the pathophysiology of emphysema.

Alveolar walls are destroyed causing an increase in dead space ⟶ _____

_____

In later stage emphysema, carbon dioxide elimination is ⟶ _____
    impaired

_____

As the alveolar walls break down, the pulmonary capillary bed is reduced, causing increased pulmonary
    blood flow

⟱

_____   ⟶   _____

_____

⟱

Cardiac failure _____

Examining Associations

Compare the pathophysiologic changes and symptomatology for panlobular *and* centrilobular *emphysema.*

Panlobular   **Centrilobular**

_____   _____

_____   _____

_____   _____

_____   _____

_____   _____

Clinical Situations

CASE STUDY: Emphysema

Lois, who has had emphysema for 25 years, is admitted to the hospital with a diagnosis of
bronchitis.

1. During assessment, the nurse notes the presence of a "barrel chest," which the nurse knows is caused by:
    a. a compensatory expansion of the   c. "air trapping" in the lungs.
       bronchial airway.   d. a progressive increase in vital capacity.
    b. a decrease in intrapleural pressure.

2. The nurse recognizes the need to be alert for the major presenting symptom of emphysema, which is:
    a. bradypnea.   c. expiratory wheezing.
    b. dyspnea.   d. fatigue.

3. Arterial blood gas measurements that are consistent with a diagnosis of emphysema are:
   a. pH, 7.32; PaO_2, 70 mm Hg; $PaCO_2$, 50 mm Hg.
   b. pH, 7.37; PaO_2, 90 mm Hg; $PaCO_2$, 42 mm Hg.
   c. pH, 7.39; PaO_2, 80 mm Hg; $PaCO_2$, 35 mm Hg.
   d. pH, 7.40; PaO_2, 85 mm Hg; $PaCO_2$, 42 mm Hg.

4. Lois is being medicated with a bronchodilator to reduce airway obstruction. Nursing actions include observing for the side effect of:
   a. dysrhythmias.
   b. central nervous system excitement.
   c. tachycardia.
   d. all of the above.

5. Diaphragmatic breathing is recommended for Lois because it does all of the following *except*:
   a. decrease respiratory rate.
   b. decrease tidal volume.
   c. increase alveolar ventilation.
   d. reduce functional residual capacity.

6. Oxygen is prescribed for Lois. The nurse knows that the most effective delivery system is:
   a. a rebreathing bag that delivers oxygen at a concentration greater than 60%.
   b. an oxygen mask set a 8 L/min.
   c. a nasal cannula set at 6 L/min.
   d. a Venturi mask that delivers a predictable oxygen flow at about 24%.

25

Respiratory Care Modalities

I. Interpretation, Completion, and Comparison

Multiple Choice. Read each question carefully. Circle your answer.

1. The nurse knows that hypoxemia can be detected by noting a decrease in:
a. PaO_2.
b. PAO_2.
c. pH.
d. PcO_2.

2. A patient with bradycardia and hypotension would most likely exhibit:
a. anemic hypoxia.
b. circulatory hypoxia.
c. histotoxic hypoxia.
d. hypoxic hypoxia.

3. Carbon monoxide poisoning results in:
a. anemic hypoxia.
b. histoxic hypoxia.
c. hypoxic hypoxia.
d. stagnant hypoxia.

4. Decreased gas exchange at the cellular level resulting from a toxic substance is classified as:
a. circulatory
b. histotoxic.
c. hypoxemic.
d. hypoxic.

5. Oxygen therapy administered to a pulmonary patient who retains carbon dioxide:
a. can cause a dangerous rise in $PaCO_2$ levels.
b. can suppress ventilation.
c. should bring the patient's PO_2 level to 60–70 mm Hg.
d. is able to accomplish all of the above mechanisms.

6. When oxygen therapy is being used, "No Smoking" signs are posted, because oxygen:
a. is combustible.
b. is explosive.
c. prevents the dispersion of smoke particles.
d. supports combustion.

7. A patient has been receiving 100% oxygen therapy by way of a nonrebreather mask for several days. He complains of tingling in his fingers and shortness of breath. He is extremely restless and states that he has pain beneath his breastbone. The nurse should suspect:
a. oxygen-induced hypoventilation.
b. oxygen toxicity.
c. oxygen-induced atelectasis.
d. all of the above.

8. Oxygen concentrations of 70% can usually be delivered with the use of:
a. a nasal cannula.
b. an oropharyngeal catheter.
c. a partial rebreathing mask.
d. a Venturi mask.

9. The method of oxygen administration primarily used for patients with chronic obstructive pulmonary disease (COPD) is:
   a. a nasal cannula.
   b. an oropharyngeal catheter.
   c. a nonrebreathing mask.
   d. a Venturi mask.

10. Intermittent positive-pressure breathing differs from incentive spirometry in all the following ways *except*:
    a. it is a mechanical aid to lung expansion.
    b. it is used to encourage hyperinflation.
    c. it produces a forced flow of air into the lungs during inhalation.
    d. it provides for the breathing of air or oxygen.

11. To help a patient use a mininebulizer, the nurse should encourage the patient to do all of the following *except*:
    a. hold his or her breath at the end of inspiration for a few seconds.
    b. cough frequently.
    c. take rapid, deep breaths.
    d. frequently evaluate his or her progress.

12. To assist a patient with the use of an incentive spirometer, the nurse should:
    a. make sure the patient is in a flat, supine position.
    b. tell the patient to try not to cough during and after each session, because doing so will cause pain.
    c. set an unrealistic goal so that the patient will try to maximize effort.
    d. encourage the patient to take approximately 10 breaths per hour between treatments, while awake.

13. Nursing actions associated with postural drainage include:
    a. encouraging the patient to cough after the procedure.
    b. auscultating the lungs before and after the procedure.
    c. encouraging the patient to exhale through pursed lips.
    d. all of the above.

14. When using percussion to aid in secretion removal, the nurse should avoid:
    a. the sternum and spine.
    b. the liver and kidneys.
    c. the spleen and female breast area.
    d. all of the above areas.

15. Percussion is accomplished by continuing the process for:
    a. 3 to 5 minutes while the patient uses diaphragmatic breathing.
    b. 10 to 15 minutes while the patient uses diaphragmatic breathing.
    c. 3 to 5 minutes while the patient breathes normally.
    d. 10 to 15 minutes while the patient breathes normally.

16. When vibrating the patient's chest, the nurse applies vibration:
    a. while the patient is inhaling.
    b. during both inhalation and exhalation.
    c. while the patient is exhaling.
    d. while the patient is holding the breath.

17. The purpose of pursed lips during exhalation is to:
    a. prolong exhalation.
    b. slow down the respiratory rate to allow for maximum lung expansion during inspiration.
    c. widen the airways.
    d. do all of the above.

18. Signs of an upper airway obstruction include:
    a. drawing in of the upper chest, sternum, and intercostal spaces.
    b. prolonged contraction of the abdominal muscles.
    c. tracheal tug.
    d. all of the above.

19. The suggested sequence of nursing actions for management of an upper airway obstruction is:
    a. clear airway, extend head, lift chin, use cross-finger technique, and perform a Heimlich maneuver.
    b. extend head, lift chin, clear airway, and perform a Heimlich maneuver.
    c. extend head, clear airway, lift chin, and insert airway.
    d. lift chin, clear airway, and perform a Heimlich maneuver.

20. Nursing management of a patient with an endotracheal tube includes:
    a. ensuring oxygen administration with high humidity.
    b. repositioning the patient every 2 hours.
    c. suctioning the oropharynx as needed.
    d. all of the above.

21. When suctioning secretions from a tracheostomy tube, it is helpful to first instill:
    a. less than 1 mL of sterile normal saline solution.
    b. 1 to 2 mL of sterile normal saline solution.
    c. 3 to 5 mL of sterile normal saline solution.
    d. 6 to 8 mL of sterile normal saline solution.

22. When suctioning a tracheostomy tube, the nurse needs to remember that each aspiration should not exceed:
    a. 15 seconds.
    b. 30 seconds.
    c. 45 seconds.
    d. 60 seconds.

23. Choose the blood gas sequence that indicates a need for mechanical ventilation.
    a. Decreasing PO_2, decreasing PCO_2, normal pH.
    b. Increasing PO_2, decreasing PCO_2, increasing pH.
    c. Decreasing PO_2, increasing PCO_2, decreasing pH.
    d. Increasing PO_2, decreasing PCO_2, decreasing pH.

24. The most commonly used positive-pressure ventilator currently is the:
    a. chest cuirass.
    b. time-cycled ventilator.
    c. pressure-cycled ventilator.
    d. volume-cycled ventilator.

25. With positive-pressure ventilation, positive intrathoracic pressure:
    a. increases venous return and decreases cardiac output.
    b. decreases venous return and increases cardiac output.
    c. decreases venous return and decreases cardiac output.
    d. increases venous return and increases cardiac output.

26. The term used to describe thoracic surgery in which an entire lung is removed is:
    a. lobectomy.
    b. pneumonectomy.
    c. segmentectomy.
    d. wedge resection.

27. Preoperatively, the patient who is scheduled for thoracic surgery needs to know that postoperatively:
    a. chest tubes and drainage bottles may be necessary.
    b. he or she will be turned frequently and will be asked to cough and breathe deeply.
    c. oxygen will be administered to facilitate breathing if the need arises.
    d. all of the above treatments will be incorporated into a plan of care.

28. The water seal used in a disposable chest drainage system is effective if the water seal chamber is filled to the level of:
    a. 0.5 cm H_2O.
    b. 1.0 cm H_2O.
    c. 1.5 cm H_2O.
    d. 2.0 cm H_2O.

Fill-In. *Read each statement carefully. Write your response in the space provided.*

1. Oxygen transport to the tissues is dependent on four factors: _____, _____, _____, and _____.

2. The concentration of oxygen in room air is _____%.

3. A patient with a PaO_2 of 60 to 95 mm Hg would be expected to have an oxygen saturation level of _____% to _____%.

4. For a patient with COPD, the stimulus for respiration is: _____.

5. Four examples of low-flow oxygen delivery systems are: _____, _____, _____, and _____.

6. The oxygen flow rate for a nasal cannula should not exceed _____ to _____ L/min.

7. Positive-pressure ventilators work by: _____

8. Explain what is meant when the patient is said to be "bucking the ventilator":

_____

Complete the Chart

Look at the following figure of a disposable chest drainage system, and label the figure using the terms provided.

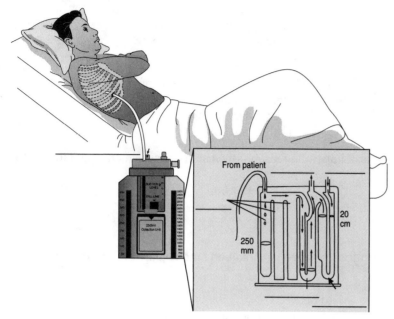

suction control
water seal
vent
drainage collection chambers
suction source
ventilation source

Example of a disposable chest drainage system

II. Critical Thinking Questions and Exercises

Clinical Problem Applications

Read the following case studies. Circle the correct answer.

CASE STUDY: Pneumonectomy: Preoperative Concerns

Mrs. Miley, a 66-year-old widow, is admitted to the clinical area as a preoperative patient scheduled for a pneumonectomy for lung cancer.

1. Nursing assessment during the admission history and physical examination includes obtaining data about the patient's:
a. breathing patterns during exertion.
b. cardiac status during exercise.
c. smoking history.
d. history relevant to all of the above.

2. The nurse knows that medical clearance for surgery is based primarily on evaluation of the:
a. cardiopulmonary system.
b. endocrine system.
c. neurologic system.
d. renal–urinary system.

3. A battery of preoperative tests are ordered. The nurse evaluates the serum creatinine level because it reflects:
a. cardiac status.
b. endocrine status.
c. pulmonary function.
d. renal function.

4. The nurse knows that Mrs. Miley's functional lung capacity can be assessed by evaluating:
a. arterial blood gases.
b. blood urea nitrogen levels.
c. chest radiographs.
d. serum protein levels.

CASE STUDY: Pneumonectomy: Postoperative Concerns

Mrs. Miley was returned to the clinical area after being in the intensive care unit. She is recovering from a right pneumonectomy.

1. The major postoperative nursing objective is to:
   a. maintain a patent airway.
   b. provide for maximum remaining lung expansion.
   c. provide rehabilitative measures.
   d. recognize early indicators of complications.

2. Mrs. Miley had a central venous pressure line in place. Readings were to be taken to detect:
   a. hypothermia.
   b. hypovolemia.
   c. hypoxemia.
   d. hypoxia.

3. Pulmonary edema is a potential danger owing to the possible rapid infusion of intravenous fluids and a reduced vascular bed. Early symptoms of pulmonary edema include:
   a. dyspnea.
   b. frothy sputum.
   c. crackles (rales).
   d. all of the above.

4. The nurse should always be alert for signs of impending respiratory insufficiency, which would include all of the following *except*:
   a. bradycardia.
   b. dyspnea.
   c. hypertension.
   d. tachypnea.

CASE STUDY: Ventilator Patient

Mr. Brown, a 25-year-old man with a drug overdose, has been maintained on a volume-cycled ventilator for 3 weeks.

1. A major nursing assessment for Mr. Brown would be:
   a. breath sounds.
   b. nutritional needs.
   c. psychological status.
   d. spontaneous ventilatory efforts.

2. Positive-pressure ventilation can alter cardiac function. The nurse assesses for indicators of hypoxia and hypoxemia, which would include all of the following *except*:
   a. bradycardia and bradypnea.
   b. diaphoresis and oliguria.
   c. restlessness and confusion.
   d. transient hypertension.

3. A primary nursing intervention for Mr. Brown is maintaining optimal gas exchange. This can be accomplished by:
   a. conservative use of analgesics so that pain is relieved, yet the respiratory drive is not decreased.
   b. daily monitoring of fluid balance to prevent fluid overload.
   c. frequent repositioning to diminish the pulmonary effects of immobility.
   d. all of the above measures.

4. The nurse wants to determine early whether Mr. Brown is "bucking" his ventilator (breathing out during the ventilator's mechanical inspiratory phase) so that he or she can initiate preventive measures if necessary. The nurse should assess for signs and symptoms related to:
   a. hypercarbia.
   b. hypoxia.
   c. inadequate minute volume.
   d. all of the above.

CASE STUDY: Weaning from Ventilator

Mr. O'Day, a 71-year-old trauma victim, is to be weaned from his ventilator.

1. Before weaning, Mr. O'Day's ventilatory capacity should be such that he:
   a. can maintain an inspiratory force of at least 20 cm H_2O pressure.
   b. has a PaO_2 greater than 60% and an FiO_2 less than 40%.
   c. is able to generate a minimum vital capacity of 10 to 15 mL/kg of body weight.
   d. is capable of all of the above.

2. Criteria to determine if Mr. O'Day's endotracheal tube could be removed include:

a. active pharyngeal and laryngeal gag reflexes.

b. adequate spontaneous ventilation.

c. voluntary cough mechanisms.

d. all of the above.

3. Mr. O'Day will be weaned from oxygen when he can breathe room air and maintain a PaO_2 in the range of:

a. 40–50 mm Hg.

b. 50–60 mm Hg.

c. 60–70 mm Hg.

d. 70–100 mm Hg.

UNIT 6

Cardiovascular, Circulatory, and Hematologic Function

26

Assessment of Cardiovascular Function

I. Interpretation, Completion, and Comparison

Multiple Choice. Read each question carefully. Circle your answer.

1. The nurse who is caring for a patient with pericarditis undersands that there is inflammation involving the:
   a. thin fibrous sac encasing the heart.
   b. inner lining of the heart and valves.
   c. heart's muscle fibers.
   d. exterior layer of the heart.

2. The coronary arteries arise from the:
   a. aorta near the origin of the left ventricle.
   b. pulmonary artery at the apex of the right ventricle.
   c. pulmonary vein near the left atrium.
   d. superior vena cava at the origin of the right atrium.

3. The pacemaker for the entire myocardium is the:
   a. atrioventricular junction.
   b. bundle of His.
   c. Purkinje fibers.
   d. sinoatrial node.

4. The intrinsic pacemaker rate of ventricular myocardial cells is:
   a. more than 80 bpm.
   b. 60 to 80 bpm.
   c. 40 to 60 bpm.
   d. fewer than 40 bpm.

5. So that blood may flow from the right ventricle to the pulmonary artery, all of the following conditions must be met *except* that:
   a. the atrioventricular valves must be closed.
   b. the pulmonic valve must be open.
   c. right ventricular pressure must be less than pulmonary arterial pressure.
   d. right ventricular pressure must rise with systole.

6. Heart rate is stimulated by all of the following *except*:
   a. excess thyroid hormone.
   b. increased levels of circulating catecholamines.
   c. the sympathetic nervous system.
   d. the vagus nerve.

7. Stroke volume of the heart is determined by:
   a. the degree of cardiac muscle strength (precontraction).
   b. the intrinsic contractility of the cardiac muscle.
   c. the pressure gradient against which the muscle ejects blood during contraction.
   d. all of the above factors.

8. A nonmodifiable risk factor for atherosclerosis is:
a. stress.
b. obesity.
c. positive family history.
d. hyperlipidemia.

9. The difference between the systolic and the diastolic pressure is called the:
a. pulse pressure.
b. auscultatory gap.
c. pulse deficit.
d. Korotkoff sound.

10. If the sphygmomanometer cuff is too small for the patient, the blood pressure reading will probably be:
a. falsely elevated.
b. falsely decreased.
c. an accurate reading.
d. significantly different with each reading.

11. The first heart sound is generated by:
a. closure of the aortic valve.
b. closure of the atrioventricular valves.
c. opening of the atrioventricular valves.
d. opening of the pulmonic valve.

12. Exercise stress testing is a noninvasive procedure that can be used to assess certain aspects of cardiac function. After the test, the patient is instructed to:
a. rest for a time.
b. avoid stimulants.
c. avoid extreme temperature changes.
d. do all of the above.

13. Postcatheterization nursing measures for a patient who has had a cardiac catheterization include:
a. assessing the peripheral pulses in the affected extremity.
b. checking the insertion site for hematoma formation.
c. evaluating temperature and color in the affected extremity.
d. all of the above.

Fill-In. *Read each statement carefully. Write your response in the space provided.*

1. Distinguish between the functions of the atrioventricular and the semilunar valves.

_____

_____

2. Briefly explain depolarization as it relates to cardiac physiology.

_____

_____

3. Estimate cardiac output for an adult heart rate of 76 bpm with an average stroke volume of 70 mL per beat.

_____

_____

4. Describe Starling's law of the heart.

_____

_____

5. List several physiologic effects on the cardiovascular system that are associated with the aging process.

_____

_____

6. Two specific enzymes traditionally used to analyze an acute myocardial infarction (MI) are

_____ and _____. The newest enzyme is _____, which has been

found to have several benefits over the others.

7. List several purposes of cardiac catheterization.

_____

_____

8. Describe selective angiography.

_____

_____

9. Discuss the implications of a low central venous pressure reading.

_____

_____

10. Identify possible complications of pulmonary artery monitoring.

_____

_____

Matching. _Match the anatomic term in Column II with its associated function in Column I._

Column I

1. _____separates the right and left atria

2. _____is located at the juncture of the superior vena cava and the right atrium

3. _____supports the heart in the mediastinum

4. _____sits between the right ventricle and the pulmonary artery

5. _____distributes venous blood to the lungs

6. _____is embedded in the right atrial wall near the tricuspid valve

Column II

a. parietal pericardium

b. pulmonary artery

c. bicuspid valve

d. pulmonic valve

e. sinatrial node

f. atrioventricular node

Copyright © 2004 by Lippincott Williams and Wilkins. Study Guide to Accompany
Smeltzer/Bare, Brunner and Suddarth's Textbook of Medical Surgical Nursing, tenth edition by Mary Jo Boyer.

Comparison. *Complete the following crossword puzzle using terminology associated with coronary atherosclerosis.*

Down

1. A principal blood lipid

2. A risk factor that causes pulmonary damage

4. The functional lesion of atherosclerosis

5. Biochemical substances, soluble in fat, that accumulate within a blood vessel

6. A risk factor that is endocrine in origin

9. A risk factor associated with a type A personality

10. A risk factor related to weight gain

14. A recommended dietary restriction risk factor for heart disease

Across

3. For persons of this sex, the incidence of coronary heart disease increases steadily with age

6. Influences amount of fat ingested

7. A symptom of myocardial ischemia

8. An unmodifiable risk factor

11. Myocardial manifestation of coronary artery disease

12. A risk factor related to patterns of daily activity

13. A part of blood vessels

15. A lifestyle habit that is considered a modifiable

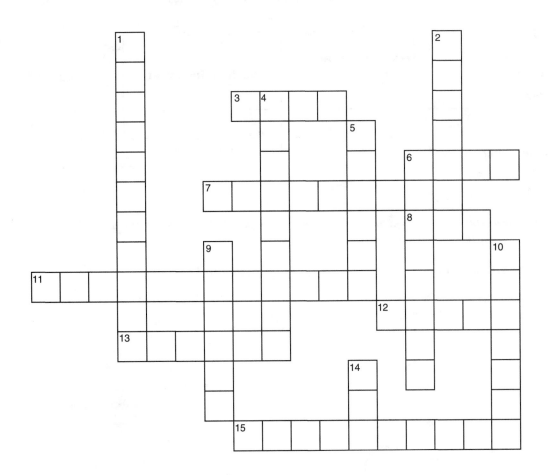

II. Critical Thinking Questions and Exercises

Analyzing Comparisons

Read each analogy. Fill in the space provided with the best response.

1. The pulmonary artery: lungs :: Aorta: _____.

2. Epicardium: outer layer of cells lining the heart :: _____: the heart muscle itself.

3. Apical area of the heart: fifth intercostal space :: Erb's point:

_____.

4. The first heart sound: closure of the mitral and tricuspid valves :: The second heart sound: closure of

_____

_____.

5. Murmurs: malfunctioning valves :: Friction rubs: _____.

Examining Associations

Compare and contrast the characteristics of chest pain specific to pericarditis, to pulmonary pain, and to esophageal pain.

Type of Pain	Pain Character, Location, Duration, and Radiation	Precipitating Events	Nursing Measures
Pericarditis			
Pain of pulmonary origin			
Esophageal pain			

Interpreting Data

Refer to the illustration in Table 26–2, page 657, depicting the pain pathway of myocardial infarction and angina pectoris. Answer the associated questions.

Myocardial Infarction

Angina Pectoris

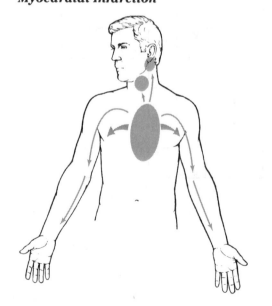
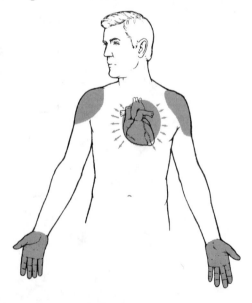

Name nursing assessment data that are relevant to record/report about the pain location, character, radiation, and duration.

_____ _____

_____ _____

_____ _____

_____ _____

Describe relevant precipitation events that would help with collaborative diagnosis.

_____ _____

_____ _____

_____ _____

Describe relevant nursing interventions based on pain assessment.

_____ _____

_____ _____

_____ _____

Clinical Applications

CASE STUDY: Cardiac Assessment for Chest Pain

Mr. Anderson is a 45-year-old executive with a major oil firm. Lately he has experienced frequent episodes of chest pressure that are relieved with rest. He has requested a complete physical examination. The nurse conducts an initial cardiac assessment.

1. The nurse immediately inspects the patient's skin. She observes a bluish tinge around the patient's lips. She knows that this is an indication of:
   a. central cyanosis.
   b. pallor.
   c. peripheral cyanosis.
   d. xanthelasma.

2. The nurse takes a baseline blood pressure measurement after the patient has rested for 10 minutes in a supine position. The reading that reflects a reduced pulse pressure is:
   a. 140/90 mm Hg.
   b. 140/100 mm Hg.
   c. 140/110 mm Hg.
   d. 140/120 mm Hg.

3. Five minutes after the initial blood pressure measurement was taken, the nurse assesses additional readings with the patient in a sitting and then in a standing position. The reading indicative of an abnormal postural response would be:
   a. lying, 140/110; sitting, 130/110; standing, 135/106 mm Hg.
   b. lying, 140/110; sitting, 135/112, standing, 130/115 mm Hg.
   c. lying, 140/110; sitting, 135/100, standing, 120/90 mm Hg.
   d. lying, 140/110; sitting, 130/108, standing, 125/108 mm Hg.

4. The nurse returns Mr. Anderson to the supine position and measures for jugular vein distention. The finding that would initially indicate an abnormal increase in the volume of the venous system would be obvious distention of the veins with the patient at:
   a. 15 degrees.
   b. 25 degrees.
   c. 35 degrees.
   d. 45 degrees.

5. The nurse auscultates the apex of the heart by placing a stethoscope over:
   a. Erb's point.
   b. the fifth intercostal space.
   c. the pulmonic area.
   d. the tricuspic area.

27

Management of Patients With Dysrhythmias and Conduction Problems

I. Interpretation, Completion, and Comparison

Multiple Choice. Read each question carefully. Circle your answer.

1. The heart is under the control of the autonomic nervous system. Stimulation of the parasympathetic system results in:
   a. slowed heart rate.
   b. lowered blood pressure.
   c. reduction in the force of contraction.
   d. all of the above.

2. The total time for ventricular depolarization and repolarization is represented on an electrocardiogram(ECG) reading as the:
   a. QRS complex.
   b. QT interval.
   c. ST segment.
   d. TP interval.

3. Ventricular rhythm can be determined by examining the _____ on an ECG strip.
   a. PP interval
   b. QT interval
   c. RR interval
   d. TP interval

4. The PR interval on an ECG strip that reflects normal sinus rhythm would be between:
   a. 0.05 and 0.10 seconds.
   b. 0.12 and 0.20 seconds.
   c. 0.15 and 0.30 seconds.
   d. 0.25 and 0.40 seconds.

5. Characteristics of sinus bradycardia include all of the following *except*:
   a. a P wave precedes every QRS complex.
   b. every QRS complex is normal.
   c. the rate is 40 to 60 bpm.
   d. the rhythm is altered.

6. A dysrhythmia common in normal hearts and described by patients as "my heart skipped a beat" is:
   a. premature atrial complex.
   b. atrial flutter.
   c. sinus tachycardia.
   d. ventricular fibrillation.

7. A saw-tooth P wave is seen on an ECG strip with:
   a. sinus bradycardia.
   b. atrial flutter.
   c. atrioventricular nodal reentry.
   d. premature junctional complex.

8. Atrial fibrillation is associated with a heart rate up to:
    a. 300 bpm.
    b. 400 bpm.
    c. 500 bpm.
    d. 600 bpm.

9. Atrioventricular (AV) nodal reentry tachycardia is characterized by an atrial rate:
    a. of 100 bpm.
    b. between 100 and 150 bpm.
    c. between 150 and 250 bpm.
    d. more than 250 bpm.

10. Ventricular bigeminy refers to a conduction defect in which:
    a. conduction is primarily from the AV node
    b. every other beat is premature.
    c. rhythm is regular but fast.
    d. the rate is between 150 and 250 bpm.

11. With ventricular tachycardia:
    a. conduction originates in the ventricle.
    b. electrical defibrillation is used immediately.
    c. the P wave usually is normal.
    d. the ventricular rate is twice the normal atrial rate.

12. Ventricular fibrillation is associated with an absence of:
    a. heartbeat.
    b. palpable pulse.
    c. respirations.
    d. all of the above.

13. First-degree AV block is characterized by:
    a. a variable heart rate, usually fewer than 60 bpm.
    b. an irregular rhythm.
    c. delayed conduction, producing a prolonged PR interval.
    d. P waves hidden with the QRS complex.

14. A conduction abnormality whereby no atrial impulse travels through the AV node is known as:
    a. first-degree AV block.
    b. second-degree AV block, type 1.
    c. second-degree AV block, type 2.
    d. third-degree AV block.

15. When assessing vital signs in a patient with a permanent pacemaker, the nurse needs to know the:
    a. date and time of insertion.
    b. location of the generator.
    c. model number.
    d. pacer rate.

16. Cardioversion is used to terminate dysrhythmias. With cardioversion, the:
    a. amount of voltage used should exceed 400 W-sec.
    b. electrical impulse can be discharged during the T wave.
    c. machine should be set to deliver a shock during the QRS complex.
    d. above statements are all true.

17. When electrical defibrillation is used:
    a. between 20 and 25 lb of pressure should be exerted on each paddle in order to ensure good skin contact.
    b. the defibrillator should discharge at 100 W-sec per kilogram of body weight.
    c. the discharge shock needs to be timed to the T wave.
    d. all of the above are necessary.

18. Candidates for implantable cardioverter defibrillation (ICD) are patients at high risk who have:
    a. experienced syncope secondary to ventricular tachycardia.
    b. survived sudden cardiac death.
    c. sustained ventricular tachycardia.
    d. experienced one or more of the above.

19. The nurse needs to teach the patient with an automatic ICD that he or she must:
    a. avoid magnetic fields such as metal detection booths.
    b. call for emergency assistance if he or she feels dizzy.
    c. record events that trigger a shock sensation.
    d. be compliant with all of the above.

Fill-In. *Read each statement carefully. Write your response in the space provided.*

1. Name the four sites of origin of the impulses that are used to name dysrythmias: _____,
_____, _____, and _____.

2. Describe the normal electrical conduction through the heart.

_____

_____

3. Name several causes of sinus tachycardia.

_____

_____

4. Sinus tachycardia occurs when the ventricular and atrial rate are greater than _____.

5. List a rate and rhythm characteristic that is necessary to diagnose ventriular tachycardia:

_____ and _____.

6. List three potential collaborative problems that a nurse would choose for a patient with a dysrhythmia:

_____, _____, and _____.

7. Describe the difference between demand and fixed pacemakers.

_____

_____

8. Describe the placement of the electrode paddles used for defibrillation on a patient's chest.

_____

_____

_____

Unscramble the letters used to answer each statement, and write the word in the space provided.

1. A term used to decribe an irregular or erratic heart rhythm:_____

S H R I C H M D T Y Y

2. The ability of the cardiac muscle to initiate an electrical impulse:_____

T A Y O I T A T I C M U

3. The ability of the cardiac muscle to transmit electrical impulses:_____

O U V T I C N Y I T D C

4. A term used to describe the electrical stimulation of the heart:_____

N O I P T R A D O L Z A E I

5. Stage of conduction in which the ventricles relax:_____

T S L D I A E O

Clinical Situations

Graph Analysis

Analyze the following ECG graphs and answer the questions below them.

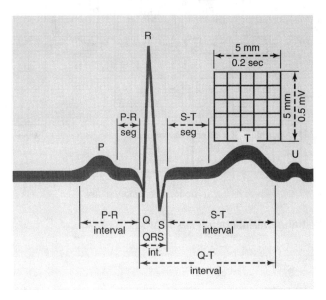

ECG graph and commonly measured complex components. Each small box represents 0.04 seconds on the horizontal axis and 1 mm or 0.1 millivolt on the vertical axis. The PR inverval is measured from the beginning of the P wave to the beginning of the QRS *complex*; the QRS *complex* is measured from the beginning of the Q wave to the end of the S wave; the QT interval is measured from the beginning of the Q wave to the end of the T wave.

1. Look at the above graphic recording of cardiac electrical activity. For each action below, choose a wave deflection that corresponds to it, and write the appropriate letter or letters on the line provided.

    a. _____ ventricular muscle repolarization

    b. _____ time required for an impulse to travel through the atria and the conduction system to the Purkinje fibers

    c. _____ atrial muscle depolarization

    d. _____ ventricular muscle depolarization

    e. _____ early ventricular repolarization of the ventricles

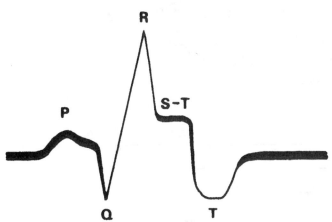

2. Consider the above graphic recording, and identify three alterations that are consistent with myocardial ischemia and infarction hours to days after the attack.

    a. _____

    b. _____

    c. _____

Analyze the graphic recording for each of the following dysrhythmias and describe the altered deflection.

1.

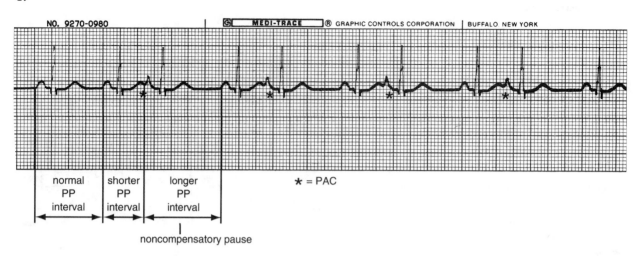

Premature atrial complexes (PACs).

_____

_____

_____

2.

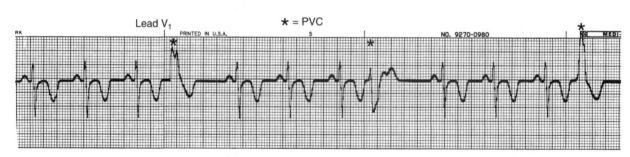

Multifocal PVCs in quadrigimeny.

_____

_____

_____

3.

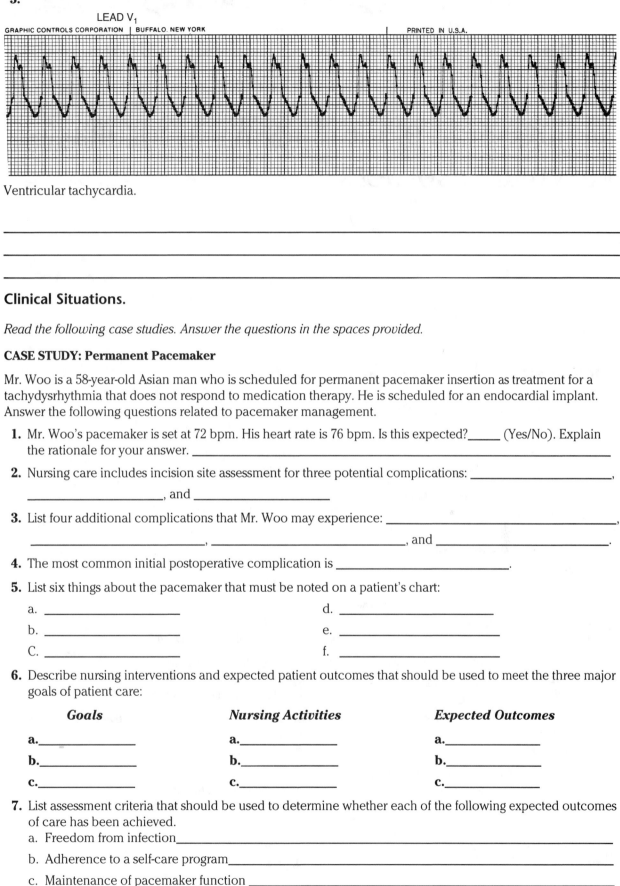

LEAD V$_1$

GRAPHIC CONTROLS CORPORATION | BUFFALO. NEW YORK | PRINTED IN U.S.A.

Ventricular tachycardia.

_____

_____

_____

Clinical Situations.

Read the following case studies. Answer the questions in the spaces provided.

CASE STUDY: Permanent Pacemaker

Mr. Woo is a 58-year-old Asian man who is scheduled for permanent pacemaker insertion as treatment for a tachydysrhythmia that does not respond to medication therapy. He is scheduled for an endocardial implant. Answer the following questions related to pacemaker management.

1. Mr. Woo's pacemaker is set at 72 bpm. His heart rate is 76 bpm. Is this expected?_____ (Yes/No). Explain the rationale for your answer. _____

2. Nursing care includes incision site assessment for three potential complications: _____,

   _____, and _____

3. List four additional complications that Mr. Woo may experience: _____,

   _____, _____, and _____.

4. The most common initial postoperative complication is _____.

5. List six things about the pacemaker that must be noted on a patient's chart:

   a. _____   d. _____

   b. _____   e. _____

   C. _____   f. _____

6. Describe nursing interventions and expected patient outcomes that should be used to meet the three major goals of patient care:

Goals	*Nursing Activities*	*Expected Outcomes*
a._____	**a.**_____	**a.**_____
b._____	**b.**_____	**b.**_____
c._____	**c.**_____	**c.**_____

7. List assessment criteria that should be used to determine whether each of the following expected outcomes of care has been achieved.

   a. Freedom from infection_____

   b. Adherence to a self-care program_____

   c. Maintenance of pacemaker function _____

28

Management of Patients With Coronary Vascular Disorders

I. Interpretation, Completion, and Comparison

Multiple Choice. *Read each question carefully. Circle your answer.*

1. The most common heart disease in the United States is:
   a. angina pectoris.
   b. coronary atherosclerosis.
   c. myocardial infarction.
   d. valvular heart disease.

2. Lumen narrowing with atherosclerosis is caused by:
   a. atheroma formation on the intima.
   b. scarred endothelium.
   c. thrombus formation.
   d. all of the above.

3. A healthy level of serum cholesterol would be a reading of:
   a. 160–200 mg/dL.
   b. 210–240 mg/dL.
   c. 250–275 mg/dL.
   d. 280–300 mg/dL.

4. A strong negative risk factor for heart disease is:
   a. cholesterol, 280mg/dL.
   b. LDL, 160 mg/dL.
   c. HDL, 60 mg/dL.
   d. a ratio of LDL to HDL, 4.5–1.0.

5. Hypertension is repeated blood pressure measurements exceeding:
   a. 110/80 mm Hg.
   b. 120/80 mm Hg.
   c. 130/90 mm Hg.
   d. 140/90 mm Hg.

6. The incidence of coronary artery disease tends to be equal for men and women after the age of:
   a. 45 years.
   b. 50 years.
   c. 56 years.
   d. 65 years.

7. The pain of angina pectoris is produced primarily by:
   a. coronary vasoconstriction.
   b. movement of thromboemboli.
   c. myocardial ischemia.
   d. the presence of atheromas.

8. A common side effect of nitroglycerin is:
   a. musculoskeletal weakness.
   b. hypertension.
   c. bradycardia.
   d. headache.

9. The nurse advises a patient that sublingual nitroglycerin should alleviate angina pain within:
  a. 3–4 minutes.
  b. 10–15 minutes.
  c. 30 minutes.
  d. 60 minutes.

10. Patient education includes telling someone who takes nitroglycerin sublingually that he or she should go quickly to the nearest emergency room if the person has taken _____ tablets at 5-minute intervals, without relief.
  a. more than 1
  b. 2 or more
  c. 3 or more
  d. more than 4

11. The scientific rationale supporting the administration of beta-adrenergic blockers is the drugs' ability to:
  a. block sympathetic impulses to the heart.
  b. elevate blood pressure.
  c. increase myocardial contractility.
  d. induce bradycardia.

12. An antidote for propranolol hydrochloride (a beta-adrenergic blocker) for bradycardia is:
  a. digoxin.
  b. atropine.
  c. protamine sulfate.
  d. sodium nitroprusside.

13. In the United States, more than 1 million people will have an acute myocardial infarction every year. Of these 1 million, _____ will die.
  a. 10%–15%
  b. 25%
  c. 30%–40%
  d. 60%

14. The most common site of myocardial infarction is the:
  a. left atrium.
  b. left ventricle.
  c. right atrium.
  d. right ventricle.

15. Choose an incorrect statement about myocardial infarction pain. It is:
  a. relieved by rest and inactivity.
  b. substernal in location.
  c. sudden in onset and prolonged in duration.
  d. viselike and radiates to the shoulders and arms.

16. Myocardial cell damage can be reflected by high levels of cardiac enzymes. The most specific index of all cardiac enzymes is:
  a. alkaline phosphatase.
  b. creatine kinase (CK-MB).
  c. myoglobin.
  d. troponin.

17. The most common vasodilator used to treat myocardial pain is:
  a. amyl nitrite.
  b. Inderal.
  c. nitroglycerine.
  d. Pavabid HCl.

18. The most common thrombolytic agent that increases plasminogen activator is:
  a. Activase.
  b. Eminase.
  c. Reteplase.
  d. Streptokinase.

19. An intravenous analgesic frequently administered to relieve chest pain associated with myocardial infarction is:
  a. meperidine hydrochloride.
  b. hydromorphone hydrochloride.
  c. morphine sulfate.
  d. codeine sulfate.

20. The need for surgical intervention of coronary artery disease is determined by the:
  a. amount of stenosis in the coronary arteries.
  b. myocardial area served by the stenotic artery.
  c. occurrence of previous infarction related to the affected artery.
  d. all of the above.

21. A candidate for percutaneous transluminal coronary angioplasty (PTCA) is a patient with coronary artery disease who:
  a. has compromised left ventricular function.
  b. has had angina longer than 3 years.
  c. has at least 70% occlusion of a major coronary artery.
  d. has questionable left ventricular function.

22. A goal of dilation in PTCA is an increase in the artery's lumen size to at least:

    a. 20%.   c. 60%.

    b. 35%.   d. 80%.

23. The nurse expects a postoperative PTCA patient to be discharged:

    a. the same day as surgery.   c. 3 days later.

    b. within 24 hours of the procedure.   d. after 1 week.

24. Possible postoperative PTCA complications for which a nurse needs to be alert to assess for clinical symptoms include:

    a. abrupt closure of the artery.   c. coronary artery spasm.

    b. arterial dissection.   d. all of the above.

25. One of the most important and immediate postoperative PTCA complications for which the nurse needs to assess is:

    a. bleeding.   c. hypertension.

    b. depression.   d. hypoventilation.

26. A candidate for traditional coronary artery bypass grafting must meet which of the following criteria:

    a. blockage that cannot be treated by PTCA.   c. unstable angina.

    b. greater than 50% blockage in the left   d. all of the above.
       coronary artery.

27. According to the critical care pathway outlined for coronary artery bypass graft (CABP), the nurse knows that postoperative teaching must occur before discharge on about the _____ day.

    a. second   c. seventh

    b. fourth   d. tenth

28. The most common nursing diagnosis for patients awaiting cardiac surgery is:

    a. activity intolerance.   c. decreased cardiac output.

    b. fear related to the surgical procedure.   d. anginal pain.

29. Extremity paresthesia, dysrhythmias (peaked T waves), and mental confusion after cardiac surgery are signs of electrolyte imbalance related to the level of:

    a. calcium.   c. potassium.

    b. magnesium.   d. sodium.

30. A complication after cardiac surgery that is associated with an alteration in preload is:

    a. cardiac tamponade.   c. hypertension.

    b. elevated central venous pressure.   d. hypothermia.

31. The most common dysrthymia seen after cardiac surgery is:

    a. bradycardia.   c. tachycardia.

    b. ectopic beats.   d. all of the above.

Fill-In. *Read each statement carefully. Write your response in the space provided.*

1. The most prevalent type of cardiovascular disease in the United States for men and women of all ethnic and racial groups is _____.

2. The most frequently occurring sign of myocardial ischemia is _____.

3. More than 50% of people with coronary artery disease have the risk factor of _____.

4. List four modifiable risk factors that are considered major causes of coronary artery disease.

    a. _____   c. _____

    b. _____   d. _____

5. Management of coronary heart disease requires a therapeutic range of cholesterol and lipoproteins. An acceptable blood level of cholesterol is _____ with a ratio of low-density lipoprotein (LDL) to high density lipoprotein (HDL) at _____. The desired level of LDL should be _____ mg/dL; the HDL level should be greater than _____ mg/dL.

6. The American Heart Association recommends that an average American diet contain about _____% fat.

7. Intractable angina is chest pain described as _____.

8. Patients with severe cardiac ischemia who are not candidates for coronary artery bypass grafting may benefit from a new and experimental procedure called _____, in which channels are created in the heart muscle.

9. Postpericardiotomy syndrome can be diagnosed by assessment of the following five symptoms:

a. _____   d. _____

b. _____   e. _____

c. _____

II. Critical Thinking Questions and Exercises

Discussion and Analysis

1. Explain how cigarette smoking contributes to the development of coronary artery disease.
2. Explain the use of hormone replacement therapy for coronary artery disease prevention.

Examining Associations

Examine the association between the items in each cluster and identify the common factor.

1. Abdominal aortic aneurysm, carotid artery disease, diabetes, existing coronary artery disease, and peripheral arterial disease

_____

2. Abdominal obesity, elevated triglycerides, low level of HDL, hypertension, and impaired function of insulin

_____

3. Age, cholesterol level, systolic blood pressure, levels of LDL and HDL, and cigarette smoking

_____

4. Cholesterol abnormalities, cigarette smoking, diabetes mellitus, and hypertension

_____

5. Total cholesterol, LDL, HDL, and triglycerides

_____

Identifying Patterns

Review the figure below and answer the following questions.

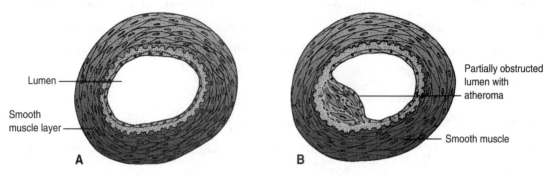

Cross section of a normal and an atherosclerotic artery. (*A*) Cross-section of normal artery in which the lumen is fully patent, or open. (*B*) Cross-section of artery with diminished patency resulting from atheroma.

1. Describe the underlying pathophysiology that causes a normal artery (A) to narrow because of atheroma deposits.

   _____

   _____

2. An atheroma is described as:

   _____

3. A possible complication of rupture or hemorrhage of the lipid core into the plaque is:

   _____.

4. A thrombus is a dangerous complication of atherosclerosis because it can lead to: _____ and

   _____.

Supporting Arguments

Offer a supporting rationale for your response.

1. Explain, supported with a scientific base to your rationale, why cigarette smoking contributes to the severity of coronary heart disease for each of these three factors:

Factor	*Scientific Rationale*
a. increased CO levels	a. _____ _____
b. increased catecholamines	b. _____ _____
c. increased platelet adhesion	c. _____ _____

2. Argue in support of using calcium channel blockers for treatment of angina.

   _____

   _____

Clinical Situations

Read the following case studies. Circle the correct answer.

CASE STUDY: Angina Pectoris

Ermelina, a 64-year-old retired secretary, is admitted to the medical-surgical area for management of chest pain caused by angina pectoris.

1. The nurse knows that the basic cause of angina pectoris is believed to be:
 a. dysrhythmias triggered by stress.
 b. insufficient coronary blood flow.
 c. minute emboli discharged through the narrowed lumens of the coronary vessels.
 d. spasms of the vessel walls owing to excessive secretion of epinephrine (adrenaline).

2. The medical record lists a probable diagnosis of chronic stable angina. The nurse knows that Ermelina's pain:
 a. has increased progressively in frequency and duration.
 b. is incapacitating.
 c. is relieved by rest and is predictable.
 d. usually occurs at night and may be relieved by sitting upright.

3. Ermelina has nitroglycerin at her bedside to take PRN. The nurse knows that nitroglycerin acts in all of the following ways *except*:
 a. causing venous pooling throughout the body.
 b. constricting arterioles to lessen peripheral blood flow.
 c. dilating the coronary arteries to increase the oxygen supply.
 d. lowering systemic blood pressure.

4. Ermelina took a nitroglycerin tablet at 10:00 AM, after her morning care. It did not relieve her pain, so she repeated the dose. Ten minutes later and still in pain, she calls the nurse, who should:
 a. administer a prn dose of diazepam (Valium), try to calm her, and recommend that she rest in a chair with her legs dependent to encourage venous pooling.
 b. assist her to the supine position, give her oxygen at 6 L/min, and advise her to rest in bed.
 c. help her to a comfortable position, give her oxygen at 2 L/min, and call her physician.
 d. suggest that she take double her previous dose after 5 minutes and try to sleep to decrease her body's need for oxygen.

CASE STUDY: Decreased Myocardial Tissue Perfusion

Mr. Lillis, a 46-year-old bricklayer, is brought to the emergency department by ambulance with a suspected diagnosis of myocardial infarction. He appears ashen, is diaphoretic and tachycardiac, and has severe chest pain. The nursing diagnosis is decreased cardiac output, related to decreased myocardial tissue perfusion.

1. The nurse knows that the most critical time period for his diagnosis is:
 a. the first hour after symptoms begin.
 b. within 24 hours after the onset of symptoms.
 c. within the first 48 hours after the attack.
 d. between the third and fifth day after the attack.

2. The nurse needs to look for symptoms associated with one of the major causes of sudden death during the first 48 hours, which is:
 a. cardiogenic shock.
 b. pulmonary edema.
 c. pulmonary embolism.
 d. ventricular rupture.

3. Mr. Lillis is transferred to a telemetry unit after 6 days in the cardiac care unit, where he was treated for an anterior wall myocardial infarction. The nurse expects Mr. Lillis to be able to do all of the following *except*:
 a. isometric exercises.
 b. self-care activities.
 c. sit in a chair several times a day.
 d. walk within his room.

4. The nurse is aware that ischemic tissue remains sensitive to oxygen demands, because scar formation is not seen until the:

a. second week.

b. third week.

c. sixth week.

d. eighth week.

5. Mr. Lillis needs to be advised that myocardial healing will not be complete for about:

a. 2 months.

b. 4 months.

c. 6 months.

d. 8 months.

6. For discharge planning, Mr. Lillis is advised to:

a. avoid large meals.

b. exercise daily.

c. restrict caffeine-containing beverages.

d. do all of the above.

29

Management of Patients With Structural, Infectious, and Inflammatory Cardiac Disorders

I. Interpretation, Comparison, and Completion

Multiple Choice. Read each question carefully. Circle your answer.

1. Incomplete closure of the tricuspid valve results in a backward flow of blood from the:
   a. aorta to the left ventricle.
   b. left atrium to the left ventricle.
   c. right atrium to the right ventricle.
   d. right ventricle to the right atrium.

2. Backward flow of blood from the left ventricle to the left atrium is through the:
   a. aortic valve.
   b. mitral valve.
   c. pulmonic valve.
   d. tricuspid valve.

3. The pathophysiology of mitral stenosis is consistent with:
   a. aortic stenosis.
   b. left ventricular failure.
   c. right atrial hypertrophy.
   d. all of the above.

4. The presence of a water-hammer pulse (quick, sharp strokes that suddenly collapse) is diagnostic for:
   a. aortic regurgitation.
   b. mitral insufficiency.
   c. tricuspid insufficiency.
   d. tricuspid stenosis.

5. Severe aortic stenotic disease is consistent with all of the following *except*:
   a. increased cardiac output.
   b. left ventricular hypertrophy.
   c. pulmonary edema.
   d. right-sided heart failure.

6. The most common valvuloplasty procedure is the:
   a. balloon valvuloplasty.
   b. annuloplasty.
   c. chordoplasty.
   d. commissurotomy.

7. Xenographs, used for valve replacement, have a viability of about:
   a. 2 years.
   b. 4 years.
   c. 8 years.
   d. 12 years.

8. The most commonly occurring cardiomyopathy is:
   a. congestive or dilated.   c. idiopathic.
   b. hypertrophic.   d. restrictive.

9. Probably the most helpful diagnostic test to identify cardiomyopathy is:
   a. serial enzyme studies.   c. echocardiogram.
   b. cardiac catheterization.   d. phonocardiogram.

10. Rheumatic endocarditis is an inflammatory reaction to:
   a. group A streptococcus.   c. *Serratia marcescens.*
   b. *Pseudomonas aeruginosa.*   d. *Staphylococcus aureus.*

11. The causative microorganism for rheumatic endocarditis can be accurately identified only by:
   a. a throat culture.   c. roentgenography.
   b. an echocardiogram.   d. serum analysis.

12. Clinical manifestations of infective endocarditis may include:
   a. embolization.   c. heart murmurs.
   b. focal neurologic lesions.   d. all of the above.

13. The characteristic sign of pericarditis is:
   a. a friction rub.   c. fever.
   b. dyspnea.   d. hypoxia.

14. A serious consequence of pericarditis is:
   a. cardiac tamponade.   c. hypertension.
   b. decreased venous pressure.   d. left ventricular hypertrophy.

Fill In. *Read each statement carefully. Write your response in the space provided.*

1. Describe mitral valve prolapse syndrome.

_____

_____

2. If dysrhythmias occur with mitral valve prolapse syndrome, the nurse advises the patient to avoid:

_____, _____, and _____

3. A nurse, using auscultation to identify aortic regurgitation, would place the stethoscope _____

and expect to hear _____.

4. With aortic stneosis, the patient should receive _____ to prevent endocarditis.

5. List four potential complications or collaborative problems for patients with cardiomyopathy:

_____, _____, _____, and _____.

6. Prompt treatment of streptococcal pharyngitis with _____ can prevent almost all attacks of:

_____.

7. Briefly describe the pathophysiology of endocarditis, beginning with the formation of a vegetation.

_____

_____

8. Infective endocarditis is usually caused by the following bacteria: _____, _____,

_____, and _____.

9. Briefly describe the pathophysiology of myocarditis.

_____

_____

10. Describe the anatomic landmark for auscultation of a pericardial friction rub.

_____

_____

Matching. Match the pathophysiology listed in Column II with the valvular disorder listed in Column I.

Column I

1. ____ mitral valve prolapse

2. ____ mitral stenosis

3. ____ mitral regurgitation

4. ____ aortic valve stenosis

5. ____ aortic regurgitation

Column II

a. leaflet malformation prevents complete closure

b. can be caused by rheumatic endocarditis

c. characterized by "water-hammer" pulse

d. blood seeps backward into left atrium

e. thickening and contracture of mitral valve cusps

II. Critical Thinking Questions and Exercises

Discussion and Analysis

1. Describe what a nurse would expect to hear when using auscultation to listen to the heart of a patient with mitral valve prolapse.

2. Explain how left ventricular hypertrophy develops from mitral valve insufficiency.

3. Describe the pathophysiology of aortic regurgitation.

4. Describe the characteristic sound of the murmur heard with aortic stenosis.

5. Explain the pathophysiology of all cardiomyopathies.

Identifying Patterns

1. Outline the pathophysiologic sequence of events that occurs when mitral valve stenosis leads to right ventricular failure.

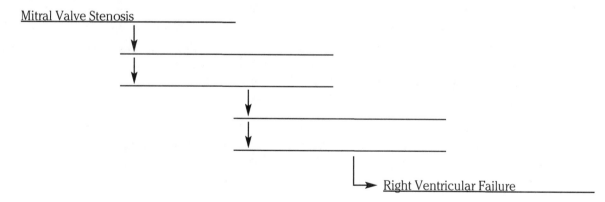

Mitral Valve Stenosis

Right Ventricular Failure

Clinical Situations

Read the following case studies. Fill in the blanks below or circle the correct answer.

CASE STUDY: Infective Endocarditis

Mr. Fontana, a 60-year-old executive, is admitted to the hospital with a diagnosis of infective endocarditis. Pertinent history includes a previous diagnosis of mitral valve prolapse. A physical examination at his physician's office before admission reveals complaints of anorexia, joint pain, intermittent fever, and a 10-lb weight loss in the past 2 months.

1. The nurse knows, prior to assessment, that Mr. Fontana's vague clinical symptoms are characteristic of an

   insidious disease onset that develops from one of three conditions: _____,

   _____, or _____.

2. While examining Mr. Fontana's eyes during the admission assessment, the nurse notes conjunctival hemorrhages with pale centers caused by emboli in the nerve fiber of the eye. These are known as:
   a. Roth's spots.
   b. Osler's nodes.
   c. Janeway's lesions.
   d. Heberden's nodes.

3. The nurse also assesses for central nervous system manifestations of the infectious disease. She looks for

   symptoms such as: _____, _____, _____, and

   _____.

4. The primary objective of medical management is: _____.

5. Serial blood cultures identified *Streptococcus viridans* as the causative organism, and parenteral antibiotic treatment was initiated. The nurse expects that Mr. Fontana will probably remain on the antibiotic intravenous infusion for:
   a. 7 days.
   b. 2 weeks.
   c. 4 to 6 weeks.
   d. 8 to 12 weeks.

6. Even with successful treatment, organ damage can occur. Cardiac complications may include:

   _____, _____, _____, and

   _____.

7. Mr. Fontana needs to be advised that prophylactic antibiotic therapy is also recommended for:
   a. tooth extraction.
   b. bronchoscopy.
   c. cystoscopy.
   d. all of the above

CASE STUDY: Acute Pericarditis

Mrs. Russell is a 46-year-old Caucasian who developed symptoms of acute pericarditis secondary to a viral infection. Diagnosis was based on the characteristic sign of a friction rub and pain over the pericardium.

1. Based on knowledge of pericardial pain, the nurse suggests the following body position to relieve the pain symptoms:
   a. flat in bed with feet slightly higher than the head
   b. Fowler's
   c. right side-lying
   d. semi-Fowler's

2. Based on assessment data, the major nursing diagnosis is: _____.

3. Initial nursing intervention includes maintenance of bed rest until the following symptom disappears:
   a. fever
   b. friction rub
   c. pain
   d. all of the above

4. Identify three drug classifications that are commonly prescribed for management or treatment:

_____, _____, and _____.

5. Name the anatomic landmarks used to auscultate for a pericardial friction rub:

_____

6. List the two major expected patient outcomes for nursing management of a patient with pericarditis:

_____ and _____.

30

Management of Patients With Complications From Heart Disease

I. Interpretation, Completion, and Comparison

Multiple Choice. Read each question carefully. Circle your answer.

1. The multilumen pulmonary artery catheter allows the nurse to measure hemodynamic pressures at various points in the heart. When the tip enters the small branches of the pulmonary artery, the nurse can assess all of the following measurements *except*:
   a. central venous pressure (CVP).
   b. pulmonary artery capillary pressure (PACP).
   c. pulmonary artery obstructive pressure (PAOP).
   d. pulmonary artery wedge pressure (PAWP).

2. Hemodynamic monitoring by means of a multilumen pulmonary artery catheter can provide detailed information about:
   a. preload.
   b. afterload.
   c. cardiac output.
   d. all of the above.

3. Nursing measures in hemodynamic monitoring include assessing for localized ischemia caused by inadequate arterial flow. The nurse should:
   a. assess the involved extremity for color and temperature.
   b. check for capillary filling.
   c. evaluate pulse rate.
   d. do all of the above.

4. The most frequent cause for hospitalization for people older than 65 years of age is:
   a. angina pectoris.
   b. congestive heart failure.
   c. hypertension.
   d. pulmonary edema.

5. The primary cause of heart failure is:
   a. arterial hypertension.
   b. coronary atherosclerosis.
   c. myocardial dysfunction.
   d. valvular dysfunction.

6. The dominant function in cardiac failure is:
   a. ascites.
   b. hepatomegaly.
   c. inadequate tissue perfusion.
   d. nocturia.

7. The treatment for cardiac failure is directed at:
   a. decreasing oxygen needs of the heart.
   b. increasing the cardiac output by strengthening muscle contraction or decreasing peripheral resistance.
   c. reducing the amount of circulating blood volume.
   d. all of the above.

8. A primary classification of medications used in the treatment of systolic heart failure is:
   a. ACE inhibitors.
   b. beta-blockers.
   c. diuretics.
   d. calcium channel blockers.

9. An example of a potassium-sparing diuretic that might be prescribed for a person with congestive heart failure is:
   a. Aldactone.
   b. Mykrox.
   c. Zaroxolyn.
   d. Lasix.

10. Digitalis toxicity can occur when serum digitalis levels are in the range of:
    a. 0.25–0.50 mg/dL.
    b. 0.50–1.0 mg/dL.
    c. 1.0–2.0 mg/dL.
    d. 2.5–3.5 mg/dL.

11. The primary underlying disorder of pulmonary edema is:
    a. decreased left ventricular pumping.
    b. decreased right ventricular elasticity.
    c. increased left atrial contractility.
    d. increased right atrial resistance.

12. Pulmonary edema is characterized by:
    a. elevated left ventricular end-diastolic pressure.
    b. a rise in pulmonary venous pressure.
    c. increased hydrostatic pressure.
    d. all of the above alterations.

13. With pulmonary edema, there is usually an alteration in:
    a. afterload.
    b. contractility.
    c. preload.
    d. all of the above.

14. A commonly prescribed diuretic that is given intravenously to produce a rapid diuretic effect is:
    a. Bumex.
    b. Lasix.
    c. Mykrox.
    d. Zaroxolyn.

15. A popular catecholamine that when given intravenously can rapidly increase cardiac contractility is:
    a. Bumex.
    b. Dobutrex.
    c. Primacor.
    d. Natricor.

16. Morphine is given in acute pulmonary edema to redistribute the pulmonary circulation to the periphery by decreasing:
    a. peripheral resistance.
    b. pulmonary capillary pressure.
    c. transudation of fluid.
    d. all of the above.

17. A recommended position for a patient in acute pulmonary edema is:
    a. prone, to encourage maximum rest, thereby decreasing respiratory and cardiac rates.
    b. semi-Fowler's, to facilitate breathing and promote pooling of blood in the sacral area.
    c. Trendelenburg, to drain the upper airways of congestion.
    d. upright with the legs down, to decrease venous return.

18. Cardiogenic shock is pump failure that occurs primarily as the result of:
    a. coronary artery stenosis.
    b. left ventricular damage.
    c. myocardial ischemia.
    d. right atrial flutter.

19. Classic signs of cardiogenic shock include all of the following *except*:
    a. bradycardia.
    b. cerebral hypoxia.
    c. hypotension.
    d. oliguria.

20. A clinical manifestation of pericardial infusion is:
    a. widening pulse pressure.
    b. a decrease in venous pressure.
    c. shortness of breath.
    d. an increase in blood pressure.

21. The most reliable sign of cardiac arrest is:
- a. absence of a pulse.
- b. cessation of respirations.
- c. dilation of the pupils.
- d. inaudible heart sounds.

22. Brain damage occurs with cessation of circulation after an approximate interval of:
- a. 2 minutes.
- b. 4 minutes.
- c. 6 minutes.
- d. 8 minutes.

23. The drug of choice during cardiopulmonary resuscitation to suppress ventricular dysrhythmias is:
- a. atropine.
- b. epinephrine.
- c. lidocaine.
- d. morphine.

Matching. *Match the type of congestive failure listed in Column II with its associated pathophysiology in Column I.*

Column I

1. _A_ fatigability

2. _b_ dependent edema

3. _A_ pulmonary congestion predominates

4. _b_ distended neck veins JUD

5. _b_ ascites

6. _A_ dyspnea from fluid in alveoli

7. _A_ orthopnea

8. _b_ hepatomegaly

9. _A_ cough that may be blood-tinged

10. _b_ nocturia

Column II

a. left-sided cardiac failure

b. right-sided cardiac failure

Fill-In. *Read each statement carefully. Write your response in the space provided.*

1. Distinguish between the terms *preload* and *afterload*.

Preload: _____

Afterload: _____

2. Explain the meaning of CO = HR × SV. _____

3. Name two factors that determine preload: _____ and _____.

4. Two noninvasive tests are used to assess cardiac hemodynamics: _____ for right ventricular preload and _____ for left ventricular preload.

5. List four common etiologic factors that cause myocardial dysfunction: _____, _____, _____, and _____.

6. List four common side effects of diuretics: _____, _____, _____, and _____.

7. List six symptoms indicative of hypokalemia:

a. _____　　　　　e. _____

b. _____　　　　　f. _____

c. _____

d. _____

II. Critical Thinking Questions and Exercises

Identifying Patterns

Complete the following outline that depicts the pathophysiology of pulmonary edema, beginning with decreased left ventricular pumping ability and ending with hypoxemia and death if not treated.

Pathophysiology of Pulmonary Edema

Decreased Left Ventricular Pumping

Death if not treated

Clinical Situations

Read the following case study. Fill in the blanks or circle the correct answer.

CASE STUDY: Pulmonary Edema

Mr. Wolman is to be discharged from the hospital to home. He is 79 years old, lives with his wife, and has just recovered from mild pulmonary edema secondary to congestive heart failure.

1. The most common cause of pulmonary edema is: _____.

2. The sequence of pathophysiologic events is triggered by:
   a. elevated left ventricular end-diastolic pressure.
   b. elevated pulmonary venous pressure.
   c. increased hydrostatic pressure.
   d. impaired lymphatic drainage.

3. The nurse advises Mr. Wolman to rest frequently at home. This advice is based on the knowledge that rest:
   a. decreases blood pressure.
   b. increases the heart reserve.
   c. reduces the work of the heart.
   d. does all of the above.

4. The nurse reminds Mr. Wolman to sleep with two pillows to elevate his head about 10 inches. This position is recommended because:
   a. preload can be increased, thus enhancing cardiac output.
   b. pulmonary congestion can be reduced.
   c. venous return to the lungs can be improved, thus reducing peripheral edema.
   d. all of the above can help relieve his symptoms.

5. Mr. Wolman takes 0.25 mg of digoxin once a day. The nurse should tell him about signs of digitalis toxicity, which include:
   a. anorexia.
   b. bradycardia and tachycardia.
   c. nausea and vomiting.
   d. all of the above.

6. Mr. Wolman also takes Lasix (40 mg) twice a day. He is aware of signs related to hypokalemia and supplements his diet with foods high in potassium, such as:
   a. bananas.
   b. raisins.
   c. orange juice.
   d. all of the above.

31

Assessment and Management of Patients With Vascular and Peripheral Circulation Problems

I. Interpretation, Completion, and Comparison

Multiple Choice. Read each question carefully. Circle your answer.

1. The most important factor in regulating the caliber of blood vessels, which determines resistance to flow, is:
   a. hormonal secretion.
   b. independent arterial wall activity.
   c. the influence of circulating chemicals.
   d. the sympathetic nervous system.

2. Clinical manifestations of acute venous insufficiency include all of the following *except*:
   a. cool and cyanotic skin.
   b. initial absence of edema.
   c. sharp pain that may be relieved by the elevation of the extremity.
   d. full superficial veins.

3. With peripheral arterial insufficiency, leg pain during rest can be reduced by:
   a. elevating the limb above heart level.
   b. lowering the limb so that it is dependent.
   c. massaging the limb after application of cold compresses.
   d. placing the limb in a plane horizontal to the body.

4. Probably the strongest risk factor for the development of atherosclerotic lesions is:
   a. cigarette smoking.
   b. lack of exercise.
   c. obesity.
   d. stress.

5 Saturated fats are strongly implicated in the causation of atherosclerosis. Saturated fats include all of the following *except*:
   a. corn oil.
   b. eggs and milk.
   c. meat and butter.
   d. solid vegetable oil.

6. The American diet is known to be high in fat. The amount of calories typically supplied by fat in most diets is _____ of the total caloric intake.
   a. 20%
   b. 40%
   c. 60%
   d. 80%

7. Buerger's disease is characterized by all of the following except:
   a. arterial thrombus formation and occlusion.
   b. lipid deposits in the arteries.
   c. redness or cyanosis in the limb when it is dependent.
   d. venous inflammation and occlusion.

7. The most outstanding symptom of Buerger's disease is:
   a. a burning sensation.
   b. cramping in the feet.
   c. pain.
   d. paresthesia.

9. The most common cause of all thoracic aortic aneurysms is:
   a. a congenital defect in the vessel wall.
   b. atherosclerosis.
   c. infection.
   d. trauma.

10. Diagnosis of a thoracic aortic aneurysm is done primarily by:
   a. computed tomography.
   b. sonography.
   c. radiography.
   d. all of the above.

11. A nurse who suspects the presence of an abdominal aortic aneurysm should look for the presence of:
   a. a pulsatile abdominal mass.
   b. low back pain.
   c. lower abdominal pain.
   d. all of the above.

12. To save a limb that is affected by occlusion of a major artery, surgery must be initiated before necrosis develops, which is usually:
   a. within the first 4 hours.
   b. between 6 and 10 hours.
   c. between 12 and 24 hours.
   d. within 1 to 2 days.

13. Raynaud's disease is a form of:
   a. arterial vessel occlusion caused by multiple emboli that develop in the heart and are transported through the systemic circulation.
   b. arteriolar vasoconstriction, usually on the fingertips, that results in coldness, pain, and pallor.
   c. peripheral venospasm in the lower extremities owing to valve damage resulting from prolonged venous stasis.
   d. phlebothrombosis related to prolonged vasoconstriction resulting from overexposure to the cold.

14. A significant cause of venous thrombosis is:
   a. altered blood coagulation.
   b. stasis of blood.
   c. vessel wall injury.
   d. all of the above.

15. Clinical manifestations of deep vein obstruction include:
   a. edema and pain.
   b. pigmentation changes.
   c. ulcerations.
   d. all of the above.

16. When administering anticoagulant therapy, the nurse needs to monitor the clotting time to make certain that it is within the therapeutic range of:
   a. one to two times the normal control.
   b. two to three times the normal control.
   c. 3.5 times the normal control.
   d. 4.5 times the normal control.

17. When caring for a patient who has started anticoagulant therapy with warfarin (Coumadin), the nurse knows not to expect therapeutic benefits for:
   a. at least 12 hours.
   b. the first 24 hours.
   c. 2 to 3 days.
   d. 3 to 5 days.

18. Knowing the most serious complication of venous insufficiency, the nurse would assess the patient's lower extremities for signs of:
   a. rudor.
   b. cellulitis.
   c. dermatitis.
   d. ulceration.

19. A nurse should teach a patient with chronic venous insufficiency to do all of the following *except*:
   a. avoid constricting garments.
   b. elevate the legs above the heart level for 30 minutes every 2 hours.
   c. sit as much as possible to rest the valves in the legs.
   d. sleep with the foot of the bed elevated about 6 inches.

20. Nursing measures to promote a clean leg ulcer include:
    a. applying wet-to-dry saline solution dressings, which would remove necrotic debris when changed.
    b. flushing out necrotic material with hydrogen peroxide.
    c. using an ointment that would treat the ulcer by enzymatic débridement.
    d. all of the above.

21. The physician prescribed a Tegapore dressing to treat a venous ulcer. The nurse knows that the ankle-brachial index (ABI) must be _____ for the circulatory status to be adequate.
    a. 0.10
    b. 0.25
    c. 0.35
    d. 0.50

22. A varicose vein is caused by:
    a. phlebothrombosis.
    b. an incompetent venous valve.
    c. venospasm.
    d. venous occlusion.

23. Postoperative nursing management for vein ligation and stripping include all of the following *except*:
    a. dangling the legs over the side of the bed for 10 minutes every 4 hours for the first 24 hours.
    b. elevating the foot of the bed to promote venous blood return.
    c. maintaining elastic compression of the leg continuously for about 1 week.
    d. starting the patient ambulating 24 to 48 hours after surgery.

Matching. *Match the type of vessel insufficiency listed in Column II with its associated symptoms listed in Column I.*

Column I

1. ____A____ intermittent claudication
2. ____b____ paresthesia
3. ____A____ dependent rubor
4. ____A____ cold, pale extremity
5. ____b____ ulcers of lower legs and ankles
6. ____b____ muscle fatigue and cramping
7. ____A____ diminished or absent pulses
8. ____A____ reddish blue discoloration with dependency

Column II

a. arterial insufficiency
b. venous insufficiency

II. Critical Thinking Questions and Exercises

Examining Associations

Read each analogy. Fill in the space provided with the best response.

1. Rudor : reddish-blue discoloration:: Claudication : cramp-like pain in the extremities with exercise.

2. International normalized ratio (INR): the measurement of anticoagulant levels :: Ankle-brachial index (ABI): _____.

3. The intima: inner layer of the arterial wall:: _____: outer layer of connective tissue.

4. The right lymphatic duct: lymphatic fluid delivery to the right side of the head and neck:: The thoracic duct: _____.

5. Arterial pressure: 100 mm Hg:: Venous pressure: _____.

6. Hydrostatic pressure: force generted by blood pressure :: Osmotic pressure: _____.

Clinical Applications

Read the following case study. Circle the correct answer.

CASE STUDY: Peripheral Arterial Occlusive Disease

Fred, a 43-year-old construction worker, has a history of hypertension. He smokes two packs of cigarettes a day, is nervous about the possibility of being unemployed, and has difficulty coping with stress. His current concern is calf pain during minimal exercise, which decreases with rest.

1. The nurse assesses Fred's symptoms as being associated with peripheral arterial occlusive disease. The nursing diagnosis is probably:
   a. alteration in tissue perfusion related to compromised circulation.
   b. dysfunctional use of extremities related to muscle spasms.
   c. impaired mobility related to stress associated with pain.
   d. impairment in muscle use associated with pain on exertion.

2. The nurse knows that the hallmark symptom of peripheral arterial occlusion disease is:
   a. intermittent claudication.
   b. phlebothrombosis.
   c. postphlebitis syndrome.
   d. thrombophlebitis.

3. Additional symptoms to support the nurse's diagnosis include all of the following *except*:
   a. blanched skin appearance when the limb is elevated.
   b. diminished distal pulsations.
   c. reddish-blue discoloration of the limb when it is dependent.
   d. warm and rosy coloration of the extremity after exercise.

4. The pain associated with this condition commonly occurs in muscle groups ___I don't level below stenosis or occul___

5. The pain is due to the irritation of nerve endings by the build-up of ___muscle metabolytes___ and ___Lactic Acid___

6. Pain is experienced when the arterial lumen narrows to about:
   a. 15%.
   b. 25%.
   c. 35%.
   d. 50%.

7. The nurse notices that several minutes after Jack's leg is dependent, the vessels remain dilated. This is evidenced by the coloring of the skin, which the nurse describes as:
   a. rosy.
   b. rubor.
   c. pallor.
   d. cyanotic.

8. The nurse is asked to determine ABI. The right posterior tibial reading is 75 mm Hg, and the brachial systolic pressure is 150 mm Hg. The ABI would be:
   a. 0.25.
   b. 0.50.
   c. 0.65.
   d. 0.80.

9. In health teaching, the nurse should suggest methods to increase arterial blood supply, which include:
   a. a planned program involving systematic lowering of the extremity below heart level.
   b. Buerger-Allen exercises.
   c. graded extremity exercises.
   d. all of the above.

Complete the outline below, which depicts the pathophysiology of atherosclerosis, beginning with the direct results of atherosclerosis in the arteries and ending with fibrotic tissue formation.

Pathophysiology of Atherosclerosis

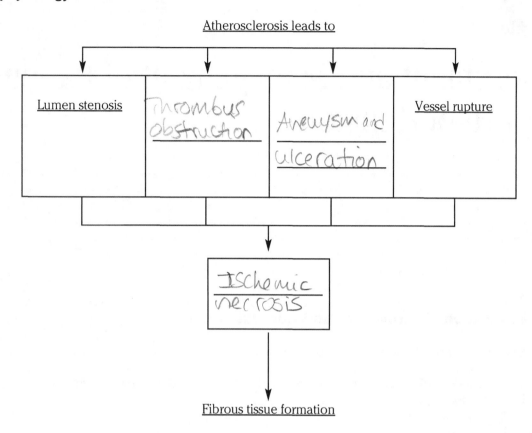

Atherosclerosis leads to

Lumen stenosis | Thrombus obstruction | Aneuysm and ulceration | Vessel rupture

Ischemic necrosis

Fibrous tissue formation

32

Assessment and Management of Patients With Hypertension

I. Interpretation, Completion, and Comparison

Multiple Choice. Read each question carefully. Circle your answer.

1. Hypertension is defined as persistent blood pressure levels in which the systolic pressure is above ____ and the diastolic is above ____.
   a. 110/60
   b. 120/70
   c. 130/80
   d. 140/90

2. The percentage of adults in the United States who have hypertension is approximately:
   a. 10%.
   b. 15%.
   c. 25%.
   d. 40%.

3. The incidence of hypertension is highest in the ____ section of the United States.
   a. northeastern
   b. southeastern
   c. northwestern
   d. southwestern

4. The desired systolic reading for hypertensive treatment for a person with diabetes mellitus is:
   a. 120 mm Hg.
   b. 130 mm Hg.
   c. 140 mm Hg.
   d. 150 mm Hg.

5. Pharmacologic therapy for patients with uncomplicated hypertension would include the administration of:
   a. ACE inhibitors.
   b. alpha-blockers.
   c. beta-blockers.
   d. calcium antagonists.

6. A characteristic symptom of damage to the vital organs as a result of hypertension is:
   a. angina.
   b. dyspnea.
   c. epitaxis.
   d. all of the above.

7. An expected nursing diagnosis for a patient with hypertension is:
   a. heart failure.
   b. knowledge deficit.
   c. myocardial infarction.
   d. renal insufficiency.

8. The percentage of patients with hypertension who discontinue their drug therapy within 1 year after its initiation is estimated to be:

a. 15%.

b. 30%.

c. 50%.

d. 75%.

9. One of the most significant concerns for medical and nursing management of hypertension is:

a. complications from medications.

b. insufficient information.

c. noncompliance with recommended therapy.

d. uncontrolled dietary management.

10. Blood pressure control is initially achieved by approximately _____ of patients when they actively participate in their care.

a. 10%

b. 25%

c. 45%

d. 70%

Fill-In. *Read each statement carefully. Write your response in the space provided.*

1. Blood pressure is the product of _____ multiplied by _____.

2. Cardiac output is the product of _____ multiplied by _____.

3. Approximately _____% of the population has primary hypertension, a class of hypertension with an unidentified cause.

4. Prolonged hypertension can cause significant damage to blood vessels in four "target organs":

a. _____

b. _____

c. _____

d. _____

5. List six consequences of prolonged, uncontrolled hypertension on the body and its systems.

a. _____

b. _____

c. _____

d. _____

e. _____

f. _____

6. Structural and functional changes in the heart and blood vessels that occur with aging and cause hypertension are:

_____, _____, _____, and

_____.

7. Give three examples of conditions that can trigger a hypertensive emergency in which blood pressure must be immediately lowered: _____, _____, and _____

II. Critical Thinking Questions and Exercises

Discussion and Analysis

1. Discuss in detail several hypotheses about the pathophysiologic basis for elevated blood pressure.

2. Explain how lifestyle changes and medications can control, not cure, hypertension.

Identifying Patterns

Complete the following schematic: "Pathophysiology of Hypertension Secondary to Renal Dysfunction"

Pathophysiology of Essential Hypertension

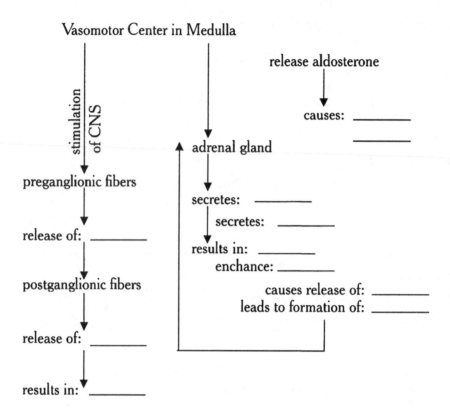

Clinical Applications

Read the following case study. Circle the correct answers.

CASE STUDY: Secondary Hypertension

Georgia, 30 years old, is diagnosed as having secondary hypertension when serial blood pressure recordings show her average reading to be 170/100 mm Hg. Her hypertension is the result of renal dysfunction.

1. The kidneys help maintain the hypertensive state in essential hypertension by:

   a. increasing their elimination of sodium in response to aldosterone secretion.

   b. releasing renin in response to decreased renal perfusion.

   c. secreting acetylcholine, which stimulates the sympathetic nervous system to constrict major vessels.

   d. doing all of the above.

2. Renal pathology associated with essential hypertension can be identified by:

   a. a urine output greater than 2000 mL in 24 hours.

   b. a urine specific gravity of 1.005.

   c. hyponatremia and decreased urine osmolality.

   d. increased blood urea nitrogen and creatinine levels.

3. Georgia is prescribed spironolactone (Aldactone), 50 mg once every day. The nurse knows that spironolactone:
   a. blocks the reabsorption of sodium, thereby increasing urinary output.
   b. inhibits renal vasoconstriction, which prevents the release of renin.
   c. interferes with fluid retention by inhibiting aldosterone.
   d. prevents the secretion of epinephrine from the adrenal medulla.

4. Health education for Georgia includes advising her to:
   a. adhere to her dietary regimen.
   b. become involved in a regular program of exercise.
   c. take her medication as prescribed.
   d. do all of the above.

33

Assessment and Management of Patients With Hematologic Disorders

I. Interpretation, Completion, and Comparison

Multiple Choice. Read each question carefully. Circle your answer.

1. An elderly patient presents to the physician's office with a complaint of exhaustion. The nurse, aware of the most common hematologic condition affecting the elderly, knows to check the patient's:
   a. white blood cell count.
   b. red blood cell count.
   c. thrombocyte count.
   d. levels of plasma proteins.

2. A nurse who cares for a patient who has experienced bone marrow aspiration or biopsy should be aware of the most serious hazard of:
   a. hemorrhage.
   b. infection.
   c. shock.
   d. splintering of bone fragments.

3. A person can usually tolerate a gradual reduction in hemoglobin until the level reaches:
   a. 5.0–5.5 g/dL.
   b. 4.0–4.5 g/dL.
   c. 3.0–3.5 g/dL.
   d. 2.0–2.5 g/dL.

4. A patient with chronic renal failure is being examined by the nurse practitioner for anemia. The nurse knows to review the laboratory data for a decreased hemoglobin level, red blood cell count, and:
   a. decreased level of erythropoietin.
   b. decreased total iron-binding capacity.
   c. increased mean corpuscular volume.
   d. increased reticulocyte count.

5. During a routine assessment of a patient diagnosed with anemia, the nurse notes the patient's beefy red tongue. The nurse knows that this is a sign of _____ anemia.
   a. autoimmune
   b. folate deficiency
   c. iron deficiency
   d. megaloblastic

6. The most frequent symptom and complication of anemia is:
   a. bleeding gums.
   b. ecchymosis.
   c. fatigue.
   d. jaundice.

7. The nurse begins to design a nutritional packet of information for a patient diagnosed with iron deficiency anemia. The nurse would recommend an increased intake of:
a. fresh citrus fruits.
b. milk and cheese.
c. organ meats.
d. whole-grain breads.

8. A physician prescribes one tablet of ferrous sulfate daily for a 15-year-old girl who experiences heavy flow during her menstrual cycle. The nurse advises the patient and her mother that this over-the-counter preparation must be taken for _____ months for iron replenishment to occur.
a. 1–2   b. 3–5   c. 6–12   d. longer than 12

9. The recommended parenteral route for administering iron preparations to treat anemia is:
a. deep gluteal intramuscular injection, using the Z-track method.
b. intermittent infusion.
c. intramuscular injection in the deltoid so that muscle contraction can help dissipate the medication.
d. subcutaneous injection with weekly site rotation.

10. The cause of aplastic anemia may:
a. be related to drugs, chemicals, or radiation damage.
b. be idiopathic.
c. result from certain infections.
d. be related to all of the above.

11. A nurse should know that a diagnosis of hemolytic anemia is associated with all of the following except:
a. abnormality in the circulation of plasma.
b. decrease in the reticulocyte count.
c. defect in the erythrocyte.
d. elevated indirect bilirubin.

12. Absence of intrinsic factor is associated with a vitamin B_{12} deficiency, because the vitamin cannot bind to be transported for absorption in the:
a. duodenum.
b. ileum.
c. jejunum.
d. stomach.

13. A diagnostic sign of pernicious anemia is:
a. a smooth, sore, red tongue.
b. exertional dyspnea.
c. pale mucous membranes.
d. weakness.

14. The Schilling test is used to diagnose:
a. aplastic anemia.
b. iron deficiency anemia.
c. megaloblastic anemia.
d. pernicious anemia.

15. A nurse expects an adult patient with sickle cell anemia to have a hemoglobin value of:
a. near 3 g/dL.
b. near 5 g/dL.
c. between 5 and 7 g/dL.
d. between 7 and 10 g/dL.

16. Sickle-shaped erythrocytes cause:
a. cellular blockage in small vessels.
b. decreased organ perfusion.
c. tissue ischemia and infarction.
d. all of the above.

17. A person with sickle cell trait would:
a. be advised to avoid fluid loss and dehydration.
b. be protected from crisis under ordinary circumstances.
c. experience hemolytic jaundice.
d. have chronic anemia.

18. Polycythemia vera is characterized by bone marrow overactivity, resulting in the clinical manifestations of:
a. angina.
b. claudication.
c. thrombophlebitis.
d. all of the above.

19. The common feature of the leukemias is:
a. a compensatory polycythemia stimulated by thrombocytopenia.
b. an unregulated accumulation of white cells in the bone marrow, which replace normal marrow elements.
c. increased blood viscosity, resulting from an overproduction of white cells.
d. reduced plasma volume in response to a reduced production of cellular elements.

20. Nursing assessment for a patient with leukemia should include observation for:
    a. fever and infection.
    b. dehydration.
    c. petechiae and ecchymoses.
    d. all of the above.

21. The major cause of death in patients with acute, myeloid leukemia is believed to be:
    a. anemia.
    b. dehydration.
    c. embolis.
    d. infection.

22. Multiple myeloma:
    a. can be diagnosed by roentgenograms that show bone lesion destruction.
    b. is a malignant disease of plasma cells that affects bone and soft tissue.
    c. is suspected in any person who evidences albuminuria.
    d. is associated with all of the above.

23. In the normal blood-clotting cycle, the final formation of a clot will occur:
    a. during the platelet phase.
    b. during the vascular phase.
    c. when fibrin reinforces the platelet plug.
    d. when the plasmin system produces fibrinolysis.

24. Bleeding and petechiae do not usually occur with thrombocytopenia until the platelet count falls below $50,000/mm^3$. The normal value for blood platelets is:
    a. $50,000–100,000/mm^3$.
    b. $100,000–150,000/mm^3$.
    c. between $150,000$ and $350,000/mm^3$.
    d. greater than $350,000/mm^3$.

25. Hemophilia is a hereditary bleeding disorder that:
    a. has a higher incidence among males.
    b. is associated with joint bleeding, swelling, and damage.
    c. is related to a genetic deficiency of a specific blood-clotting factor.
    d. is associated with all of the above.

26. Hypoprothrombinemia, in the absence of gastrointestinal or biliary dysfunction, may be caused by a deficiency in vitamin:
    a. A.
    b. B_{12}.
    c. C.
    d. K.

27. A potential blood donor would be rejected if he or she:
    a. had a history of infectious disease exposure within the past 2 to 4 months.
    b. had had close contact with a hemodialysis patientwithin the past 6 months.
    c. had donated blood within the past 3 to 6 months.
    d. had received a blood transfusion 9 to 12 months before the blood donation time.

28. The recommended minimum hemoglobin level for a woman to donate blood is:
    a. 8.0 g/dL.
    b. 10.5 g/dL.
    c. 12.5 g/dL.
    d. 14 g/dL.

Fill-In. *Read each statement carefully. Write your response in the space provided.*

1. The volume of blood in humans is about _____ L.

2. Blood cell formation (hematopoiesis) occurs in the _____.

3. Red bone marrow activity is confined in adults to the _____, _____,

_____, and _____

4. The principal function of the erythrocyte is to: _____.

5. Each 100 mL of blood should normally contain _____ g of hemoglobin.

6. The average life span of a circulating red blood cell is _____ days.

7. The major function of leukocytes is to _____.

8. Plasma proteins consist primarily of _____ and _____.

9. The two most common areas used for bone marrow aspirations in an adult are _____ and
_____.

10. Distinguish between *primary* and *secondary* polycythemia.

_____

_____

Complete the following scramblegram by circling the word or words that answer each statement below.

F	I	B	R	I	N	O	G	E	N	A	N	O	E	L
B	D	H	E	M	O	S	T	A	S	I	S	P	R	M
F	R	S	S	C	M	P	R	H	S	G	T	H	Y	I
I	E	W	C	V	R	T	C	E	L	L	S	A	T	P
B	E	A	B	B	T	L	D	E	F	I	J	G	H	R
R	S	W	A	O	H	O	A	S	V	T	S	O	R	K
I	F	T	P	N	R	K	L	B	J	N	M	C	O	L
N	E	U	T	R	O	P	H	I	L	S	K	Y	C	B
F	W	O	D	C	M	F	N	K	G	H	A	T	Y	O
A	H	B	E	R	B	S	J	C	T	C	B	O	T	N
H	E	M	A	T	O	P	O	I	E	S	I	S	E	E
E	M	N	E	E	C	F	M	F	G	P	S	I	S	M
M	O	N	O	C	Y	T	E	S	P	L	A	S	M	A
O	S	C	G	D	T	K	L	A	I	E	L	K	A	R
G	T	O	A	H	E	E	I	J	B	E	B	A	J	R
L	A	G	P	E	S	F	R	M	C	N	U	L	B	O
O	S	G	T	I	J	D	S	A	N	M	M	S	L	W
B	I	H	E	O	A	G	H	H	D	O	I	I	T	L
I	S	D	A	U	O	U	L	M	E	S	N	P	U	M
N	A	S	E	L	Y	M	P	H	O	C	Y	T	E	S

Definition of Terms

1. The fluid portion of blood

2. Another term for platelets

3. The mature form of white blood cells

4. The process of continually replacing blood cells

5. The site of blood cell formation

6. Makes up 95% of the mass of the red blood cell

7. The ingestion and digestion of bacteria by neutrophils

8. The largest classification of leukocytes

9. A clotting factor present in plasma

10. A plasma protein primarily responsible for the maintenance of fluid balance

11. The site of activity for most macrophages

12. The process of stopping bleeding from a severed blood vessel

13. A protein that forms the basis of blood clotting

14. Integral component of the immune system

15. The term for red blood cell

16. The letters used for the term reticuloendothelial system

17. The balance between clot formation and clot dissolution

18. A term used to describe T lymphocytes

II. Critical Thinking Questions and Exercises

Clinical Situations

Read the following case studies. Fill in the blanks or circle the correct answer.

CASE STUDY: Sickle Cell Crises

Tonika, a 15-year-old with sickle cell disease, is admitted to the hospital for treatment of sickle cell crises.

1. Based on knowledge of the etiology of sickle cell anemia, the nurse expects the patient to be of _____ descent.
   a. African   c. Middle Eastern
   b. Indian   d. Mediterranean

2. The nurse understands that the shape of the red blood cell is altered with this disease. Instead of being

   round, biconcave, and disc-like in appearance, it can be described as _____, _____,

   _____, and _____.

3. On assessment, the nurse notes that the patient's face and skull bones are enlarged. She knows this is a

   compensatory response to: _____.

4. The severe pain that occurs during sickle cell crises is the result of: _____.

5. The nurse understands that Tonika's abdominal pain is probably caused by involvement of the _____, the most common organ responsible for sequestration crises in young adults:
   a. kidney   c. pancreas
   b. liver   d. spleen

6. Nursing interventions are focused on five goals: _____, _____,

   _____, _____, and _____.

CASE STUDY: Leukemia

John is a 51-year-old accountant recently diagnosed with acute myeloid leukemia.

1. Acute myeloid leukemia affects the _____.

2. A bone marrow specimen is diagnostic if it shows an excess of: _____.

3. A characteristic symptom that results from insufficient red blood cell production is:

a. bleeding tendencies.

b. fatigue.

c. susceptibility to infection.

d. all of the above.

4. Survival rates for those who receive treatment average:

a. 6 months.

b. 1 year.

c. 2 years.

d. 5 years.

5. The major form of therapy that frequently results in remission is:

a. bone marrow transplantation.

b. chemotherapy.

c. radiation.

d. surgical intervention.

CASE STUDY: Hodgkin's Disease

Ian, a 24-year-old graduate student, was recently diagnosed as having Hodgkin's disease. He sought medical attention because of an annoying pruritus and a small enlargement on the right side of his neck.

1. Ian's disease is classified as Hodgkin's paragranuloma. The nurse knows that this classification is associated with:

a. a minimal degree of cellular differentiation in the affected nodes.

b. an excessive production of the Reed-Sternberg cell, the diagnostic atypical cell of Hodgkin's disease.

c. nodular sclerosis, which reflects advanced malignancy.

d. replacement of the involved lymph nodes by tumor cells.

2. A positive diagnosis of Hodgkin's disease depends on:

a. enlarged, firm, and painful lymph nodes.

b. histologic analysis of an enlarged lymph node.

c. progressive anemia.

d. the presence of generalized pruritus.

3. Ian's diagnosis of stage I Hodgkin's disease implies that the disease:

a. has disseminated diffusely to one or more extrahepatic sites.

b. involves multiple nodes and is confined to one side of the diaphragm.

c. is limited to a single node or a single intralymphatic organ or site.

d. is present above and below the diaphragm and may include spleen involvement.

4. The nurse expects that Ian's course of treatment will involve:

a. a combination of chemotherapy and radiation.

b. a drug regimen of nitrogen mustard, vincristine, and a steroid.

c. chemotherapy with vincristine alone.

d. radiotherapy to the specific node over a space of 4 weeks.

CASE STUDY: Transfusion

Jerry is to receive one unit of packed red cells because he has a hemoglobin level of 8 g/dL and a diagnosis of gastrointestinal bleeding.

1. Before initiating the transfusion, the nurse needs to check:

a. for the abnormal presence of gas bubbles and cloudiness in the blood bag.

b. that the blood has been typed and cross-matched.

c. that the recipient's blood numbers match the donor's blood numbers.

d. all of the above.

2. Administration technique should include all of the following *except*:

a. adding 50 to 100 mL of 0.9% NaCl to the packed cells to dilute the solution and speed up delivery of the transfusion.

b. administering the unit in combination with dextrose in water if the patient needs additional carbohydrates.

c. administering the unit of blood over 1 to 2 hours.

d. squeezing the bag of blood every 20 to 30 minutes during administration to mix the cell.

3. The nurse is aware that a transfusion reaction, if it occurs, will probably occur:

a. 1 to 2 minutes after the infusion begins.

b. during the first 15 to 30 minutes of the transfusion.

c. after half the solution has been infused.

d. several hours after the infusion, when the body has assimilated the new blood components into the general circulation.

4. If a transfusion reaction occurs, the nurse should:

a. call the physician and wait for directions based on the specific type of reaction.

b. stop the transfusion immediately and keep the vein patent with a saline or dextrose solution.

c. slow the infusion rate and observe for an increase in the severity of the reaction.

d. slow the infusion and request a venipuncture for retyping to start a second transfusion.

UNIT 7
Digestive and Gastrointestinal Function

34

Assessment of Digestive and Gastrointestinal Function

I. Interpretation, Completion, and Comparison

Multiple Choice. *Read each question carefully. Circle your answer.*

1. Reflux of food into the esophagus from the stomach is prevented by contraction of the:
   a. ampulla of Vater.
   b. cardiac sphincter.
   c. ileocecal valve.
   d. pyloric sphincter.

2. The digestion of starches begins in the mouth with the secretion of the enzyme:
   a. lipase.
   b. pepsin.
   c. ptyalin.
   d. trypsin.

3. The stomach, which derives its acidity from hydrochloric acid, has a pH of approximately:
   a. 1.0.
   b. 3.5.
   c. 5.0.
   d. 7.5.

4. Intrinsic factor is a gastric secretion necessary for the intestinal absorption of vitamin _____, without which pernicious anemia develops.
   a. B_1
   b. B_{12}
   c. C
   d. K

5. During the initial assessment of a patient complaining of increased stomach acid related to stress, the nurse knows that the physician will want to consider the influence of the neuroregulator:
   a. gastrin.
   b. cholecystokinin.
   c. norepinephrine.
   d. secretin.

6. Pancreatic secretions into the duodenum:
   a. are stimulated by hormones released in the presence of chyme as it passes through the duodenum.
   b. have an alkaline effect on intestinal contents.
   c. increase the pH of the food contents.
   d. all of the above.

7. Bile, which emulsifies fat, enters the duodenum through the:
   a. cystic duct.
   b. common bile duct.
   c. common hepatic duct.
   d. pancreatic duct.

8. Secretin is a gastrointestinal hormone that:
   a. causes the gallbladder to contract.
   b. influences contraction of the esophageal and pyloric sphincters.
   c. regulates the secretion of gastric acid.
   d. stimulates the production of bicarbonate in pancreatic juice.

9. The major carbohydrate that tissues use for fuel is:
   a. fructose.
   b. galactose.
   c. glucose.
   d. sucrose.

10. It usually takes _____ for food to enter the colon.
   a. 2 or 3 hours after a meal is eaten
   b. 4 or 5 hours after a meal is eaten
   c. 6 or 7 hours after a meal is eaten
   d. 8 or 9 hours after a meal is eaten

11. When completing a nutritional assessment of a patient who is admitted for a gastrointestinal disorder, the nurse notes a recent history of dietary intake. This is based on the knowledge that a portion of digested waste products can remain in the rectum for _____ days after a meal is digested.
   a. 1   b. 2   c. 3   d. 4

12. Obstruction of the gastrointestinal tract leads to:
   a. increased force of intestinal contraction.
   b. distention above the point of obstruction.
   c. pain and a sense of bloating.
   d. all of the above.

13. A nurse who is investigating a patient's statement about duodenal pain should assess the:
   a. epigastric area and consider possible radiation of pain to the right subscapular region.
   b. hypogastrium in the right or left lower quadrant.
   c. left lower quadrant.
   d. periumbilical area, followed by the right lower quadrant.

14. Abdominal pain associated with indigestion is usually:
   a. described as crampy or burning.
   b. in the left lower quadrant.
   c. less severe after an intake of fatty foods.
   d. relieved by the intake of coarse vegetables, which stimulate peristalsis.

15. Consequences of diarrhea include all of the following except:
   a. acidosis.
   b. decreased bicarbonate.
   c. electrolyte imbalance.
   d. hyperkalemia.

16. The nurse has been directed to position a patient for an examination of the abdomen. She knows to place the patient in the:
   a. prone position with pillows positioned to alleviate pressure on the abdomen.
   b. semi-Fowler's position with the left leg bent to minimize pressure on the abdomen.
   c. supine position with the knees flexed to relax the abdominal muscles.
   d. reverse Trendelenburg position to facilitate the natural propulsion of intestinal contents.

17. The nurse auscultates the abdomen to assess bowel sounds. She documents five to six sounds heard in less than 30 seconds. She documents that the patient's bowel sounds are:
   a. normal.
   b. hypoactive.
   c. hyperactive.
   d. none of the above.

18. A gastric analysis with stimulation that results in an excess of gastric acid being secreted could be diagnostic of:
   a. chronic atrophic gastritis.
   b. a duodenal ulcer.
   c. gastric carcinoma.
   d. pernicious anemia.

19. Before a gastroscopy, the nurse should inform the patient that:
   a. he or she must fast for 6 to 12 hours before the examination.
   b. his or her throat will be sprayed with a local anesthetic.
   c. after gastroscopy, he or she cannot eat or drink until the gag reflex returns (1–2 hrs).
   d. all of the above will be necessary.

20. A flexible sigmoidoscope permits examination of the lower bowel for:
   a. 5 to 10 inches.
   b. 10 to 15 inches.
   c. 16 to 20 inches.
   d. 25 to 35 inches.

21. A fiberoptic colonoscopy is most frequently used for a diagnosis of:
- a. bowel disease of unknown origin.
- b. cancer.
- c. inflammatory bowel disease.
- d. occult bleeding.

22. For adults who are older than 50 years of age and at low risk for colorectal cancer, the recommended screening is a:
- a. flexible signoidoscopy every 3 years.
- b. colonoscopy every 10 years.
- c. fecal occult blood test annually.
- d. colonoscopy every 2 years.

23. Magnetic resonance imaging (MRI) is contraindicated for patients who have:
- a. permanent pacemakers.
- b. artificial heart valves.
- c. implanted insulin pumps.
- d. all of the above.

24. Patient preparation for esophageal manometry requires the withholding of specific medications such as:
- a. anticholinergics.
- b. calcium channel blockers.
- c. sedatives.
- d. all of the above.

Matching. Match the major digestive enzyme in Column II with its associated digestive action listed in Column I.

Column I	Column II
1. ____ helps convert protein into amino acids	**a.** amylase
2. ____ facilitates the production of dextrins and maltose	**b.** maltase
3. ____ digests protein and helps form polypeptides	**c.** sucrase
4. ____ digests carbohydrates and helps form fructose	**d.** lactase
5. ____ glucose is a product of this enzyme's action	**e.** pepsin
6. ____ helps form galactose	**f.** trypsin

Fill-In. Complete the following.

Next to each diagnostic test, list one or more patient-preparation activities that the nurse must monitor and/or document.

Diagnostic Test	Patient Preparation
1. Barium enema	**a.** _____
	b. _____
	c. _____
	d. _____
	e. _____
2. Gastric analysis	**a.** _____
	b. _____
	c. _____
3. Upper gastrointestinal fiberscopic examination	**a.** _____
	b. _____
	c. _____
4. Fiberoptic colonoscopy	**a.** _____
	b. _____
	c. _____
	d. _____

35

Management of Patients With Oral and Esophageal Disorders

I. Interpretation, Completion, and Comparison

Multiple Choice. Read each question carefully. Circle your answer.

1. A nurse knows that adequate nutrition is related to good dental health. As part of health assessment, a nurse also knows that about _____ of adults 45 to 64 years of age have severe peridontal disease.
   a. 5%   b. 10%   c. 15%   d. 25%

2. Actinic cheilitis is a lip lesion that results from sun exposure and can lead to squamous cell carcinoma. It is evidenced by:
   a. erythema.   c. white hyperkeratosis.
   b. fissuring.   d. all of the above.

3. A common disease of oral tissue characterized by painful, inflamed, and swollen gums is:
   a. candidiasis.   c. herpes simplex.
   b. gingivitis.   d. periodontitis.

4. A common lesion of the mouth that is also referred to as a canker sore is:
   a. aphthous stomatitis.   c. leukoplakia buccalis.
   b. candidiasis.   d. lichen planus.

5. The incidence of most dental caries is directly related to an increase in the dietary intake of:
   a. fat.   c. salt.
   b. protein.   d. sugar.

6. Postoperative nursing care for drainage of a dentoalveolar or periapical abscess includes all of the following except:
   a. soft diet after 24 hours.   c. external heat by pad or compress to hasten the resolution of the inflammatory swelling.
   b. fluid restriction for the first 48 hours because the gums are swollen and painful.   d. warm saline mouthwashes every 2 hours while awake.

7. Preventive orthodontics for malocclusion can start as early as age:
   a. 3 years.
   b. 5 years.
   c. 7 years.
   d. 9 years.

8. The most commonly inflamed salivary gland is the:
   a. buccal.
   b. parotid.
   c. sublingual.
   d. submaxillary.

9. Neoplasms of the salivary glands:
   a. are normally malignant and are treated by surgical excision.
   b. commonly recur, and recurrences are more malignant than the original tumor.
   c. are usually always treated with radiation.
   d. are characterized by all of the above.

10. The most common site for cancer of the oral cavity is the:
    a. lip.
    b. mouth.
    c. pharynx.
    d. tongue.

11. The typical lesion in oral cancer can be described as:
    a. an indurated ulcer.
    b. a warty growth.
    c. a white or red plaque.
    d. a painful sore.

12. A nurse inspects the Stensen duct of the parotid gland to determine inflammation and possible obstruction. The nurse would examine the oral cavity in the area of the:
    a. buccal mucosa next to the upper molars.
    b. dorsum of the tongue.
    c. roof of the mouth next to the incisors.
    d. posterior segment of the tongue near the uvula.

13. Usually the first symptom associated with esophageal disease is:
    a. dysphagia.
    b. malnutrition.
    c. pain.
    d. regurgitation of food.

14. The nurse suspects that a patient who presents with the symptom of food "sticking" in the lower portion of the esophagus may have the motility disorder known as:
    a. achalasia.
    b. diffuse spasm.
    c. gastroesophageal reflex.
    d. hiatal hernia.

15. A hiatal hernia involves:
    a. an extension of the esophagus through the diaphragm.
    b. an involution of the esophagus, which causes a severe stricture.
    c. a protrusion of the upper stomach into the lower portion of the thorax.
    d. a twisting of the duodenum through an opening in the diaphragm.

16. Intervention for a person who has swallowed strong acid includes all of the following except:
    a. administering an irritant that will stimulate vomiting.
    b. aspirating secretions from the pharynx if respirations are affected.
    c. neutralizing the chemical.
    d. washing the esophagus with large volumes of water.

17. Cancer of the esophagus occurs primarily in:
    a. black men older than 50 years of age.
    b. black women after menopause.
    c. white men 30 to 40 years old.
    d. white women older than 60 years of age.

18. A common postoperative complication of esophageal surgery for cancer is:
    a. aspiration pneumonia.
    b. hemorrhage.
    c. incompetence of the suture line, resulting in fluid seepage.
    d. the dumping syndrome.

Matching. Match the abnormality listed in Column II with its associated symptomatology of the lip, mouth, or gums listed in Column I.

Column I

1. ____ ulcerated and painful, white papules

2. ____ reddened area or rash associated with itching

3. ____ painful, inflamed, swollen gums

4. ____ white overgrowth of horny layer of epidermis

5. ____ shallow ulcer with a red border and white or yellow center

6. ____ hyperkeratotic white patches usually in buccal mucosa

7. ____ reddened circumscribed lesion that ulcerates and becomes encrusted

8. ____ white patches with rough, hairlike projections usually found on the tongue

Column II

a. actinic chelitis

b. leukoplakia

c. chancre

d. canker sore

e. gingivitis

f. lichen planus

g. contact dermatitis

h. hairy leukoplakia

I. Critical Thinking Questions and Exercises

Applying Concepts

Refer to the figure below, and answer the following questions related to a neck-dissection procedure.

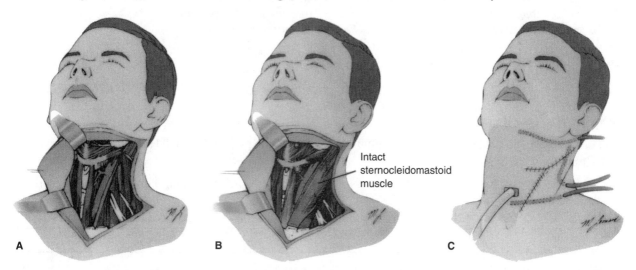

A   B   C

(A) A classic radical neck dissection in which the sternocleidomastoid and smaller muscles are removed. All tissue is removed, from the ramus of the jaw to the clavicle. The jugular vein has also been removed. The functional neck dissection (B) is similar but preserves the sternocleidomastoid muscle, internal jugular vein, and the spinal accessory nerve. The wound is closed (C), and portable suction drainage tubes are in place.

Read each question carefully. Either circle the answer or write the best response in the space provided.

1. A radical neck dissection (see A) is often performed to help prevent _____, the primary reason for death from neck malignancies.

2. Two common morbidities associated with a radical neck dissection are _____ and _____.

3. Reconstructive techniques involve grafts that normally use the _____ muscle.

4. List three postoperative complications expected when someone has surgery to the neck area (see A and B):
   _____, _____, and _____.

5. Two collaborative, postoperative nursing problems may be: _____ and _____.

6. After a radical neck dissection, a patient is placed in Fowler's position to:
   a. decrease venous pressure on the skin flaps.
   b. facilitate swallowing.
   c. increase lymphatic drainage.
   d. accomplish all of the above.

7. Postoperatively, a finding that should be immediately reported is:
   a. temperature of 99°F.
   b. pain.
   c. stridor.
   d. localized wound tenderness.

8. A nurse who is caring for a patient who has had radical neck surgery notices an abnormal amount of serosanguineous secretions in the wound suction unit during the first postoperative day. An expected normal amount of drainage is:
   a. between 40 and 80 mL.
   b. approximately 80 to 120 mL.
   c. between 120 and 160 mL.
   d. greater than 160 mL.

9. A major potential complication is hemorrhage from the:
   a. brachial artery.
   b. carotid artery.
   c. innominate artery.
   d. vertebral artery.

10. Postoperatively, the nurse observes excessive drooling. She assesses for damage to the:
    a. facial nerve.
    b. hypoglossal nerve.
    c. spinal accessory nerve.
    d. auditory nerve.

Clinical Situations

Read the following case studies. Fill in the blanks or circle the correct answer.

CASE STUDY: Mandibular Fracture

William, a 17-year-old student, suffered a mandibular fracture while playing football. He is scheduled for jaw repositioning surgery.

1. Preoperatively, the nurse explains the surgical procedure for treatment of a mandibular fracture. Describe the procedure that would be used.

   _____

   _____

2. Postoperatively, the nurse should immediately position William:
   a. flat on his back to facilitate lung expansion during inspiration.
   b. on his side with his head slightly elevated to prevent aspiration.
   c. supine with his head to the side to promote the drainage of secretions.
   d. with his head lower than his trunk to prevent aspiration of fluids.

3. Postoperatively, the nurse's primary goal is to maintain:
   a. adequate nutrition.
   b. an open airway.
   c. jaw immobilization.
   d. oral hygiene.

4. What would you tell the patient to explain why nasogastric suctioning is needed?

_____

_____

5. For emergency use, which of the following should be available at the head of the bed?
a. a nasogastric suction tube
b. a nasopharyngeal suction catheter
c. a wire cutter or scissors
d. an oxygen cannula

6. A recommended initial postoperative diet for William would be:
a. bland pureed.
b. clear liquid.
c. full liquid.
d. semisoft.

7. William must be instructed not to chew food until the ____ postoperative week.
a. third
b. fourth
c. fifth
d. eighth

8. What essential item must be sent home with William when he is discharged?

_____

CASE STUDY: Cancer of the Mouth

Edith, a 64-year-old mother of two, has been a chain smoker for 20 years. During the past month she noticed a dryness in her mouth and a roughened area that is irritating. She mentioned her symptoms to her dentist, who referred her to a medical internist.

1. Based on the patient's health history, the nurse suspects oral cancer. Describe what the nurse would expect the lesion to look like.

_____

2. During the health history the nurse noted that Edith did not mention a late-occurring symnptom of mouth cancer, which is:
a. drainage.
b. fever.
c. odor.
d. pain.

3. On physical examination, Edith evidenced changes associated with cancer of the mouth, such as:
a. a sore, roughened area that has not healed in 3 weeks.
b. minor swelling in an area adjacent to the lesion.
c. numbness in the affected area of the mouth.
d. all of the above.

4. To confirm a diagnosis of carcinoma of the mouth, a physician would order:
a. a biopsy.
b. a staining procedure.
c. exfoliative cytology.
d. roentgenography.

5. List three therapies that are considered effective for treatment.

a. _____

b. _____

c. _____

36

Gastrointestinal Intubation and Special Nutritional Modalities

I. Interpretation, Completion, and Comparison

Multiple Choice. Read each question carefully. Circle your answer.

1. The Levin tube, a commonly used nasogastric tube, has circular markings at specific points. The tube should be inserted to:
   a. a length of 50 cm (20 in).
   b. a point that equals the distance from the nose to the xiphoid process.
   c. the midpoint between a 50-cm marking and the distance measured from the tip of the nose to the xiphoid process.
   d. the distance determined by measuring from the tragus of the ear to the xiphoid process.

2. When continuous or intermittent suction is used with a nasogastric tube, the goal is to have the amount of suction in the gastric mucosa reduced to:
   a. 30–40 mm Hg.
   b. 60 mm Hg.
   c. 70–80 mm Hg.
   d. 100–120 mm Hg.

3. It is essential for the nurse who is managing a gastric sump tube to:
   a. maintain intermittent or continuous suction at a rate greater than 120 mm Hg.
   b. keep the vent lumen above the patient's midline to prevent gastric content reflux.
   c. irrigate only through the vent lumen.
   d. do all of the above.

4. A nasoenteric tube used for decompression is a:
   a. Cantor tube.
   b. Moss tube.
   c. Gastric-Sump Salem.
   d. Sengstaken-Blakemore.

5. Nasoenteric tubes usually remain in place until:
   a. bowel sounds are present.
   b. flatus is passed.
   c. peristalsis is resumed.
   d. all of the above mechanisms occur.

6. A commonly used double-lumen decompression tube is the:
   a. Cantor tube.
   b. Harris tube.
   c. Levin tube.
   d. Miller-Abbott tube.

7. A nurse prepares a patient for insertion of a nasoenteric tube. The nurse positions the patient:
  a. in high Fowler's position.
  b. flat in bed.
  c. on his or her right side.
  d. in semi-Fowler's position with his or her head turned to the left.

8. A nasoenteric-decompression tube can be safely advanced 2 to 3 inches every:
  a. 1 hour.
  b. 2 hours.
  c. 4 hours.
  d. 8 hours.

9. Symptoms of oliguria, lethargy, and hypothermia in a patient would indicate to the nurse that the patient may be experiencing the initial common potential complication of nasoenteric intubation, which is:
  a. a cardiac dysrhythmia.
  b. fluid volume deficit.
  c. mucous membrane irritation.
  d. pulmonary complications.

10. Osmosis is the process whereby:
  a. particles disperse throughout a liquid medium to achieve an equal concentration throughout.
  b. particles move from an area of greater concentration to an area of lesser concentration to establish equilibrium.
  c. water moves through a membrane from a dilute solution to a more concentrated solution to achieve equal osmolality.
  d. water moves through a membrane from an area of higher osmolality to an area of lesser osmolality to establish equilbrium.

11. Residual content is checked before each tube feeding. A feeding would be delayed and the patient reassessed if the residual were:
  a. about 50 mL.
  b. between 50 and 80 mL.
  c. about 100 mL.
  d. greater than 150 mL.

12. The dumping syndrome occurs when high-carbohydrate foods are administered over a period of less than 20 minutes. A nursing measure to prevent or minimize the dumping syndrome is to administer the feeding:
  a. at a warm temperature to decrease peristalsis.
  b. by bolus to prevent continuous intestinal distention.
  c. with about 100 mL of fluid to dilute the high carbohydrate concentration.
  d. with the patient in semi-Fowler's position to decrease transit time influenced by gravity.

13. Gastrostomy feedings are preferred to nasogastric feedings in the comatose patient, because the:
  a. gastroesophageal sphincter is intact, lessening the possibility of regurgitation.
  b. digestive process occurs more rapidly as a result of the feeding's not having to pass through the esophagus.
  c. feedings can be administered with the patient in the recumbent position.
  d. the patient cannot experience the deprivational stress of not swallowing.

14. Initial fluid nourishment after a gastrostomy usually consists of:
  a. distilled water.
  b. 10% glucose and tap water.
  c. milk.
  d. high-calorie liquids.

15. When administering a bolus gastrostomy feeding, the receptacle should be held no higher than:
  a. 9 in.   b. 18 in.   c. 27 in.   d. 36 in.

16. The basic hyperalimentation solution consists of _____ glucose.
  a. 10%   b. 25%   c. 35%   d. 50%

17. The preferred route for infusion of parenteral nutrition is the:
  a. brachial vein.
  b. jugular vein.
  c. subclavian vein.
  d. superior vena cava.

18. The most common infectious organism for patients receiving parenteral nutrition is:
  a. *Candida albicans.*
  b. *Klebsiella pneumoniae.*
  c. *Staphylococcus aureus.*
  d. *Staphyloccus epidermidis.*

19. Patients who are receiving total parenteral nutrition should be observed for signs of hyperglycemia, which would include:
a. diuresis.
b. lethargy.
c. stupor.
d. all of the above.

Matching. *Match the description of the type of nasogastric, nasoenteric, and regular feeding tube in Column II with its appropriate name listed in Column I.*

Column I

1. _____ Harris

2. _____ Sengstaken-Blakemore

3. _____ Miller-Abbott

4. _____ Levin

5. _____ Cantor

6. _____ Gastric-Sump Salem

7. _____ Moss

8. _____ Dubhoff or Keofeed II

Column II

a. double-lumen, rubber decompression tube about 10 feet in length

b. triple-lumen nasogastric tube that also has a duodenal lumen for postoperative feedings

c. nasoenteric feeding tube about 6 feet in length

d. single-lumen, rubber, nasoenteric decompression tube that contains a mercury-weighted bag

e. single-lumen, plastic or rubber nasogastric tube about 4 feet in length

f. double-lumen, plastic nasogastric tube about 120 cm in length

g. mercury-weighted, single-lumen nasoenteric tube about 180 cm in length

h. triple-lumen, rubber nasogastric tube (two lumens are used to inflate the gastric and esophageal balloons)

II. Critical Thinking Questions and Exercises

Read the following case studies. Fill in the blanks or circle the correct answer.

CASE STUDY: Cantor Tube

Martin, a 69-year-old widower who lives alone, has been diagnosed as having an obstruction of the small intestine. The physician has requested nursing assistance for insertion of a Cantor tube.

1. Before insertion of the Cantor tube, the nurse should:
a. assist Martin to high Fowler's position and help him hyperextend his neck.
b. explain the purpose of the tube.
c. screen Martin to ensure privacy.
d. do all of the above.

2. Martin needs to be informed that the procedure may involve:
a. having him hold ice chips in his mouth for a few minutes.
b. mouth breathing or panting during passage of the tube.
c. the spraying of his oropharynx with tetracaine (Pontocaine) to dull the nasal passages and gag reflex.
d. all of the above.

3. After the tube has passed the pyloric sphincter, nursing responsibilities include advancing the tube:
a. 1 inches every hour.
b. 1 inches every 4 hours.
c. 2–3 inches every hour.
d. 2–3 inches every 4 hours.

4. The nurse knows that tube placement can be verified by checking the pH of aspirated secretions. If the tube were in the intestines, the pH reading would be approximately:
   a. 2.0.   b. 3.0.   c. 5.0.   d. 6.0.

5. Fluid volume deficit is a potential problem with nasoenteric intubation. Indicators of fluid volume deficit include all of the following *except*:
   a. the body temperature of 102°F.   c. lethargy and exhaustion.
   b. dry mucous membranes.   d. oliguria.

CASE STUDY: Dumping Syndrome

Nancy is 37 years old, 5 ft 7 in tall, and weighs 140 lb. She receives 250 mL of Osmolite (liquid nutrition) over a 15-minute period every 4 hours through a nasogastric tube. Nancy has had esophageal surgery for carcinoma.

1. Nancy tells the nurse that she has diarrhea. The nurse suspects Nancy is experiencing the dumping syndrome. The nurse also knows that she needs to eliminate other possible causes, such as: _____,

   _____, _____, and _____.

2. The nurse reviews Nancy's chart to see what medications she is receiving, because she knows that certain drugs increase the frequency of the syndrome in some patients. List several of these medications.

   _____

   _____

3. Because of the dumping syndrome, the physician reduces Nancy's current rate of infusion by 50%. The nurse should adjust the rate of the gastrostomy feeding to _____mL/min.
   a. 8   b. 10   c. 12   d. 16

4. The nurse notes a residual gastric content of 50 mL. She should:
   a. delay the feeding for 2 hours and reassess.   c. notify the physician.
   b. discard the 50 mL and administer the next   d. return the solution through the tube and
      feeding.   administer the next feeding.

CASE STUDY: Total Parenteral Nutrition

Penny is 30 years old and single. She is 5 ft 7 in tall, weighs 150 pounds, and is receiving parenteral nutrition solution at the rate of 3 L per day. Her postoperative condition warrants receiving nutrients by the intravenous route.

1. The nurse knows that, to spare body protein, Penny's daily calorie intake must be:
   a. about 500 calories per day.   c. around 800 calories per day.
   b. approximately 1500 calories per day.   d. equal to 1000 calories per day.

2. The nurse estimates Penny's caloric intake for each 1000 mL of total parenteral nutrition to yield a glucose concentration of _____calories.
   a. 500   b. 800   c. 1000   d. 1500

3. Penny's infusion rate is 120 mL/hour. Her rate has slowed because of positional body changes. To compensate, the nurse could safely increase Penny's rate for 8 hours to _____mL/hour.
   a. 100   b. 125   c. 138   d. 146

4. The nurse should observe Penny for signs of rapid fluid intake, which may include:
   a. chills   c. nausea
   b. fever   d. all of the above

5. The nurse weighs Penny daily. After 7 days, Penny's weight gain is abnormal at:
   a. 3.5 lb.   b. 5.0 lb.   c. 7.0 lb.   d. 12 lb.

Applying Concepts

Refer to the figure below and answer the following questions.

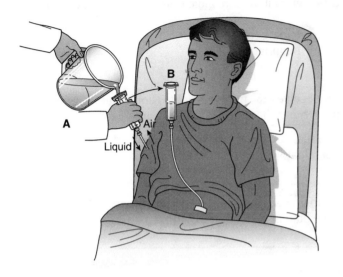

Gastrostomy feeding by gravity. (*A*) Feeding is instilled at an angle so that air does not enter the stomach. (*B*) Syringe is raised perpendicular to the stomach so that feeding can enter by gravity.

1. List three nursing diagnoses for a postoperative patient that address nursing care for a gastrotomy tube.

   a. _____

   b. _____

   c. _____

2. List three possible collaborative problems for a patient with a gastrostomy tube.

   a. _____

   b. _____

   c. _____

3. When giving an initial tube feeding, the nurse would be looking for _____ around the tube site on the abdomen.

4. A dressing over the tube outlet and the gastrostomy tube protects the skin around the incision from

   _____ and _____.

5. The syringe, filled with feeding solution, is raised perpendicular to the abdomen so that the solution can enter by gravity. How long should it take for 100 mL to instill?

   _____

6. If the solution fails to instill, the nurse could _____

   _____.

7. The syringe should not be elevated higher than 18 inches above the abdominal wall, because:

   _____

   _____.

8. Explain why the patient in the figure is sitting upright.

   _____

   _____.

37

Management of Patients With Gastric and Duodenal Disorders

1. Interpretation, Completion, and Comparison

Multiple Choice. Read each question carefully. Circle your answer.

1. Acute gastritis is often caused by:
   a. ingestion of strong acids.
   b. irritating foods.
   c. overuse of aspirin.
   d. all of the above.

2. To promote fluid balance when treating gastritis, the nurse knows that the minimal daily intake of fluids should be:
   a. 1.0 L.   b. 1.5 L.   c. 2.0 L.   d. 2.5 L.

3. The most common site for peptic ulcer formation is the:
   a. duodenum.
   b. esophagus.
   c. pylorus.
   d. stomach.

4. A symptom that distinguishes a chronic gastric ulcer from a chronic duodenal ulcer is the:
   a. absence of any correlation between the presence of the ulcer and a malignancy.
   b. normal to below-normal secretion of acid.
   c. relief of pain after food ingestion.
   d. uncommon incidence of vomiting.

5. The blood group that seems most susceptible to peptic ulcer disease is group:
   a. A.   b. B.   c. AB.   d. O.

6. *Helicobacter pylori* bacteria is present in _____ of those with duodenal ulcers.
   a. 25%   b. 50%   c. 75%   d. 95%

7. Peptic ulcers occur with the most frequency in those between the ages of:
   a. 15 and 25 years.
   b. 20 and 30 years.
   c. 40 and 60 years.
   d. 60 and 80 years.

8. A diagnostic clinical manifestation of Zollinger-Ellison syndrome is:
   a. diarrhea.
   b. hypercalcemia.
   c. steatorrhea.
   d. tetany.

9. A characteristic associated with peptic ulcer pain is a:
   a. burning sensation localized in the back or midepigastrium.
   b. feeling of emptiness that precedes meals from 1 to 3 hours.
   c. severe gnawing pain that increases in severity as the day progresses.
   d. combination of all of the above.

10. The best time to administer an antacid is:
   a. with the meal.
   b. 30 minutes before the meal.
   c. 1 to 3 hours after the meal.
   d. immediately after the meal.

11. A Billroth I procedure is a surgical approach to ulcer management whereby:
   a. a partial gastrectomy is done with anastomosis of the stomach segment to the duodenum.
   b. a sectioned portion of the stomach is joined to the jejunum.
   c. the antral portion of the stomach is removed and a vagotomy is performed.
   d. the vagus nerve is cut and gastric drainage is established.

12. The most common complication of peptic ulcer disease is:
   a. hemorrhage.
   b. intractable ulcer.
   c. perforation.
   d. pyloric obstruction.

13. Nursing interventions associated with peptic ulcers include:
   a. checking the blood pressure and pulse rate every 15 to 20 minutes.
   b. frequently monitoring hemoglobin and hematocrit levels.
   c. observing stools and vomitus for color, consistency, and volume.
   d. all of the above.

14. If peptic ulcer hemorrhage were suspected, an immediate nursing action would be to:
   a. place the patient supine with his or her legs elevated.
   b. prepare a peripheral and central line for intravenous infusion.
   c. assess vital signs.
   d. accomplish all of the above.

15. Pyloric obstruction can occur when the area distal to the pyloric sphincter becomes stenosed by:
   a. edema.
   b. scar tissue.
   c. spasm.
   d. all of the above.

16. Symptoms associated with pyloric obstruction include all of the following *except*:
   a. anorexia.
   b. diarrhea.
   c. nausea and vomiting.
   d. weight loss.

17. Morbid obesity is a term applied to people who are more than:
   a. 20 lb above ideal body weight.
   b. 50 lb above ideal body weight.
   c. 75–80 lb above ideal body weight.
   d. 100 lb above ideal body weight.

18. Pulmonary complications frequently follow upper-abdominal incisions, because:
   a. aspiration is a common occurrence associated with postoperative injury to the pyloric sphincter or the cardiac sphincter.
   b. pneumothorax is a common complication of abdominal surgery when the chest cavity has been entered.
   c. the patient tends to have shallow respirations in an attempt to minimize incisional pain.
   d. all of the above.

19. Teaching points to help a patient with total gastric resection avoid the dumping syndrome include all of the following *except*:
   a. eating small, frequent meals.
   b. increasing the carbohydrate content of the diet to supply needed calories for energy.
   c. lying down after meals.
   d. taking fluids between meals to decrease the total volume in the stomach at one time.

Fill-In. Read each statement carefully. Write the best response in the space provided.

1. Describe an immediate treatment that can be used to treat the ingestion of corrosive acid:

_____

2. Explain why patients with gastritis due to a vitamin deficiency usually have a malabsorption of vitamin B_{12}:

_____

3. Name two conditions specifically related to peptic ulcer development:

   a. _____

   b. _____

4. List the bacillus that is commonly associated with gastric and possibly duodenal ulcers:

_____

5. List several findings characteristic of Zollinger-Ellison syndrome:

_____

_____

6. Define the term *stress ulcer:*

_____

7. Distinguish between the cause and locations of Cushing's and Curling's ulcers:

_____

8. Explain the current theory about diet modification for peptic ulcer disease:

_____

9. Name three major complications of a peptic ulcer:

   a. _____

   b. _____

   c. _____

10. Describe the clinical manifestations associated with peptic ulcer perforation:

_____

_____

II. Critical Thinking Questions and Exercises

Discussion and Analysis

1. Describe the pathophysiology of gastritis.

2. Chronic gastritis can be caused by the bacteria *H. pylori.* Describe four diagnostic tests that can be used to determine the presence of the bacteria.

Existing Inferences

Examine the figure below. Outline in detail the pathophysiology of peptic ulcer formation. Explain why specific sites are more common and what contributes to common inflammatory sites.

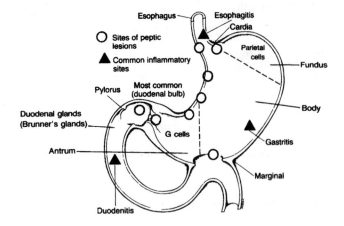

Peptic lesions may occur in the esophagus (esophagitis), stomach (gastritis), or duodenum (duodenitis). Note peptic ulcer sites and common inflammatory sites. Hydrochloric acid is formed by parietal cells in the fundus; gastrin is secreted by G cells in the antrum. The duodenal glands secrete an alkaline mucous solution.

38

Management of Patients With Intestinal and Rectal Disorders

I. Interpretation, Completion, and Comparison

Multiple Choice. Read each question carefully. Circle your answer.

1. The pathophysiology of constipation may be related to interference with:
   a. myoelectric activity of the colon.
   b. mucosal transport.
   c. processes involved in defecation.
   d. all of the above mechanisms.

2. Nursing suggestions to help a person break the constipation habit include all of the following *except*:
   a. a fluid intake of at least 2 L/day.
   b. a low-residue, bland diet.
   c. establishing a regular schedule of exercise.
   d. establishing a regular time for daily elimination.

3. The classification of moderate diarrhea refers to the quantity of daily unformed stools described as:
   a. more than two bowel movements a day.
   b. between two and four bowel movements movements a day.
   c. between three and six bowel movements a day.
   d. more than six bowel movements a day.

4. In assessing stool characteristics associated with diarrhea, the nurse knows that the presence of greasy stools suggests:
   a. disorders of the colon.
   b. inflammatory enteritis.
   c. intestinal malabsorption.
   d. small-bowel disorders.

5. Hypokalemia may occur rapidly in an elderly person who experiences diarrhea. The nurse should report a critical potassium level of _____mEq/L to the physician immediately.
   a. 3.0   b. 4.0   c. 4.5   d. 5.0

6. Malabsorption diseases may affect the ability of the digestive system to absorb the major water soluble vitamin:
   a. A.   b. B_{12}.   c. D.   d. K.

7. A positive Rovsing's sign is indicative of appendicitis. The nurse knows to assess for this indicator by palpating the:
   a. right lower quadrant.
   b. left lower quadrant.
   c. right upper quadrant.
   d. left upper quadrant.

8. The most common site for diverticulitis is the:
- a. duodenum.
- b. ileum.
- c. jejunum.
- d. sigmoid.

9. The incidence of diverticulitis in those older than 60 years of age is about:
- a. 15%.
- b. 35%.
- c. 60%.
- d. 80%.

10. Diverticulitis is clinically manifested by:
- a. a low-grade fever.
- b. a change in bowel habits.
- c. left lower quadrant pain.
- d. all of the above.

11. Common clinical manifestations of Crohn's disease are:
- a. abdominal pain and diarrhea.
- b. edema and weight gain.
- c. nausea and vomiting.
- d. obstruction and ileus.

12. A nurse suspects a diagnosis of regional enteritis when she assesses the symptoms of:
- a. abdominal distention and rebound tenderness.
- b. hyperactive bowel sounds in the right lower quadrant.
- c. intermittent pain associated with diarrhea.
- d. all of the above.

13. Nutritional management for regional enteritis consists of diet therapy that is:
- a. high in fats.
- b. high in fiber.
- c. low in protein.
- d. low in residue.

14. Remission of inflammation in ulcerative colitis is possible with:
- a. antidiarrheal medication.
- b. periods of rest after meals.
- c. steroid therapy.
- d. all of the above.

15. A problem unique to the patient with an ileostomy is that:
- a. regular bowel habits cannot be established.
- b. sexual activity is restricted.
- c. skin excoriation can occur.
- d. the collecting appliance is bulky and large.

16. Postoperative nursing management for a patient with a continent ileostomy includes all of the following *except*:
- a. checking to make certain that the rectal packing is in place.
- b. irrigating the ileostomy catheter every 3 hours.
- c. nasogastric tube feedings, 30–50 mL, every 4–6 hours.
- d. perineal irrigations after the dressings are removed.

17. Clinical manifestations associated with small-bowel obstruction include all of the following *except*:
- a. dehydration.
- b. pain that is wavelike.
- c. the passage of blood-tinged stool.
- d. vomiting.

18. The mortality rate for cancer of the colon is:
- a. less than 20%.
- b. 25% to 35%.
- c. 40% to 50%.
- d. greater than 60%.

19. Preoperatively, intestinal antibiotics are given for colon surgery to:
- a. decrease the bulk of colon contents.
- b. reduce the bacteria content of the colon.
- c. soften the stool.
- d. do all of the above.

20. For colostomy irrigation, the enema catheter should be inserted into the stoma:
- a. 1 inch.
- b. 2–3 inches.
- c. 4–6 inches.
- d. 8 inches.

21. For colostomy irrigation, the patient should be directed to hold the enema can or bag at shoulder level approximately _____ above the stoma.
- a. 6 inches.
- b. 8–16 inches.
- c. 18–24 inches.
- d. 30 inches.

22. The total quantity of irrigating solution that can be instilled at one session is:
- a. 1000 mL.
- b. 1500 mL.
- c. 2500 mL.
- d. 3000 mL.

Complete the following crossword puzzle using common terms associated with intestinal and rectal disorders..

Down

1. A tubular fibrous tract that extends from an opening beside the anus into the anal canal

2. Dilated and atonic colon caused by a fecal mass

3. A chemotherapeutic agent used to treat colon cancer

4. A food to avoid for a patient with an ileostomy

6. Straining at stool

8. Another name for regional enteritis

12. A highly reliable blood study used to diagnose colon cancer

13. Painful straining at stool

14. The most common bacteria associated with peritonitis

Across

5. Another term for fecal matter

7. An ileal outlet on the abdomen

9. Intestinal rumbling

10. Another food to avoid for a patient with an ileostomy

11. The most popular "over-the-counter" medication purchased in the United States

15. Intravenous nutrition used for inflammatory bowel disease

16. The most common complication of appendicitis

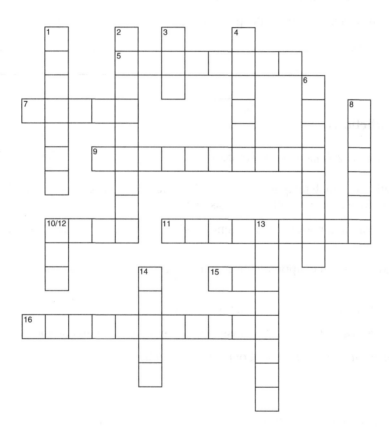

Matching. *Match the type of laxative listed in Column III with its classification in Column II. Then match the classification in Column II with its action listed in Column I.*

Column I	Column II	Column III
1. _____ magnesium ions alter stool consistency	1. _____ bulk-forming	a. Mineral oil
2. _____ surfactant action hydrates stool	2. _____ stimulant	b. Metamucil
3. _____ electrolytes induce diarrhea	3. _____ fecal softener	c. Milk of Magnesia
4. _____ polysaccharides and cellulose mix with intestinal contents	4. _____ lubricant	d. Dulcolax
	5. _____ saline agent	e. Colace
5. _____ colon is irritated and sensory nerve endings stimulated	6. _____ osmotic agent	f. Colyte
6. _____ hydrocarbons soften fecal matter		

II. Critical Thinking Questions and Exercises

Discussion and Analysis

1. Discuss the physiologic processes that result in the urge to defecate.

2. Explain the Valsalva maneuver that can occur as a complication of constipation.

3. For each of these three diseases, explain the pathophysiology of malabsorption:

Pancreatic insufficiency:_____

Zollinger-Ellison syndrome: _____

Celiac disease: _____

Recognizing Contradictions

Rewrite each statement correctly. Underline the key concepts.

1. Diarrhea is a condition in which there is an increased frequency of bowel movements (more than six per day) associated with increased amount and consistency.

2. Peritonitis, the most common reason for emergency abdominal surgery, occurs in about 10% of the population.

3. The most serious complication of appendicitis is strangulation of adjacent bowel tissue, which occurs in 5% of the cases.

4. The major cause of death from peritonitis is hypovolemia.

5. The most common areas affected in Crohn's disease are the sigmoid colon and the cecum.

6. Surgery is rarely necessary for the treatment of regional enteritis.

Clinical Situations

Read the following case studies. Fill in the blanks or circle the correct answer.

CASE STUDY: Appendicitis

Rory, an 18-year-old girl, is admitted to the hospital with a possible diagnosis of appendicitis. She had been symptomatic for several days before admission.

1. During assessment, the nurse is looking for positive indicators of appendicitis, which include all of the following *except*:
   a. a low-grade fever.
   b. abdominal tenderness on palpation.
   c. thrombocytopenia.
   d. vomiting.

2. On physical examination, the nurse should be looking for tenderness on palpation at McBurney's point, which is located in the:
   a. left lower quadrant.
   b. left upper quadrant.
   c. right lower quadrant.
   d. right upper quadrant.

3. Symptoms suggestive of acute appendicitis include:
   a. a positive Rovsing's sign.
   b. increased abdominal pain with coughing.
   c. tenderness around the umbilicus.
   d. all of the above.

4. Preparation for an appendectomy includes:
   a. an intravenous infusion.
   b. prophylactic antibiotic therapy.
   c. salicylates to lower an elevated temperature.
   d. all of the above.

CASE STUDY: Peritonitis

Sharon has peritonitis subsequent to ambulatory peritoneal dialysis. Her presenting symptoms are pain, abdominal tenderness, and nausea.

1. On assessment, the nurse should be looking for additional symptoms diagnostic of peritonitis, which include:
   a. abdominal rigidity.
   b. diminished peristalsis.
   c. leukocytosis.
   d. all of the above.

2. A central venous pressure (CVP) catheter is inserted to monitor fluid balance. The nurse's readings indicate low circulatory volume. The reading is probably between:
   a. 2 and 4 cm H_2O.
   b. 6 and 8 cm H_2O.
   c. 10 and 12 cm H_2O.
   d. 14 and 16 cm H_2O.

3. Given Sharon's CVP reading indicating hypovolemia, the nurse should assess for all of the following *except*:
   a. bradycardia.
   b. hypotension.
   c. oliguria.
   d. tachypnea.

4. With treatment, Sharon's peritonitis subsides. However, the nurse continues to assess for the common complication of:
   a. abscess formation.
   b. respiratory arrest owing to excessive pressure on the diaphragm.
   c. umbilical hernia.
   d. urinary tract infection

UNIT 8
Metabolic and Endocrine Function

39

Assessment and Management of Patients With Hepatic Disorders

I. Interpretation, Completion, and Comparison

Multiple Choice. Read each question carefully. Circle your answer.

1. The majority of blood supply to the liver, which is rich in nutrients from the gastrointestinal tract, comes from the:
   a. hepatic artery.
   b. hepatic vein.
   c. portal artery.
   d. portal vein.

2. The liver plays a major role in glucose metabolism by:
   a. producing ketone bodies.
   b. synthesizing albumin.
   c. participating in gluconeogenesis.
   d. doing all of the above.

3. The liver synthesizes prothrombin only if there is enough vitamin:
   a. A.
   b. B_{12}.
   c. D.
   d. K.

4. The substance necessary for the manufacture of bile salts by hepatocytes is:
   a. albumin.
   b. bilirubin.
   c. cholesterol.
   d. vitamin D.

5. The main function of bile salts is:
   a. albumin synthesis.
   b. fat emulsification in the intestines.
   c. lipid manufacture for the transport of proteins.
   d. urea synthesis from ammonia.

6. Hepatocellular dysfunction results in all of the following *except*:
   a. decreased serum albumin.
   b. elevated serum bilirubin.
   c. increased blood ammonia levels.
   d. increased levels of urea.

7. Jaundice becomes evident when serum bilirubin levels exceed:
   a. 0.5 mg/dL.
   b. 1.0 mg/dL.
   c. 1.5 mg/dL.
   d. 2.5 mg/dL.

8. Negative sodium balance is important for a patient with ascites. An example of food permitted on a low-sodium diet is:
   a. 1/4 cup of peanut butter.
   b. 1 cup of powdered milk.
   c. one frankfurter.
   d. two slices of cold cuts.

9. A person who consumes contaminated shellfish would probably develop:
   a. hepatitis A.
   b. hepatitis B.
   c. non-A, non-B hepatitis.
   d. hepatitis C.

10. The hepatitis virus that has the shortest average incubation period is hepatitis:
   a. A virus.
   b. B virus.
   c. C virus.
   d. D virus.

11. Immune serum globulin provides passive immunity against type A hepatitis in those not vaccinated if it is administered 2 to 7 days after exposure. Immunity is effective for about:
   a. 1 month.
   b. 2 months.
   c. 3 months.
   d. 4 months.

12. Choose the correct statement about hepatitis B vaccine.
   a. All persons at risk should receive active immunization.
   b. Evidence suggests that the human immuno-deficiency (HIV) virus may be harbored in the vaccine.
   c. It should be given only once because of its potency.
   d. One dose in the dorsogluteal muscle is recommended.

13. Indications for postexposure vaccination with hepatitis B immune globulin include:
   a. accidental exposure to HbsAg-positive blood.
   b. perinatal exposure.
   c. sexual contact with those who are positive for HbsAg.
   d. all of the above exposures.

14. The chemical most commonly implicated in toxic hepatitis is:
   a. chloroform.
   b. gold compounds.
   c. phosphorus.
   d. all of the above hepatotoxins.

15. Fulminant hepatic failure may progress to hepatic encephalopathy ____ weeks after disease onset.
   a. 2
   b. 4
   c. 6
   d. 8

16. Late symptoms of hepatic cirrhosis include all of the following *except*:
   a. edema.
   b. hypoalbuminemia.
   c. hypokalemia.
   d. hyponatremia.

17. Cirrhosis results in shunting of portal system blood into collateral blood vessels in the gastrointestinal tract. The most common site is:
   a. the esophagus.
   b. the lower rectum.
   c. the stomach.
   d. a combination of all of the above.

18. Signs of advanced liver disease include:
   a. ascites.
   b. jaundice.
   c. portal hypertension.
   d. all of the above.

19. The most common single cause of death in patients with cirrhosis is:
   a. congestive heart failure.
   b. hepatic encephalopathy.
   c. hypovolemic shock.
   d. ruptured esophageal varices.

20. The mortality rate from bleeding esophageal varices is about:
   a. 10%.
   b. 30%.
   c. 50%.
   d. 80%.

21. An indicator of probable esophageal varices is:
   a. hematemesis.
   b. a positive guaiac test.
   c. melena.
   d. all of the above.

22. Bleeding esophageal varices result in a decrease in:

a. nitrogen load from bleeding.

b. renal perfusion.

c. serum ammonia.

d. all of the above.

23. Hepatic lobectomy for cancer can be successful when the primary site is localized. Because of the regenerative capacity of the liver, a surgeon can remove up to _____ of liver tissue.

a. 25%

b. 50%

c. 75%

d. 90%

Matching. *Match the vitamin listed in Column II with the signs of deficiency due to severe chronic liver disease listed in Column I.*

Column I	Column II
1._____hypoprothrombinemia	**a.** Vitamin A
2._____beriberi and polyneuritis	**b.** Vitamin C
3._____hemorrhagic lesions of scurvy	**c.** Vitamin K
4._____night blindness	**d.** Folic Acid
5._____macrocytic anemia	**e.** Thiamine
6._____skin and neurologic changes	**f.** Fiboflavin
7._____mucous membrane lesions	**g.** Pyridoxine

II. Critical Thinking Questions and Exercises

Discussion and Analysis

1. Describe the process of *conjugation.*

2. Distinguish between hemolytic, hepatocellular, and obstructive jaundice in regard to etiology.

3. Explain the pathophysiology of hepatic encephalopathy.

4. Explain the pathophysiology of alcoholic cirrhosis.

Clinical Situations

Read the following case studies. Circle the correct answer.

CASE STUDY: Liver Biopsy

Veronica is scheduled for a liver biopsy. The staff nurse assigned to care for Veronica is to accompany her to the treatment room.

1. Before a liver biopsy, the nurse should check to see that:

a. a compatible donor blood is available.

b. hemostasis tests have been completed.

c. vital signs have been assessed.

d. all of the above have been done.

2. The nurse begins preparing Veronica for the biopsy by assisting her to the correct position, which is:

a. jackknife, with her entire back exposed.

b. recumbent, with her right upper abdomen exposed.

c. lying on her right side, with the left upper thoracic area exposed.

d. supine, with the left lateral chest wall exposed.

3. The nurse knows that the biopsy needle will be inserted into the liver between the:
   a. third and fourth ribs.
   b. fourth and fifth ribs.
   c. sixth and seventh ribs.
   d. eighth and ninth ribs.

4. Immediately before needle insertion, Veronica needs to be instructed to:
   a. breathe slowly and deeply so that rib cage expansion will be minimized during needle insertion.
   b. inhale and exhale deeply and then hold her breath at the end of expiration until the needle is inserted.
   c. pant deeply and continue panting during needle insertion so pain perception will be minimized.
   d. take a deep inspiration and not breathe for 30 to 40 seconds so that the area for needle insertion can be determined; she should then resume normal breathing for the remainder of the procedure.

5. After the biopsy, the nurse assists Veronica to:
   a. high Fowler's position, in which she can effectively take deep breaths and cough.
   b. ambulate while splinting her incision.
   c. assume the Trendelenburg position to prevent postbiopsy shock.
   d. the right side-lying position with a pillow placed under the right costal margin.

CASE STUDY: Paracentesis

Wendy is scheduled for a paracentesis because of ascites formation subsequent to cirrhosis of the liver.

1. Before the procedure, the nurse obtains several drainage bottles. She knows that the maximum amount of fluid to be aspirated at one time is:
   a. 1 L.
   b. 2 L.
   c. 3 L.
   d. 4 L.

2. The nurse helps Wendy to assume the proper position for a paracentesis, which is:
   a. recumbent so that the fluid will pool to the lower abdomen.
   b. lying on her left side so that fluid will not exert pressure on the liver.
   c. semi-Fowler's to avoid shock and provide the most comfort.
   d. upright with her feet resting on a support so that the puncture site will be readily visible.

3. After the paracentesis, Wendy should be observed for signs of vascular collapse, which include all of the following *except*:
   a. bradycardia.
   b. hypotension.
   c. oliguria.
   d. pallor.

CASE STUDY: Alcoholic or Nutritional Cirrhosis

Nathan, a 50-year-old physically disabled veteran, has lived alone for 30 years. He has maintained his independence despite chronic back pain resulting from a war injury. He has a long history of depression and limited food intake. He drinks 6 to 10 bottles of beer daily. He was recently admitted to a veteran's hospital with a diagnosis of alcoholic or nutritional cirrhosis. He was asymptomatic for ascites.

1. On assessment, the nurse notes early clinical manifestations of alcoholic or nutritional cirrhosis, which include all of the following *except*:
   a. pain caused by liver enlargement.
   b. a sharp edge to the periphery of the liver.
   c. a liver decreased in size and nodular.
   d. a firm liver.

2. An abnormal laboratory finding for Nathan is a:
   a. blood ammonia level of 35 mg/dL.
   b. serum albumin concentration of 4.0 g/dL.
   c. total serum bilirubin level of 0.9 mg/dL.
   d. total serum protein level of 5.5 g/dL.

3. Nathan is 5 ft 10 in tall and weighs 140 lb. The physician recommends 50 cal/kg for weight gain. Nathan's daily caloric intake would be approximately:
   a. 2200 cal.
   b. 2800 cal.
   c. 3200 cal.
   d. 3800 cal.

4. A recommended daily protein intake for Nathan to gain weight is:
   a. 31 to 44 g.
   b. 41 to 54 g.
   c. 51 to 64 g.
   d. 61 to 74 g.

5. The physician recommends a sodium-restricted diet. The nurse expects the suggested sodium intake to be approximately:
   a. 250 to 500 mg/24 hours.
   b. 500 to 1000 mg/24 hours.
   c. 2000 to 2500 mg/24 hours.
   d. 3000 to 3500 mg/24 hours.

CASE STUDY: Liver Transplantation

Denise, a 54-year-old mother of three, is scheduled for a liver transplantation subsequent to an extensive hepatic malignancy with multifocal tumors greater than 8 cm in diameter.

1. Denise is hopeful that her surgery will be successful. She is aware, however, that her chance of survical at 1 year is_____
   a. 10%.
   b. 30%.
   c. 50%.
   d. 80%.

2. Denise knows that a successful outcome to transplantation will be compromised by:
   a. fluid and electrolyte disturbances.
   b. malnutrition.
   c. immunosuppressive therapy.
   d. all of the above.

3. The nurse is aware that postoperatively the leading cause of death after liver transplantation is:
   a. bleeding.
   b. hypotension.
   c. infection.
   d. portal hypertension.

4. The nurse knows that a patient receiving cyclosporine to prevent rejection of a transplanted liver may develop a drug side effect of:
   a. nephrotoxicity.
   b. septicemia.
   c. thrombocytopenia.
   d. all of the above reactions.

40

Assessment and Management of Patients With Biliary Disorders

1. Interpretation, Completion, and Comparison

Multiple Choice. Read each question carefully. Circle your answer.

1. A patient is diagnosed with gallstones in the bile ducts. The nurse knows to review the results of blood work for a:
   a. serum ammonia concentration of 90 μg/dL.
   b. serum albumin concentration of 4.0 g/dL.
   c. serum bilirubin level greater than 1.0 mg/dL.
   d. serum globulin concentration of 2.0 g/dL.

2. Bile is stored in the:
   a. cystic duct.
   b. duodenum.
   c. gallbladder.
   d. common bile duct.

3. The major stimulus for increased bicarbonate secretion from the pancreas is:
   a. amylase.
   b. lipase.
   c. secretin.
   d. trypsin.

4. An action not associated with insulin is the:
   a. conversion of glycogen to glucose in the liver.
   b. lowering of blood glucose.
   c. promotion of fat storage.
   d. synthesis of proteins.

5. The nurse knows that a patient with low blood sugar would have a blood glucose level of:
   a. 55–75 mg/dL.
   b. 80–120 mg/dL.
   c. 130–150 mg/dL.
   d. 160–180 mg/dL.

6. A patient with calculi in the gallbladder is said to have:
   a. cholecystitis.
   b. cholelithiasis.
   c. choledocholithiasis.
   d. choledochotomy.

7. The obstruction of bile flow due to cholelithiasis can interfere with the absorption of vitamin:
   a. A.
   b. B_6.
   c. B_{12}.
   d. C.

8. Statistics show that there is a greater incidence of gallbladder disease for women who are:
   a. multiparous.
   b. obese.
   c. older than 40 years of age.
   d. characterized by all of the above.

9. Clinical manifestations of common bile-duct obstruction include all of the following *except*:
   a. amber-colored urine.
   b. clay-colored feces.
   c. pruritus.
   d. jaundice.

10. The diagnostic procedure of choice for cholelithiasis is:
    a. radiography.
    b. oral cholecystography.
    c. cholecystography.
    d. ultrasonography.

11. Pharmacologic therapy is frequently used to dissolve small gallstones. It takes about _____ months of medication with UDCA or CDCA for stones to dissolve:
    a. 1 to 2
    b. 3 to 5
    c. 6 to 8
    d. 6 to 12

12. Chronic pancreatitis, commonly described as autodigestion of the pancreas, is often not detected until _____ of the exocrine and endocrine tissue is destroyed.
    a. 10% to 25%
    b. 30% to 50%
    c. 60% to 75%
    d. 80% to 90%

13. Mild acute pancreatitis is characterized by:
    a. edema and inflammation.
    b. pleural effusion.
    c. sepsis.
    d. disseminated intravascular coagulapathy.

14. A major symptom of pancreatitis that brings the patient to medical care is:
    a. severe abdominal pain.
    b. fever.
    c. jaundice.
    d. mental agitation.

15. The nurse should assess for an important *early indicator* of acute pancreatitis, which is an increased:
    a. serum calcium level.
    b. serum lipase level.
    c. white cell count.
    d. urine amylase level.

16. Nursing measures for pain relief for aute pancreatitis include:
    a. encouraging bed rest to decrease the metabolic rate.
    b. teaching the patient about the correlation between alcohol intake and pain.
    c. withholding oral feedings to limit the release of secretin.
    d. all of the above.

17. The analgesic of choice for severe pancreatic pain is:
    a. codeine.
    b. Demerol.
    c. Percodan.
    d. morphine.

18. The risk for pancreatic cancer is directly proportional to:
    a. age.
    b. dietary intake of fat.
    c. cigarette smoking.
    d. presence of diabetes mellitus.

19. With pancreatic carcinoma, insulin deficiency is suspected when the patient evidences:
    a. an abnormal glucose tolerance.
    b. glucosuria.
    c. hyperglycemia.
    d. all of the above.

20. Clinical manifestations associated with a tumor of the head of the pancreas include:
    a. clay-colored stools.
    b. dark urine.
    c. jaundice.
    d. all of the above.

21. A nurse should monitor blood glucose levels for a patient who is diagnosed as having hyperinsulinism. A value inadequate to sustain normal brain function is:
    a. 30 mg/dL.
    b. 50 mg/dL.
    c. 70 mg/dL.
    d. 90 mg/dL.

22. Zollinger-Ellison tumors are associated with hypersecretion of:
    a. aldosterone.
    b. gastric acid.
    c. insulin.
    d. vasopressin.

II. Critical Thinking Questions and Exercises

Clinical Situations

Read the following case studies. Circle the correct answer or fill in the blank space.

CASE STUDY: Cholecystectomy

Brenda, a 33-year-old obese mother of four, is diagnosed as having acute gallbladder inflammation. She is 5 ft 4 in tall and weighs 190 lb. The physician decides to delay surgical intervention until Brenda's acute symptoms subside.

1. Brenda's initial course of treatment would probably consist of:
  a. analgesics and antibiotics.
  b. intravenous fluids.
  c. nasogastric suctioning.
  d. all of the above.

2. After her acute attack, Brenda was limited to low-fat liquids. As foods are added to her diet, she needs to know that she should avoid:
  a. cooked fruits.
  b. eggs and cheese.
  c. lean meats.
  d. rice and tapioca.

3. Brenda is being medicated with chenodeoxycholic acid. The nurse needs to tell Brenda that the drug may not be effective if it is taken in conjunction with:
  a. dietry cholesterol.
  b. estrogens.
  c. oral contraceptives.
  d. any of the above.

Because Brenda's symptoms continue to recur, she is scheduled for gallbladder surgery.

1. Brenda has signed a consent form for removal of her gallbladder and ligation of the cystic duct and artery. She is scheduled to undergo a:
  a. cholecystectomy.
  b. cholecystostomy.
  c. choledochostomy.
  d. choledocholithotomy.

2. Postoperative nursing observation includes assessing for:
  a. indicators of infection.
  b. leakage of bile into the peritoneal cavity.
  c. obstruction of bile drainage.
  d. all of the above.

3. Brenda needs to know that fat restriction is usually lifted after the biliary ducts dilate to accommodate bile once held by the gallbladder. This takes about:
  a. 1 week.
  b. 2–3 weeks.
  c. 4–6 weeks.
  d. 2 months.

CASE STUDY: Chronic Pancreatitis

Carl, a 56-year-old traveling salesman, has recently been diagnosed with chronic pancreatitis.

1. The nurse knows that the major cause of chronic pancreatitis is: _____.

2. Describe the pathophysiologic sequence of the inflammatory process:

_____

3. Dysfunction of the pancreatic islet cells leads to a diagnosis of: _____.

4. A recommended surgical procedure that allows drainage of pancreatic secretions into the jejunum is:

_____

5. Long-term management requires two dietary modifications: _____ and _____.

Copyright © 2004 by Lippincott Williams and Wilkins. Study Guide to Accompany
Smeltzer/Bare, Brunner and Suddarth's Textbook of Medical Surgical Nursing, tenth edition by Mary Jo Boyer.

205

41

Assessment and Management of Patients With Diabetes Mellitus

I. Interpretation, Completion, and Comparison

Multiple Choice. Read each question carefully. Circle your answer.

1. The ethnic group with the *lowest* incidence of diabetes mellitus in the United States is the:
   a. African Americans.
   b. Caucasians.
   c. Hispanics.
   d. Native Americans.

2. As a cause of death by disease in the United States, diabetes mellitus ranks:
   a. first.
   b. second.
   c. third.
   d. fourth.

3. A patient who is diagnosed with type 1 diabetes mellitus (IDDM) would be expected to:
   a. be restricted to an American Diabetic Association diet.
   b. have no damage to the islet cells of the pancreas.
   c. need exogenous insulin.
   d. need to receive daily doses of a hypoglycemic agent.

4. Possible risk factors associated with type 1 diabetes mellitus include:
   a. an autoimmune susceptibility to diabetogenic viruses.
   b. environmental factors.
   c. the presence of human leukocyte antigen (HLA).
   d. all of the above.

5. Clinical manifestations associated with a diagnosis of type 1 diabetes mellitus include all of the following *except*:
   a. hypoglycemia.
   b. hyponatremia.
   c. ketonuria.
   d. polyphagia.

6. The nurse is asked to assess a patient for glucosuria. The nurse would secure a specimen of:
   a. blood.
   b. sputum.
   c. stool.
   d. urine.

7. Knowing that gluconeogenesis helps to maintain blood levels, a nurse should:
   a. document weight changes because of fatty acid mobilization.
   b. evaluate the patient's sensitivity to low room temperatures because of decreased adipose tissue insulation.
   c. protect the patient from sources of infection because of decreased cellular protein deposits.
   d. do all of the above.

8. A nurse is assigned to care for a patient who is suspected of having type 2 diabetes mellitus (NIDDM). Clinical manifestations for which the nurse should assess include:
   a. blurred or deteriorating vision.
   b. fatigue and muscle cramping.
   c. wounds that heal slowly or respond poorly to treatment.
   d. all of the above.

9. There seems to be a positive correlation between type 2 diabetes mellitus and:
   a. hypotension.
   b. kidney dysfunction.
   c. obesity.
   d. sex.

10. The lowest fasting plasma glucose level suggestive of a diagnosis of diabetes is:
    a. 90 mg/dL.
    b. 115 mg/dL.
    c. 126 mg/dL.
    d. 180 mg/dL.

11. The most sensitive test for diabetes mellitus is the:
    a. fasting plasma glucose test.
    b. oral glucose tolerance test.
    c. intravenous glucose test.
    d. urine glucose test.

12. A female diabetic who weighs 130 lb has an ideal body weight of 116 lb. For weight reduction, her daily caloric intake should be approximately:
    a. 1000 cal.
    b. 1200 cal.
    c. 1500 cal.
    d. 1800 cal.

13. The nurse should encourage exercise in the management of diabetes, because it:
    a. decreases total triglyceride levels.
    b. improves insulin utilization.
    c. lowers blood glucose.
    d. accomplishes all of the above.

14. Self-monitoring of blood glucose is recommended for patients with:
    a. abnormal renal glucose thresholds.
    b. hypoglycemia without warning symptoms.
    c. unstable diabetes.
    d. all of the above conditions.

15. An example of a commonly administered intermediate-acting insulin is:
    a. NHP.
    b. Iletin II.
    c. Humalog.
    d. Humulin U.

16. The nurse knows that an intermediate-acting insulin should reach its "peak" in:
    a. 1 to 2 hours.
    b. 3 to 4 hours.
    c. 4 to 12 hours.
    d. 16 to 20 hours.

17. Current insulin pumps in use today:
    a. can deliver a premeal dose (bolus) of insulin before each meal.
    b. deliver a continuous basal rate of insulin at 0.5–2.0 units/hour.
    c. prevent unexpected savings in blood glucose measurements.
    d. are capable of doing all of the above.

18. A probable candidate for diabetic management with oral antidiabetic agents is the patient who is:
    a. non–insulin-dependent.
    b. stable and not prone to ketosis.
    c. unable to be managed by diet alone.
    d. characterized by all of the above.

19. The nurse should expect that insulin therapy will be temporarily substituted for oral antidiabetic therapy if the diabetic:
    a. develops an infection with fever.
    b. suffers trauma.
    c. undergoes major surgery.
    d. develops any or all of the above.

20. The tissue area that provides the fastest absorption rate for regular insulin is believed to be the:
a. abdominal area.
b. anterior thigh.
c. deltoid area.
d. gluteal site.

21. Rotation sites for insulin injection should be separated from one another by 2.5 cm (1 in) and should be used only once every:
a. third day.
b. week.
c. 2 to 3 weeks.
d. 2 to 4 weeks.

22. Hypoglycemia, an abnormally low blood glucose concentration, occurs with a glucose level that is:
a. lower than 50–60 mg/dL.
b. between 60 and 80 mg/dL.
c. between 75 and 90 mg/dL.
d. 95 mg/dL.

23. A clinical feature that distinguishes a hypoglycemic reaction from a ketoacidosis reaction is:
a. blurred vision.
b. diaphoresis.
c. nausea.
d. weakness.

24. The nurse knows that treatment modalities for diabetic ketoacidosis should focus on management of:
a. acidosis.
b. dehydration.
c. hyperglycemia
d. all of the above.

25. The major electrolyte of concern in the treatment of diabetic ketoacidosis is:
a. calcium.
b. magnesium.
c. potassium.
d. sodium.

26. Mortality rates for patients with diabetes are positively correlated with atherosclerotic complications, especially in the coronary arteries, which account for about _____ of all deaths.
a. 10%
b. 30%
c. 40%
d. 60%

27. Macrovascular disease has a direct link with:
a. hypertension.
b. increased triglyceride levels.
c. obesity.
d. all of the above.

28. Clinical nursing assessment for a patient with microangiopathy who has manifested impaired peripheral arterial circulation includes all of the following *except*:
a. integumentary inspection for the presence of brown spots on the lower extremities.
b. observation for paleness of the lower extremities.
c. observation for blanching of the feet after the legs are elevated for 60 seconds.
d. palpation for increased pulse volume in the arteries of the lower extremities.

29. With nonproliferative (background) retinopathy, examination of the retina may reveal:
a. leakage of fluid or serum (exudates).
b. microaneurysms.
c. focal capillary single closure.
d. all of the above pathologic changes.

30. A diagnostic manifestation of proliferative retinopathy is:
a. decreased capillary permeability.
b. microaneurysm formation.
c. neovascularization into the vitreous humor.
d. the leakage of capillary wall fragments into surrounding areas.

31. A nurse caring for a diabetic with a diagnosis of nephropathy would expect to find the presence of _____ in the urinalysis report.
a. albumin
b. bacteria
c. red blood cells
d. white blood cells

32. With peripheral neuropathy, a diabetic has limited sensitivity to:
a. heat.
b. pain.
c. pressure.
d. all of the above.

33. Nursing care for a diabetic with peripheral neuropathy includes:
   a. assessing pain patterns to rule out peripheral vascular insufficiency.
   b. inspecting the feet for breaks in skin integrity.
   c. palpating the lower extremities for temperature variations.
   d. all of the above.

34. During surgery, glucose levels will rise, because there is an increased secretion of:
   a. cortisol.
   b. epinephrine.
   c. glucagon.
   d. all of the above.

35. The nurse expects that a type 1 diabetic may receive ____ of his or her usual morning dose of insulin preoperatively.
   a. 10% to 20%
   b. 25% to 40%
   c. 50% to 60%
   d. 85% to 90%

Matching. *Match the physiologic change listed in Column II with its associated term listed in Column I.*

Column I

1. ____ gluconeogenesis

2. ____ glucosuria

3. ____ glycogenolysis

4. ____ nephropathy

5. ____ retinopathy

Column II

a. Filtered glucose that the kidney cannot absorb spills over into urine.

b. Glycogen breaks down in the liver through the action of glucagon.

c. New glucose is produced from amino acids.

d. Microvascular changes develop in the eyes.

e. Small vessel disease affects the kidneys.

Fill-In. *Read each statement carefully. Write your response in the space provided.*

1. In the United States, diabetes mellitus is the leading cause of three pathologic conditions: _____, _____ and _____.

2. The renal threshold for glucose is: _____.

3. Gestational diabetes occurs in _____% of pregnant women.

4. List the five major components of management for diabetes:

_____, _____, _____, _____, and _____

5. The current recommended distribution of calories for a diabetic meal plan is _____% carbohydrates, _____% fat, and _____% protein.

6. The sulfonylureas act by _____

7. List the four main areas for insulin injection:

_____, _____, _____, and _____

8. List three major acute complications of diabetes:

_____, _____, and _____

9. Clinical manifestations characteristic of hyperglycemic hyperosmolar nonketotic syndrome would include:

_____, _____, _____ and _____.

10. Identify five possible collaborative problems that a nurse should be aware of for a patient newly diagnosed with diabetes mellitus:

_____, _____, _____,

_____, and _____

II. Critical Thinking Questions and Exercises

Discussion and Analysis

1. Explain how insulin regulation is altered in the diabetic state.

2. Describe the pathophysiologic difference between type 1 and type 2 diabetes.

3. Distinguish between the "Dawn Phenomenon" and the "Somogyi Effect."

Examining Associations

For each of the clinical characteristics listed below, choose the associated classification of diabetes mellitus. Enter "1" for type 1 (insulin-dependent) diabetes mellitus or "2" for type 2 (non–insulin-dependent) diabetes mellitus.

1. ____ Etiology includes obesity.
2. ____ Ketosis is rare.
3. ____ Patient usually thin at diagnosis.
4. ____ Patient needs insulin to preserve life.
5. ____ Patient often has islet cell antibodies.
6. ____ Patient has no islet cell antibodies.
7. ____ Onset can occur at any age .
8. ____ Usually is diagnosed after age 30 years.
9. ____ Hyperosmolar nonketotic syndrome is a complication.
10. ____ There is little or no endogenous insulin.

Identifying Patterns

In diagram format, illustrate the pathophysiologic sequence of changes that occurs with type 1 diabetes, from "decreased insulin production by beta cells" to "ketoacidosis." Any outline format is acceptable as long as a cause-and-effect sequence can be seen.

Applying Concepts

Examine Figure 41–10 below and answer the following questions.

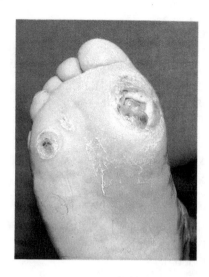

FIGURE 41–10 Neuropathic ulcers occur on pressure points in areas with diminished sensation in diabetic polyneuropathy. Pain is absent (and therefore the ulcer may go unnoticed).

1. Explain how each of the following diabetic complications leads to the formation of neuropathic ulcers and foot infections.

   a. Sensory neuropathy causes: _____

   b. Autonomic neuropathy causes: _____

   c. Motor neuropathy causes: _____

2. Appropriate foot care could prevent up to _____% of lower extremity amputations as a result of foot infections and complications.

3. Explain how peripheral vascular disease affects the progression of a foot infection and ulcer formation.

   _____

4. Explain how hyperglycemia affects the spread of a foot infection.

   _____

5. The three events that typically occur in sequence and lead to the development of a diabetic foot ulcer are:
   _____, _____, and _____.

6. List five daily activities related to foot care that a nurse should instruct a diabetic to complete.

   _____,   _____,

   _____,   _____,

   _____

7. Foot infections and ulcers may progress to the point that amputation is necessary, because:

   _____

   _____

Clinical Situations

Read the following case studies. Circle the correct answer.

CASE STUDY: Type 1 Diabetes

Albert, a 35-year-old insulin-dependent diabetic, is admitted to the hospital with a diagnosis of pneumonia. He has been febrile since admission. His daily insulin requirement is 24 units of NPH.

1. Every morning Albert is given NPH insulin at 7:30 AM. Meals are served at 8:30 AM, 12:30 PM, and 6:30 PM. The nurse expects that the NPH insulin will reach its maximum effect (peak) between the hours of:
   a. 11:30 AM and 1:30 PM.
   b. 1:30 PM and 7:30 PM.
   c. 3:30 PM and 9:30 PM.
   d. 5:30 PM and 11:30 PM.

2. A bedtime snack is provided for Albert. This is based on the knowledge that intermediate-acting insulins are effective for an approximate duration of:
   a. 6 to 8 hours.
   b. 10 to 14 hours.
   c. 16 to 20 hours.
   d. 24 to 28 hours.

3. Albert refuses his bedtime snack. This should alert the nurse to assess for:
   a. an elevated serum bicarbonate and a decreased blood pH.
   b. signs of hypoglycemia earlier than expected.
   c. symptoms of hyperglycemia during the peak time of NPH insulin.
   d. sugar in the urine.

CASE STUDY: Hypoglycemia

Betty, an 18-year-old type 1 diabetic, is unconscious when admitted to the hospital. Her daily dose of insulin has been 32 units of NPH each morning.

1. Based on knowledge of hypoglycemia, the nurse would expect that Betty's serum glucose level on admission is approximately:
   a. 50 mg/dL.
   b. 70 mg/dL.
   c. 90 mg/dL.
   d. 110 mg/dL.

2. Betty is given 1 mg of glucagon hydrochloride, subcutaneously, in the emergency department. Knowledge about the action of this drug alerts the nurse to observe for latent symptoms associated with:
   a. glucosuria.
   b. hyperglycemia.
   c. ketoacidosis.
   d. rebound hypoglycemia.

3. After Betty is medically stabilized, she is admitted to the clinical area for observation and health teaching. The nurse should make sure that Betty is aware of warning symptoms associated with hypoglycemia, such as:
   a. emotional changes.
   b. slurred speech and double vision.
   c. staggering gait and incoordination.
   d. all of the above.

4. Betty should also be taught that hypoglycemia may be prevented by:
   a. eating regularly scheduled meals.
   b. eating snacks to cover the peak time of insulin.
   c. increasing food intake when engaging in increased levels of physical exercise.
   d. doing all of the above.

CASE STUDY: Diabetic Ketoacidosis

Christine, a 64-year-old woman, is admitted to the clinical area with a diagnosis of diabetic ketoacidosis. On admission, she is drowsy yet responsive.

1. Nursing actions for a diagnosis of ketoacidosis include:
   a. monitoring urinary output by means of an indwelling catheter.
   b. evaluating serum electrolytes.
   c. testing for glucosuria and acetonuria.
   d. all of the above.

2. The nurse should expect that the rehydrating intravenous solution used will be:
   a. 0.9% saline solution.
   b. 5% dextrose in water.
   c. 10% dextrose in water.
   d. sterile water.

3. In evaluating the laboratory results, the nurse expects all of the following to indicate ketoacidosis *except:*

a. a decreased serum bicarbonate level.

b. an elevated blood glucose.

c. an increased blood urea.

d. an increased blood pH.

4. The physician notes a change in Christine's respirations. Her breathing is described as Kussmaul respirations. The nurse knows that these respirations are:

a. deep.

b. labored.

c. rapid.

d. shallow.

5. Christine is started on low-dose intravenous insulin therapy. Nursing assessment includes all of the following *except* frequent:

a. blood pressure measurements to monitor the degree of hypotension.

b. estimates of serum potassium, because increased blood glucose levels are correlated with elevated potassium levels.

c. evaluation of blood glucose levels, because glucose levels should decline as insulin levels increase.

d. elevation of serum ketones to monitor the course of ketosis.

6. As blood glucose levels approach normal, the nurse should assess for signs of electrolyte imbalance associated with:

a. hypernatremia.

b. hypercapnia.

c. hypocalcemia.

d. hypokalemia.

42

Assessment and Management of Patients With Endocrine Disorders

I. Interpretation, Completion, and Comparison

Multiple Choice. Read each question carefully. Circle your answer.

1. An example of exocrine glands are the:
   a. adrenals.
   b. ovaries.
   c. parathyroids.
   d. sweat glands.

2. The major structure balancing the rapid action of the nervous system with slower hormonal action is the:
   a. hypothalamus.
   b. pineal gland.
   c. hypophysis.
   d. thyroid gland.

3. Diabetes insipidis is a disorder related to a deficiency of:
   a. growth hormone.
   b. prolactin.
   c. oxytocin.
   d. vasopressin.

4. When thyroid hormone is administered for prolonged hypothyroidism, the nurse knows to monitor the patient for:
   a. angina.
   b. depression.
   c. mental confusion.
   d. hypoglycemia.

5. A clinical manifestation not usually associated with hyperthyroidism is:
   a. a pulse rate slower than 90 beats per minute.
   b. an elevated systolic blood pressure.
   c. muscular fatigability.
   d. weight loss.

6. Patients with hyperthyroidism are characteristically:
   a. apathetic and anorexic.
   b. calm.
   c. emotionally stable.
   d. insensitive to heat.

7. Iodine or iodide compounds are used for hyperthyroidism because they do all of the following except:
   a. decrease the basal metabolic rate.
   b. increase the vascularity of the gland.
   c. lessen the release of thyroid hormones.
   d. reduce the size of the gland.

8. The objectives of pharmacotherapy for hyperthyroidism include:
a. destroying overreactive thyroid cells.
b. preventing thyroid hormonal synthesis.
c. increasing the amount of thyroid tissue.
d. all of the above.

9. Signs of thyroid storm include all of the following *except*:
a. bradycardia.
b. delirium or somnolence.
c. dyspnea and chest pain.
d. hyperpyrexia.

10. Medical management for thyroid crisis includes:
a. intravenous dextrose fluids.
b. hypothermia measures.
c. oxygen therapy.
d. all of the above.

11. Pharmacotherapy for thyroid storm would *not* include the administration of:
a. acetaminophen.
b. iodine.
c. propylthiouracil.
d. synthetic levothyroxine.

12. The most common type of goiter is etiologically related to a deficiency of:
a. thyrotropin.
b. iodine.
c. thyroxine.
d. calcitonin.

13. A diagnosis of hyperparathyroidism can be established by all of the following signs *except*:
a. a negative reading on a Sulkowitch test.
b. a serum calcium level of 12 mg/dL.
c. an elevated level of parathyroid hormone.
d. bone demineralization seen on radiographic film.

14. A recommended breakfast for a hyperparathyroid patient would be:
a. cereal with milk and bananas.
b. fried eggs and bacon.
c. orange juice and toast.
d. pork sausage and cranberry juice.

15. The pathophysiology of hypoparathyroidism is associated with all of the following *except*:
a. a decrease in serum calcium.
b. an elevation of blood phosphate.
c. an increase in the renal excretion of phosphate.
d. a lowered renal excretion of calcium.

16. The goal of medical management for hypoparathyroidism is to:
a. achieve a serum calcium level of 9–10 mg/dL.
b. eliminate clinical symptoms.
c. reverse the symptoms of hypocalcemia.
d. accomplish all of the above.

17. Nursing management for a hypoparathyroid patient would not include:
a. maintaining a quiet, subdued environment.
b. making certain that calcium gluconate is kept at the bedside.
c. observing the patient for signs of tetany.
d. supplementing the diet with milk and milk products.

18. A pheochromocytoma is an adrenal medulla tumor that causes arterial hypertension by increasing the level of circulating:
a. catecholamines.
b. enzymes.
c. hormones.
d. glucocorticoids.

19. A positive test for overactivity of the adrenal medulla is an epinephrine value of:
a. 50 pg/mL.
b. 100 pg/mL.
c. 100 to 300 pg/mL.
d. 450 pg/mL.

20. Laboratory findings suggestive of Addison's disease include all of the following *except*:
a. a relative lymphocytosis.
b. hyperkalemia and hyponatremia.
c. hypertension.
d. hypoglycemia.

21. A positive diagnosis of Cushing's syndrome is associated with:
a. the disappearance of lymphoid tissue.
b. a reduction in circulating eosinophils.
c. an elevated cortisol level.
d. all of the above.

22. Clinical manifestations of Cushing's syndrome may be modified with a diet that is:
a. high in protein.
b. low in carbohydrates.
c. low in sodium.
d. all of the above.

23. The nurse needs to be aware that large-dose corticosteroid therapy is most effective when administered:
a. at 8:00 AM.
b. at 8:00 PM.
c. between 4:00 AM and 5:00 AM.
d. between 4:00 PM AND 6:00 PM.

24. Nursing assessment for a patient who is receiving corticosteroid therapy includes observation for the unacceptable side effect of:
a. glaucoma.
b. facial mooning.
c. potassium loss.
d. weight gain.

Matching. Match the hormonal function listed in Column II with its corresponding hormone listed in Column I.

Column I	Column II
1.___ glucagon	**a.** controls excretion of water by the kidneys
2.___ aldosterone	**b.** lowers blood sugar
3.___ oxytocin	**c.** inhibits bone resorption
4.___ somatotropin	**d.** influences metabolism that is essential for normal growth
5.___ vasopressin	**e.** supports sexual maturation
6.___ calcitonin	**f.** promotes the secretion of milk
7.___ prolactin	**g.** stimulates the reabsorption of sodium and the elimination of potassium
8.___ melatonin	**h.** promotes glycogenolysis
9.___ parathormone	**i.** increases the force of uterine contractions during parturition
10.___ insulin	

Fill-In. Read each statement carefully. Write your response in the space provided.

1. The term used to describe the regulation of hormone concentration in the bloodstream is: _____.

2. Hormones are classified three ways: _____, _____ and _____.

3. The two major hormones secreted by the posterior lobe of the pituitary gland are: _____ and

_____.

4. Oversecretion of adrenocorticotropic hormone (ACTH) or the growth hormone results in _____ disease.

5. A deficiency of antidiuretic hormone (ADH) or vasopressin can result in the disorder known as

_____.

6. The thyroid gland produces three hormones: _____, _____ and

_____.

7. The most common cause of hypothyroidism is: _____.

8. Hyperthyroidism is second only to _____ as a common endocrine disorder.

9. The most common type of hyperthyroidism is: _____.

10. The two most common medications used to treat hyperthyroidism are: _____ and

_____

11. Tetany is suggested when either of these signs are positive: _____ or _____

12. Name the three types of steroid hormones produced by the adrenal cortex:

_____, _____, and

_____

Unscramble the letters to answer each statement.

1. The master gland of the endocrine system is: _____.

| I | U | I | Y | T | P | R | T | A |

2. The pituitary gland is controlled by the: _____.

| O | A | T | M | P | U | A | S | H | H | L | Y |

3. Another name for the growth hormone is: _____.

| P | O | T | T | I | A | S | N | R | O | O | M |

4. Excessive secretion of ADH results in a syndrome that causes fluid retention, which is identified by the five letters: _____.

| H | D | A | I | S |

5. The thyroid gland depends on the uptake of _____ to synthesize its hormones.

| E | O | N | I | D | I |

6. The term used to describe "bulging eyes" found in patients with hyperthyroidism is: _____.

| H | M | P | L | O | S | E | A | X | O | H | T |

7. The term used to describe hyperirritability of the nerves and excessive muscular twitching secondary to hypocalcemia is: _____.

| Y | T | N | A | E | T |

II. Critical Thinking Questions and Exercises

Clinical Situations

Read the following case studies. Circle the correct answer.

CASE STUDY: Primary Hypothyroidism

Connie had been hospitalized for 1 week for studies to confirm a diagnosis of primary hypothyroidism.

1. Several tests were used in Connie's assessment. All of the following results are consistent with her diagnosis of hypothyroidism *except* for:
   a. an increased level of thyrotropin (TSH).
   b. a low uptake of radioactive iodine (^{131}I).
   c. a protein-bound iodine reading of 3 mg/dL.
   d. a T_3 uptake value of 45%.

2. Nursing care for Connie includes assessing for clinical manifestations associated with hypothyroidism. A manifestation not consistent with her diagnosis is a:
   a. change in her menstrual pattern.
   b. pulse rate of 58 beats per minute.
   c. temperature of 95.8°F.
   d. weight loss of 10 lb over a 2-week period.

3. The principal objective of medical management is to:

a. irradiate the gland in an attempt to stimulate hormonal secretion.

b. replace the missing hormone.

c. remove the diseased gland.

d. withhold exogenous iodine to create a negative feedback response, which will force the gland to secrete hormones.

4. Nursing comfort measures for Connie should include:

a. encouraging frequent periods of rest throughout the day.

b. offering her additional blankets to help prevent chilling.

c. using a cleansing lotion instead of soap for her skin.

d. all of the above.

5. Health teaching for Connie includes making sure that she knows that iodine-based chemotherapy is:

a. administered intravenously for 1 week so that her symptoms may be rapidly put into remission.

b. needed for life.

c. recommended for 1 to 3 months.

d. used until her symptoms disappear.

CASE STUDY: Hyperparathyroidism

Emily is 65 years old and has been complaining of continued emotional irritability. Her family described her as always being "on edge" and neurotic. After several months of exacerbated symptoms, Emily underwent a complete physical examination and was diagnosed with hyperparathyroidism.

1. Emily's clinical symptoms are all related to an increase in serum:

a. calcium.

b. magnesium.

c. potassium.

d. sodium.

2. As a nurse, you know that the normal level of the mineral identified in the previous question is:

a. 8.8–10 mg/dL.

b. 1.3–2.1 mEq/L.

c. 3.5–5.0 mEq/L.

d. 135–148 mmol/L.

3. Describe eight symptoms usually seen when hyperparathyroidism involves several body systems.

_____, _____, _____, _____,

_____, _____, _____, and _____

4. Name one of the most important organ complications of hyperparathyroidism: _____.

5. A musculoskeletal symptom found with hyperparathyroidism is:

a. deformities due to demineralization.

b. pain on weight-bearing.

c. pathologic fractures due to osteoclast growth.

d. all of the above.

6. The recommended treatment for primary hyperparathyroidism is:

a. pharmacotherapy until the elevated serum levels return to normal.

b. surgical removal of the abnormal parathyroid tissue.

c. adrenalectomy.

d. all of the above treatments.

7. Acute hypercalcemic crises can occur in hyperparathyroidism. The treament would involve immediate:

a. administration of diuretic agents to promote renal excretion of calcium.

b. phosphate therapy to correct hypophosphatemia.

c. dehydration with large volumes of intravenous fluids.

d. management with all of the above modalities.

CASE STUDY: Subtotal Thyroidectomy

Darrell, a 37-year-old father of two, has just returned to the clinical area from the recovery room. Darrell has had a subtotal thyroidectomy.

1. Postoperatively, Darrell is assisted from the stretcher to the bed. The most comfortable position for him to assume would be:

a. high Fowler's with his neck supported by a soft collar.

b. recumbent with his neck hyperextended and supported by a neck pillow.

c. recumbent with sandbags preventing his neck from rotating.

d. semi-Fowler's with his head supported by pillows.

2. Postoperative bleeding when the patient is in the dorsal position would probably be evidenced:

a. anteriorly.

b. laterally.

c. posteriorly.

d. in any of the above areas.

3. Indicators of internal bleeding include:

a. a sensation of fullness at the incision site.

b. hypotension.

c. tachycardia.

d. all of the above.

4. The nurse should assess for the common manifestation of recurrent laryngeal nerve damage, which is:

a. any voice change.

b. the inability to speak.

c. pain while speaking.

d. pain while swallowing.

5. The nurse expects Darrell's postoperative diet to be:

a. clear liquids, such as tea and carbonated beverages.

b. high in calories.

c. low in fat and protein.

d. low in minerals, especially calcium.

6. The nurse should monitor serum calcium levels for hypocalcemia, which will occur with a serum calcium level of:

a. 5 mg/dL.

b. 9 mg/dL.

c. 13 mg/dL.

d. 17 mg/dL.

UNIT **9**
Renal and Urinary Tract Function

43

Assessment of Renal and Urinary Tract Function

I. Interpretation, Completion, and Comparison

Multiple Choice. Read each question carefully. Circle your answer.

1. An abnormal constituent of urine is:
   a. creatinine.
   b. glucose.
   c. potassium.
   d. urea.

2. The normal quantity of water ingested and excreted in the urine is approximately:
   a. 0.5 L/day.
   b. 1.5 L/day.
   c. 2.5 L/day.
   d. 4.0 L/day.

3. The normal amount of sodium ingested and excreted in the urine is approximately:
   a. 2 to 3 g/day.
   b. 4 to 5 g/day.
   c. 6 to 8 g/day.
   d. 9 to 10 g/day.

4. Increased blood osmolality will result in:
   a. antidiuretic hormone (ADH) stimulation.
   b. an increase in urine volume.
   c. diuresis.
   d. less reabsorption of water.

5. A major sensitive indicator of kidney disease is the:
   a. blood urea nitrogen level.
   b. creatinine clearance level.
   c. serum potassium level.
   d. uric acid level.

6. A major manifestation of uremia is:
   a. a decreased serum phosphorus level.
   b. hyperparathyroidism.
   c. hypocalcemia with bone changes.
   d. increased secretion of parathormone.

7. Significant nursing assessment data relevant to renal function should include information about:
   a. any voiding disorders.
   b. the patient's occupation.
   c. the presence of hypertension or diabetes mellitus.
   d. all of the above.

8. Oliguria is said to be present when urinary output is:
   a. less than 30 mL/hour.
   b. about 100 mL/hour.
   c. between 300 and 500 mL/hour.
   d. between 500 and 1000 mL/hour.

9. A 24-hour urine collection is scheduled to begin at 8:00 AM. The nurse should begin the procedure:
   a. after discarding the 8:00 AM specimen.
   b. at 8:00 AM, with or without a specimen.
   c. 6 hours after the urine is discarded.
   d. with the first specimen voided after 8:00 AM.

10. The nurse should inform a patient that preparation for intravenous urography includes:
    a. a liquid restriction for 8 to 10 hours before the test.
    b. liquids before the test.
    c. enemas until clear.
    d. remaining NPO from midnight before the test.

11. Nursing responsibilities after renal angiography include:
    a. assessment of peripheral pulses.
    b. color and temperature comparisons between the involved and uninvolved extremities.
    c. examination of the puncture site for swelling and hematoma formation.
    d. all of the above.

12. A cystoscope allows visualization of the:
    a. bladder.
    b. ureteral orifices.
    c. urethra.
    d. above areas.

13. Nursing management after a renal biopsy includes:
    a. assessing for the clinical manifestations of hemorrhage.
    b. encouraging a fluid intake of 3 L every 24 hours.
    c. obtaining a sample of each voided urine to compare it with a prebiopsy specimen.
    d. all of the above.

Fill-In. *Read each statement carefully. Write the best response in the space provided.*

1. The kidneys are located in the posterior wall of the abdomen, from the _____ vertebra to the _____ vertebra.

2. The functional unit of each kidney is the _____.

3. Normal adult bladder capacity is _____mL of urine.

4. The regulation of the amount of sodium excreted depends on the hormone _____.

5. The normal urine osmolality ranges between _____ and _____.

6. When a person is dehydrated, the urine osmolality is _____.

7. Water is reabsorbed, rather than excreted, under the control of the _____.

8. The test that most accurately reflects glomerular filtration and renal excretory function is the

   _____ test.

II. Critical Thinking Questions and Exercises

Identifying Patterns

Draw the sequence of pathophysiologic events that are triggered when the blood pressure decreases and the hormone renin is released from the cells in the kidneys.

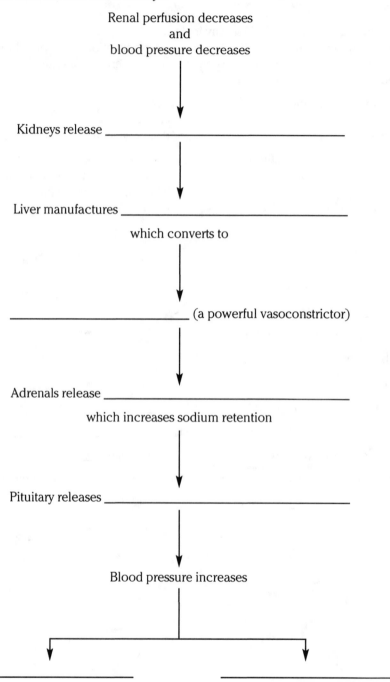

Renal perfusion decreases
and
blood pressure decreases

Kidneys release _____

Liver manufactures _____

which converts to

_____ (a powerful vasoconstrictor)

Adrenals release _____

which increases sodium retention

Pituitary releases _____

Blood pressure increases

_____   _____

44

Management of Patients With Upper or Lower Urinary Tract Dysfunction

I. Interpretation, Completion, and Comparison

Multiple Choice. Read each question carefully. Circle your answer.

1. The most accurate indicator of fluid loss or gain in an acutely ill patient is:
a. blood pressure.
b. capillary refill.
c. serum sodium levels.
d. weight.

2. The nurse notes that a patient who is retaining fluid had a 1-kg weight gain. The nurse knows this is equivalent to about:
a. 250 mL.
b. 500 mL.
c. 750 mL.
d. 1000 mL.

3. The type of incontinence that results from a sudden increase in intra-abdominal pressure is:
a. reflex incontinence.
b. stress incontinence.
c. overflow incontinence.
d. urge incontinence.

4. Fluid management as a method of behavioral therapy for incontinence requires a daily liquid intake of:
a. 0.5 mL.
b. 1.0 mL.
c. 1.5 mL.
d. 2.0 mL.

5. A spastic neurogenic bladder is associated with all of the following *except:*
a. a loss of conscious sensation and cerebral motor control.
b. a lower motor neuron lesion.
c. hypertrophy of the bladder walls.
d. reduced bladder capacity.

6. The major complication of neurogenic bladder is:
a. hypertrophy.
b. infection.
c. pain.
d. spasm.

7. The major cause of death for patients with neurologic impairment of the bladder is:
a. myocardial infarction.
b. pulmonary edema.
c. septicemia.
d. renal failure.

8. Nursing measures for the patient with neurogenic bladder include:
a. encouraging a liberal fluid intake.
b. keeping the patient as mobile as possible.
c. offering a diet low in calcium.
d. all of the above.

9. When managing a closed urinary drainage system, the nurse needs to remember not to:
  a. allow the drainage bag to touch the floor.
  b. disconnect the bag.
  c. raise the drainage bag above the level of the patient's bladder.
  d. do any of the above.

10. A sign of a possible urinary tract infection is:
  a. a negative urine culture.
  b. an output of 200 to 900 mL with each voiding.
  c. cloudy urine.
  d. urine with a specific gravity of 1.005 to 1.022.

11. A woman is taught to catheterize herself by inserting the catheter into the urethra:
  a. 1/2 to 1 in.
  b. 2 in.
  c. 3 in.
  d. 5 in.

12. The process that underlies and supports the procedure of hemodialysis is:
  a. diffusion.
  b. osmosis.
  c. ultrafiltration.
  d. all of the above processes.

13. An incomplete protein not recommended for the diet of a patient managed by long-term hemodialysis is that found in:
  a. eggs.
  b. fish.
  c. milk.
  d. nuts.

14. With peritoneal dialysis, urea and creatinine pass through the peritoneum by:
  a. active transport.
  b. diffusion and osmosis.
  c. filtration.
  d. ultrafiltration.

15. The complete peritoneal dialysis process of removing toxic substances and body wastes takes approximately:
  a. 6 to 8 hours.
  b. 9 to 11 hours.
  c. 12 to 24 hours.
  d. 36 to 48 hours.

16. At the end of five peritoneal exchanges, the patient's fluid loss was 500 mL. This loss is equal to approximately:
  a. 0.5 lb.
  b. 1.0 lb.
  c. 1.5 lb.
  d. 2 lb.

17. The chief danger after renal surgery is:
  a. abdominal distention owing to reflex cessation of intestinal peristalsis.
  b. hypovolemic shock caused by hemorrhage.
  c. paralytic ileus caused by manipulation of the colon during surgery.
  d. pneumonia caused by shallow breathing because of severe incisional pain.

18. A nephrostomy tube is inserted to:
  a. conserve and restore tissue traumatized by obstruction.
  b. provide drainage from the kidney postoperatively.
  c. provide ureter drainage when there is an interruption of the normal drainage course.
  d. do all of the above.

Matching. Match the symptom listed in Column II with its associated fluid or electrolyte imbalance listed in Column I.

Column I	Column II
1.___calcium deficit	**a.** carpopedal spasm and tetany
2.___calcium excess	**b.** muscle hypotonicity and flank pain
3.___fluid volume deficit	**c.** oliguria and weight loss
4.___fluid volume excess	**d.** positive Chvostek's sign
5.___magnesium deficit	**e.** crackles and dyspnea

6. ____potassium deficit
7. ____potassium excess
8. ____protein deficit
9. ____sodium deficit
10. ____sodium excess

f. chronic weight loss and fatigability
g. fingerprinting on the sternum
h. irritability and intestinal colic
i. rough, dry tongue and thirst
j. soft, flabby muscles and weakness

Fill-In. *Read each statement carefully. Write your response in the space provided.*

1. List three classifications of medications that cause urinary retention by inhibiting contractility.

_____, _____, and

_____

2. List four reasons for catheterization.

_____, _____,

_____, and _____

3. List several pathogens responsible for catheter-associated urinary tract infections.

_____

_____

4. List several signs and symptoms associated with catheter-induced urinary tract infections.

_____

_____

5. One leading cause of death for patients undergoing chronic hemodialysis is:_____

6. List six potential complications of dialysis treatment.

_____, _____, _____,

_____, _____, and _____

7. The most common and serious complication of continuous ambulatory peritoneal dialysis (CAPD) is:

_____

8. Two complications of renal surgery that are believed to be caused by reflex paralysis of intestinal peristalsis and manipulation of the colon or duodenum during surgery are: _____ and _____.

II. Critical Thinking Questions and Exercises

Recognizing Contradictions

Rewrite each statement correctly. Underline the key concepts.

1. About 8 million adults in the United States suffer from urinary incontinence.

2. Urinary incontinence afflicts about one third of all nursing home residents.

3. With a closed drainage system, only 20% of all patients experience bacteriuria.

4. Hemodialysis can be used as a long-term management therapy that can reverse the progress of renal disease.

5. CAPD is a good choice for home management because the process needs to be completed only once a day.

Clinical Situations

Read the following case study. Circle the correct answer.

CASE STUDY: Continuous Ambulatory Peritoneal Dialysis

Edward, a 29-year-old diabetic, chose CAPD as a way of managing his end-stage renal disease.

1. Edward chose CAPD because it helped him:
   a. avoid severe dietary restrictions.
   b. control his blood pressure.
   c. have control over his daily activities.
   d. do all of the above.

2. Using CAPD, Edward needs to dialyze himself:
   a. approximately 4 to 5 times a day with no night changes.
   b. every 3 hours while awake.
   c. every 4 hours around the clock.
   d. once in the morning and once in the evening every day.

3. Edward needs to be aware that toxic wastes are exchanged during the equilibration or dwell time, which usually lasts for:
   a. 10–15 minutes.
   b. 30 minutes.
   c. 1 hour.
   d. 2–3 hours.

4. Edward needs to be taught how to detect signs of the most serious and most common complication of CAPD, which is:
   a. an abdominal hernia.
   b. anorexia.
   c. edema.
   d. peritonitis.

5. Edward's diet should be modified to be:
   a. high in carbohydrates.
   b. high in fats.
   c. high in protein.
   d. low in bran and fiber.

45

Management of Patients With Urinary Disorders

I. Interpretation, Completion, and Comparison

Multiple Choice. *Read each question carefully. Circle your answer.*

1. The most common site of a lower urinary tract infection (UTI) is the:
   a. bladder.
   b. kidney.
   c. prostate.
   d. urethra.

2. There is an increased risk of UTIs in the presence of:
   a. altered metabolic states.
   b. immunosuppression.
   c. urethral mucosa abrasion.
   d. all of the above.

3. The most common organism responsible for UTIs in the elderly is:
   a. *Klebsiella*.
   b. *Escherichia coli*.
   c. *Proteus*.
   d. *Pseudomonas*.

4. Recent clinical trials for antibacterial agents against UTIs found the following drug to be significantly effective:
   a. Bactrim.
   b. Cipro.
   c. Macrodantin.
   d. Septra.

5. A majority of randomized studies have indicated that daily consumption of _____ juice decreases the incidence of UTIs:
   a. apple
   b. cranberry
   c. grapefruit
   d. orange

6. Health information for a female patient diagnosed as having cystitis includes all of the following *except*:
   a. cleanse around the perineum and urethral meatus (from front to back) after each bowel movement.
   b. drink liberal amounts of fluid.
   c. shower rather than bathe in a tub.
   d. void no more frequently than every 6 hours to allow urine to dilute the bacteria in the bladder.

7. Complications of chronic pyelonephritis include:
   a. end-stage renal disease.
   b. hypertension.
   c. kidney stone formation.
   d. all of the above.

8. Acute glomerulonephritis refers to a group of kidney diseases in which there is:
a. an inflammatory reaction.
b. an antigen-antibody reaction to streptococci that results in circulating molecular complexes.
c. cellular complexes that lodge in the glomeruli and injure the kidney.
d. a combination of all of the above.

9. In most cases, the major stimulus to acute glomerulonephritis is:
a. *Escherichia coli.*
b. group A streptococcal infection of the throat.
c. *Staphylococcus aureus.*
d. *Neisseria gonorrhoeae.*

10. Laboratory findings consistent with acute glomerulonephritis include all of the following *except*:
a. hematuria.
b. polyuria.
c. proteinuria.
d. white cell casts.

11. Chronic glomerulonephritis is manifested by:
a. anemia secondary to erythropoiesis.
b. hypercalcemia and decreased serum phosphorus.
c. hypokalemia and elevated bicarbonate.
d. metabolic alkalosis.

12. The major manifestation of nephrotic syndrome is:
a. hematuria.
b. hyperalbuminemia.
c. edema.
d. anemia.

13. Oliguria is a clinical sign of acute renal failure that refers to a daily urine output of:
a. 1.5 L.
b. 1.0 L.
c. less than 400 mL.
d. less than 50 mL.

14. A fall in CO_2-combining power and blood pH indicates a _____ accompanying renal function.
a. metabolic acidosis
b. metabolic alkalosis
c. respiratory acidosis
d. respiratory alkalosis

15. Hyperkalemia is a serious electrolyte imbalance that occurs in acute renal failure (ARF) and results from:
a. protein catabolism.
b. electrolyte shifts in response to metabolic acidosis.
c. tissue breakdown.
d. all of the above.

16. Potassium intake can be restricted by eliminating high-potassium foods such as:
a. butter.
b. citrus fruits.
c. cooked white rice.
d. salad oils.

17. A patient with ARF and negative nitrogen balance is expected to lose about:
a. 0.5 kg/day.
b. 1.0 kg/day.
c. 1.5 kg/day.
d. 2 kg/day.

18. The leading cause of end-stage renal disease is:
a. diabetes mellitus.
b. hypertension.
c. glomerulonephritis.
d. toxic agents.

19. In chronic renal failure (end-stage renal disease), decreased glomerular filtration leads to:
a. increased pH.
b. decreased creatinine clearance.
c. increased blood urea nitrogen (BUN).
d. all of the above.

20. Decreased levels of erythropoietin, a substance normally secreted by the kidneys, leads to _____, a serious complication of chronic renal failure.
a. anemia
b. acidosis
c. hyperkalemia
d. pericarditis

21. Recent research about the long-term toxicity of aluminum products has led physicians to recommend antacids that lower serum phosphorus, such as:
a. calcium carbonate.
b. sodium bicarbonate.
c. magaldrate.
d. milk of magnesia.

22. Dietary intervention for renal deterioration includes limiting the intake of:
   a. fluid.
   b. protein.
   c. sodium and potassium.
   d. all of the above.

23. Preoperative management for a patient who is to undergo kidney transplantation includes:
   a. bringing the metabolic state to as normal a level as possible.
   b. making certain that the patient is free of infection.
   c. suppressing immunologic defense mechanisms.
   d. all of the above.

24. Postoperative management for a recipient of a transplanted kidney includes:
   a. aseptic technique to avoid infection.
   b. hourly urinary output measurements to estimate the degree of kidney function.
   c. protective isolation while immunosuppressive drug therapy is at its maximum dosage.
   d. all of the above.

25. A major clinical manifestation of renal stones is:
   a. dysuria.
   b. hematuria.
   c. infection.
   d. pain.

26. Patients with urolithiasis need to be encouraged to:
   a. increase their fluid intake so that they can excrete 3000 to 4000 mL every day, which will help to prevent additional stone formation.
   b. participate in strenuous exercises so that the tone of smooth muscle in the urinary tract can be strengthened to help propel calculi.
   c. supplement their diet with calcium needed to replace losses to renal calculi.
   d. limit their voiding to every 6 to 8 hours so that increased volume can increase hydrostatic pressure, which will help push stones along the urinary system.

27. A patient being prescribed a diet moderately reduced in calcium and phosphorus should be taught to avoid:
   a. citrus fruits.
   b. milk.
   c. pasta.
   d. whole grain breads.

28. The usual early clinical sign of a renal tumor is:
   a. a palpable mass.
   b. painless hematuria.
   c. localized tenderness.
   d. renal colic.

29. The most common symptom of cancer of the bladder is:
   a. back pain.
   b. dysuria.
   c. gross painless hematuria.
   d. infection.

30. The predominant cause of bladder cancer is:
   a. chronic renal failure.
   b. cigarette smoking.
   c. environmental pollution.
   d. metatasis from another primary site.

31. The most effective intravesical agent for recurrent bladder cancer is:
   a. Bacille Calmette-Guérin (BCG).
   b. doxorubicin.
   c. etoglucid.
   d. thiotepa.

32. The urinary diversion whereby the patient will void from his rectum for the rest of his life is known as a:
   a. cutaneous ureterostomy.
   b. nephrostomy.
   c. suprapubic cystotomy.
   d. ureterosigmoidostomy.

33. Tuberculosis of the kidney and lower urinary tract is always:
   a. localized rather than a systemic disease.
   b. a primary infection.
   c. secondary to renal tuberculosis.
   d. subsequent to pulmonary tuberculosis.

34. All of the following statements about interstitial cystitis are correct *except*:
   a. It is associated with pain in the abdomen and perineum.
   b. It is characterized by severe voiding symptoms.
   c. It is seen in women between the ages of 40 and 50 years.
   d. It is caused by *Escherichia coli*.

Fill-In. Read each statement carefully. Write your response in the space provided.

1. The organism most commonly responsible for UTIs in women is:_____.

2. Name common signs and symptoms associated with an uncomplicated lower UTI (cystitis).

_____

_____

3. List the six clinical manifestations of acute pyelonephritis:

_____, _____, _____,

_____, _____, and _____

4. Describe the physical appearance of the urine early in the stage of acute glomerulonephritis.

_____ core colored _____

5. Name four physiologic disorders that characterize the nephrotic syndrome:

_____, _____,

_____, and _____

6. List three major conditions that cause acute renal failure. For each condition, give one to two examples.

a. _Pre renal_   Examples: _Hemmorage / sepsis_

b. _Intrarenal_   Examples: _Crushing Injuries/infection_

c. _post renal_   Examples: _Obstruction distal kidney_

7. List several clinical manifestations seen in patients with acute renal failure.

Lathary, Headache, muscle twitering, siezures

N & V, diareeha, urine Breath

8. Name several signs or symptoms seen in patients with threatened kidney transplant rejection.

_____

_____

9. List three crystalline substances known to form stones in the urinary tract:

_____, _____, and _____.

10. Identify seven complications that may occur after an ileal conduit:

_____, _____, _____, _____,

_____, _____, and _____

II. Critical Thinking Questions and Exercises

Recognizing Contradictions

Rewrite each statement correctly. Underline the key concepts.

1. The majority of hospital-acquired urinary tract infections are caused by infrequent urination secondary to dehydration.

2. Urethrovesical reflux refers to the backward flow of urine from the bladder into one or both ureters.

3. Currently, cystoscopy and intravenous pyelography are the diagnostic tests of choice for individuals with recurring urinary tract infections.

4. Glomerulonephritis is primarily a disease of the elderly, especially in those older than 70 years of age.

5. Septicemia, secondary to uremia, is the most serious life-threatening condition of acute renal failure.

6. The earliest clinical manifestation of cancer of the kidney is severe, debilitating pain.

Clinical Situations

Read the following case study. Circle the correct answer.

CASE STUDY: Acute Renal Failure

Fran is hospitalized with a diagnosis of ARF. She had been taking gentamicin sulfate for a pseudomonal infection.

1. The nurse knows that the kidney is susceptible to damage by nephrotoxic antibiotic agents, because it functions as a major excretory pathway and receives ____ of cardiac output at rest.
a. 5%
b. 15%
c. 25%
d. 45%

2. The nurse needs to assess for symptoms consistent with pathology secondary to reduced renal blood flow. Symptoms would include:
a. reduced glomerular filtration.
b. renal ischemia.
c. tubular damage.
d. all of the above.

3. During the oliguric phase of ARF, Fran's protein intake for her 156-lb body weight should be approximately:
a. 35 g/24 hours.
b. 70 g/24 hours.
c. 120 g/24 hours.
d. 156 g/24 hours.

4. While evaluating laboratory studies, the nurse expects that Fran's oliguric phase will be marked by all of the following *except*:
a. blood urea nitrogen of 10 mg/dL.
b. serum creatinine of 0.8 mg/dL.
c. serum potassium of 6 mEq/L.
d. urinary volume less than 600 mL/24 hours.

5. After the diuretic phase, the nurse should recommend a:
a. high-potassium diet.
b. high-protein diet.
c. low-carbohydrate diet.
d. low-fat diet.

6. The nurse expects the period of recovery to follow a period of oliguria and to last approximately:
a. 2 weeks.
b. 6 weeks.
c. 2 months.
d. 6–12 months.

UNIT 10
Reproductive Function

46

Assessment and Management of Female Physiologic Processes

I. Interpretation, Completion, and Comparison

Multiple Choice. *Read each question carefully. Circle your answer.*

1. The menstrual cycle is dependent on hormone production. The hormone responsible for stimulating progesterone is:
   a. androgens.
   b. estradiol.
   c. the follicle-stimulating hormone.
   f. the luteinizing hormone.

2. A neighbor tells you that she has had vaginal bleeding for the past several days. She is postmenopausal and has not had a menstrual period for the past 4 years. You recommend that she:
   a. see her gynecologist or physician as soon as possible.
   b. mention the bleeding episode to her physician at her next appointment.
   c. disregard this bleeding episode, because it is probably normal.
   d. use a birth control method, because she may be fertile with her next ovulation.

3. An annual pelvic examination should begin at age:
   a. 14 years.
   b. 18 years.
   c. 21 years.
   d. 25 years.

4. During an internal vaginal examination, the nurse practitioner notes a frothy and malodorous discharge. She suspects it is caused by the bacteria:
   a. *Candida*.
   b. *Eschar*.
   c. *Trichomonas*.
   d. *E. coli*.

5. The results of a patient's cytologic test for cancer (Pap test) were interpreted as class II. The nurse explains that a class II finding indicates:
   a. squamous cell abnormalities.
   b. malignancy.
   c. suggestive but not conclusive malignancy.
   d. the absence of atypical or abnormal cells.

6. Newer classifications are being used to describe the findings of the cytologic smear. For example, a high-grade, squamous, intraepithelial lesion corresponds to type:
   a. I.
   b. II.
   c. III.
   d. IV.

7. After a cervical cone biopsy, the patient needs to be instructed to:
   a. leave the packing in place for 18 to 24 hours.
   b. report any excessive bleeding.
   c. delay sexual intercourse until healing occurs.
   d. do all of the above.

8. The normal menstrual cycle usually lasts 4 to 5 days with a loss of about _____ of blood.
   a. 30 mL   b. 60 mL   c. 90 mL   d. 120 mL

9. To prevent toxic shock syndrome, the nurse advises the 15-year-old girl to change tampons every _____ hours.
   a. 2–3   b. 4–6   c. 8   d. 12

10. A middle-aged woman experiencing dyspareunia can use ____ to diminish the discomfort.
   a. ibuprofen   c. K-Y jelly
   b. petroleum jelly   d. aspirin

11. A nutritional recommendation for postmenopausal women would be dietary increase in:
   a. calcium.   c. salt.
   b. iron.   d. vitamin K.

12. Premenstrual syndrome (PMS) may be caused by estrogen rising and progesterone decreasing during the phase of the menstrual cycle known as:
   a. follicular.   c. ovulation.
   b. luteal.   d. premenstrual.

13. In educating a patient with PMS about changing her dietary practices, the nurse would recommend that she increase her intake of:
   a. magnesium.   c. iron.
   b. vitamin D.   d. zinc.

14. Pain at the time of the regular menstrual flow is referred to as:
   a. dysmenorrhea.   c. menorrhagia.
   b. amenorrhea.   d. metrorrhagia.

15. In the United States, the percentage of pregnancies that are unplanned is about:
   a. 20%.   b. 30%.   c. 50%.   d. 80%.

16. The most common side effect of the implantable contraceptive, Norplant, is:
   a. breast cancer.   c. thrombophlebitis.
   b. irregular bleeding.   d. upper-arm pain at insertion site.

17. Statistically, use of the calendar rhythm method as a means of contraception yields a pregnancy rate of:
   a. less than 10%.   c. about 40%.
   b. between 10% and 20%.   d. about 80%.

18. Spontaneous abortion occurs in 10% to 20% of conceptions. Spontaneous abortion occurs most commonly at:
   a. 4 weeks.   c. 8–12 weeks.
   b. 4–6 weeks.   d. 16 weeks.

19. The highest incidence of ectopic pregnancy occurs in the:
   a. cervix.   c. fallopian tube.
   b. interstitial tissue.   d. abdominal area.

20. The incidence of recurrence of an ectopic pregnancy is:
   a. 5%.   c. 20%.
   b. 7%–15%.   d. 25%–40%.

Fill-In. *Read each statement carefully. Write your response in the space provided.*

1. Identify the normal range in years during which menopause usually begins.

_____

2. List seven danger signals that any woman should report to a health care professional:

_____, _____, _____, _____,

_____, _____, and _____

3. The most accurate outpatient procedure for evaluating a woman for endometrial cancer is _____.

4. Menopause puts a woman at risk for four serious conditions: _____, _____,

_____ and _____.

5. List eight major symptoms a woman with premenstrual syndrome (PMS) may experience:

_____, _____, _____, _____,

_____, _____, _____, and _____

6. Explain why amenorrhea occurs with anorexia and bulimia.

_____

_____

7. Describe the physiologic basis for "the pill" as a contraceptive.

_____

_____

8. Identify some risk factors that would absolutely contraindicate the use of oral contraceptives.

_____

_____

9. Explain how an injection of Depo-Provera works.

_____

10. Explain how the emergency use of estrogen or estrogen and a progestin can prevent pregnancy.

_____

_____

11. Describe in vitro fertilization.

_____

_____

_____

Matching. Match the term in Column II with its corresponding definition in Column I.

Column I

1. _____painful sexual intercourse

2. _____bladder protruding into the vagina

3. _____beginning of menstration

4. _____description of ovaries and fallopian tubes

5. _____painful menstration

6. _____implantation of endometrial tissue in other areas of the pelvis

7. _____pain on movement of the cervix

8. _____absence of menstrual flow

Column II

a. adnexa

b. amenorrhea

c. chandelier sign

d. cystocele

e. dysmenorrhea

f. dyspaneunia

g. endometriosis

h. menarche

II. Critical Thinking Questions and Exercises

Recognizing Contradictions

Rewrite each statement correctly. Underline the key concepts.

1. When conducting a health assessment, the nurse knows that about 10% of women have been victims of incest.

2. Women born to mothers who took diethylstilbestrol (DES) during their pregnancy have a higher than average chance of suffering miscarriage.

3. A cervical cone biopsy may be done without anesthesia because the cervix is less sensitive to pain.

4. Magnetic resonance imaging (MRI) exposes the patient to radiation and is more expensive than other pelvic diagnostic aids.

5. Estrogen prepares the uterus for implantation of the fertilized ovum.

6. Progesterone can cause painful cramps during ovulation because it causes myometrial contractility and arteriolar vasospasm.

7. More than 1 million yearly pregnancies in the United States are unintended.

8. An abortion drug, methotrexate, can be used during the second trimester.

Extracting Inferences

Refer to Figure 46–9 when answering the following questions about ectopic pregnancies.

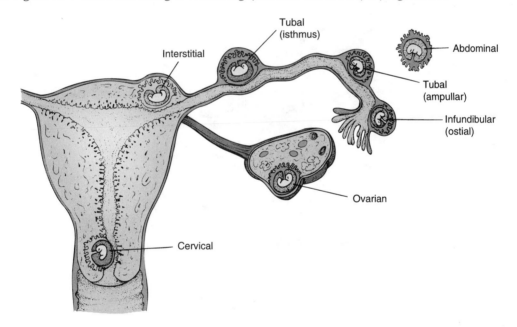

FIGURE 46–9   Sites of ectopic pregnancy.

1. Explain what occurs after the ovum is fertilized to cause an ectopic pregnancy.

_____

_____

2. List several possible causes of ectopic implantation.

_____

_____

_____

3. Look at the ovum implanted in the tubal (isthmus) area. What symptoms would you expect the woman to exhibit before tubal rupture occurs?

_____

_____

4. Name three possible surgical options to treat ectopic pregnancies.

a. _____   b. _____   c. _____.

5. Postoperative medical management would include assessing the level of beta-HCG to _____

_____.

6. Potential maternal complications for ectopic pregnancies are: _____ and _____.

47

Management of Patients With Female Reproductive Disorders

I. Interpretation, Completion, and Comparison

Multiple Choice. *Read each question carefully. Circle your answer.*

1. Conditions that increase a woman's chances of developing candidiasis include:
   a. pregnancy.
   b. diabetes mellitus.
   c. antibiotic therapy.
   d. all of the above.

2. Metronidazole (Flagyl) is the recommended treatment for a vaginal infection caused by:
   a. *Candida albicans*.
   b. *Escherichia coli*.
   c. *Streptococcus*.
   d. *Trichomonas vaginalis*.

3. Nursing interventions for the relief of pain and discomfort for a woman with a vulvovaginal infection include:
   a. warm perineal irrigations.
   b. sitz baths.
   c. cornstarch for chafed inner thighs.
   d. all of the above.

4. The most common sexually transmitted disease among young, sexually active populations is:
   a. candidiasis.
   b. human papillomavirus.
   c. endocervicitis.
   d. salpingitis.

5. To prevent the occurrence of toxic shock syndrome (TSS), women should be advised to do all of the following *except*:
   a. avoid the use of superabsorbent tampons.
   b. change tampons frequently.
   c. avoid the use of diaphragms.
   d. alternate the use of tampons with sanitary pads.

6. The bacterium responsible for mucopurulent cervicitis is:
   a. chlamydia.
   b. gonorrhea.
   c. staphylococcus.
   d. pseudomonas.

7. The incidence of chlamydia infections in the United States is:
   a. 5%.
   b. 10%.
   c. 20%.
   d. 40%.

8. The majority of women diagnosed with pelvic inflammatory disease (PID) annually in the United States are:
a. 16–24 years of age.
b. 25–30 years of age.
c. 35–45 years of age.
d. post-menapausal.

9. Women who are HIV positive and are considering getting pregnant need to know that there is a _____ chance of perinatal transmission.
a. 10%   b. 25%   c. 50%   d. 100%

10. Mrs. Jakes has had a pessary inserted for long-term treatment of a prolapsed uterus. As part of your teaching plan, you would advise Mrs. Jakes to:
a. see her gynecologist to remove and clean the pessary at regular intervals.
b. keep the insertion site clean and dry.
c. avoid sexual intercourse.
d. avoid climbing stairs as much as possible.

11. Mrs. Schurman, who has been diagnosed as having endometriosis, asks for an explanation of the disease. The best response for the nurse is to explain that:
a. she has developed an infection in the lining of her uterus.
b. tissue from the lining of the uterus has implanted in areas outside the uterus.
c. the lining of the uterus is thicker than usual, causing heavy bleeding and cramping.
d. the lining of the uterus is too thin because endometrial tissue has implanted outside the uterus.

12. The highest frequency of endometriosis is found in the:
a. cervix.
b. cul-de-sac.
c. ovaries.
d. ureterovesical peritoneum.

13. Mrs. Schurman's treatment involves taking oral danazol (Danocrine), 800 mg/day, for 9 months. Danazol is:
a. a gonadotropin that decreases ovarian and pituitary stimulation.
b. an antigonadotropin that increases pituitary stimulation and decreases ovarian stimulation.
c. a gonadotropin that decreases pituitary stimulation and increases ovarian stimulation.
d. an antigonadotropin that decreases pituitary and ovarian stimulation.

14. Risk factors commonly associated with cancer of the cervix include:
a. chronic cervical infections.
b. exposure to diethylstilbestrol (DES) in utero.
c. multiple sexual partners.
d. all of the above.

15. By incidence, cervical cancer is the ____ most common female reproductive cancer.
a. first
b. second
c. third
d. fourth

16. The two chief symptoms of early carcinoma of the cervix are:
a. leukoplakia and metrorrhagia.
b. dyspareunia and foul-smelling vaginal discharge.
c. "strawberry" spots and menorrhagia.
d. leukorrhea and irregular vaginal bleeding or spotting.

17. Using the International Classification of Carcinoma of the Uterine Cervix, a stage II Pap smear result indicates:
a. cancer in situ.
b. vaginal invasion.
c. pelvic wall invasion.
d. bladder extension.

18. A postmenopausal woman who has irregular uterine or vaginal bleeding should be encouraged by a nurse to:
a. stop taking her Premarin (hormonal therapy).
b. see her gynecologist as soon as possible.
c. disregard this phenomenon because it is common during this life stage.
d. mention it to her physician during her next annual examination.

19. Cancer of the uterus, the most common pelvic neoplasm in women, ranks ____ among cancers for women.
a. first
b. second
c. third
d. fourth

20. Women who experience postmenopausal bleeding have a ____ chance of developing cancer of the uterus.
   a. 10%
   b. 20%
   c. 35%
   d. 75%

21. The most common symptom of cancer of the vulva is:
   a. a foul-smelling discharge.
   b. bleeding.
   c. pain.
   d. pruritus.

22. The primary treatment for vulvar malignancy is:
   a. chemotherapy creams.
   b. laser vaporization.
   c. radiation.
   d. wide excision.

23. Postoperative nursing care for a simple vulvectomy should include:
   a. cleansing the wound daily.
   b. offering a low-residue diet.
   c. positioning the patient with pillows.
   d. all of the above.

24. Ovarian cancer ranks ____ as the cause of cancer deaths related to the female reproductive system.
   a. first
   b. second
   c. third
   d. fourth

25. A diagnosis of stage III ovarian cancer indicates that growth involves:
   a. only the ovaries.
   b. the ovaries with pelvic extension.
   c. metastases outside the pelvis.
   d. distant metastases.

26. Radiation therapy is the treatment of choice for:
   a. ovarian cancer.
   b. squamous cell carcinoma of the cervix.
   c. uterine carcinoma.
   d. vaginal wall cancer.

Complete the following scramblegram by circling the word or words that answer each statement below. Terms may be written in any direction.

A	E	E	T	D	A	C	Y	C	L	O	V	I	R
H	L	B	K	E	M	O	M	C	M	U	R	S	C
C	E	D	H	R	A	L	I	T	L	K	L	P	H
V	C	P	A	M	D	E	C	V	Y	L	M	R	A
P	O	A	L	O	N	G	O	S	G	B	E	O	D
B	T	P	U	I	M	D	S	C	A	R	N	L	S
Y	S	S	T	D	Y	L	T	N	L	I	O	A	M
M	Y	M	S	N	M	F	A	B	F	L	R	P	Y
O	C	E	I	R	A	C	T	G	O	T	R	S	T
T	R	A	F	O	S	F	I	Y	E	B	H	E	I
C	E	R	T	S	C	I	N	O	J	K	A	L	R
E	W	D	R	B	D	B	E	P	I	S	G	C	A
R	B	G	B	F	C	R	A	R	M	D	I	B	P
E	R	C	L	M	D	O	I	O	E	S	A	N	I
T	D	S	E	P	T	I	C	S	H	O	C	K	L
S	H	E	R	M	H	D	R	J	R	A	T	H	L
Y	B	A	G	A	C	S	Y	A	T	B	O	L	U
H	B	H	M	D	M	T	P	C	K	T	I	D	N

Definition of Terms

1. Intense burning and inflammation of the vulva

2. A preferred treatment for candidiasis

3. The recommended treatment for trichomoniasis

4. The drug of choice for herpes genitalis

5. A potential complication of toxic shock syndrome

6. The downward displacement of the bladder toward the vaginal orifice

7. This test is used for diagnosis of cervical cancer

8. Term used to describe the surgical procedure in which the uterus, cervix, and ovaries are removed

9. A term to describe vaginal bleeding

10. Another name for benign tumors of the uterus

11. In utero exposure to this drug increases the incidence of vaginal cancer

12. A risk factor for uterine cancer

13. Exercises that strengthen the pelvic muscles

14. An opening between two hollow organs

15. Displacement of the uterus into the vaginal canal

16. Cysts that arise from parts of the ovum

II. Critical Thinking Questions and Exercises

Discussion and Analysis

1. Explain why a decrease in estrogen can lead to vaginal infections.

2. Explain the extent of organ involvement with pelvic inflammatory disease.

3. Describe the typical profile of a women diagnosed with AIDS.

Clinical Situations

Read the following case studies. Fill-in the blanks or circle the correct answer.

Maryanne, a 19-year-old college student, has recently noticed increased vaginal discharge.

CASE STUDY: Bacterial Vaginosis

1. After examination, the nurse prepares a wet mount (vaginal smear). When potassium hydroxide solution is added to the smear, a fishy odor is noted. Maryanne probably has a nonspecific vaginitis known as:
   a. bacterial vaginosis.
   b. candidiasis.
   c. trichomoniasis.
   d. atropic vaginitis.

2. A characteristic symptom of bacterial vaginosis is:
   a. a scanty to minimal discharge.
   b. a fishlike odor.
   c. painful menstruation.
   d. a greenish discharge between periods.

3. Metronidazole is prescribed to be taken twice a day for 1 week. While taking this medication, Maryanne should be instructed to:
   a. avoid dairy products.
   b. avoid sunlight.
   c. avoid alcohol.
   d. lie down flat for at least 30 minutes after inserting the medication.

4. If Maryanne's vaginal infection recurs, the nurse should recommend that:
   a. her sexual partner be tested and treated.
   b. she refrain from sexual intercourse.
   c. she avoid the use of tampons.
   d. she take only showers and no tub baths for awhile.

5. An appropriate nursing diagnosis for Maryanne is:
   a. Altered Comfort—pain and discomfort related to burning or itching from the infectious process.
   b. Self-care Deficit related to inability to perform activities of daily living.
   c. Altered Comfort related to *Gardnerella*-associated vaginitis.
   d. Altered Comfort related to candidiasis.

CASE STUDY: Herpes Genitalis

Paige, a 37-year-old mother of one, has just been recently diagnosed with herpes genitalis.

1. Herpes genitalis, a sexually transmitted disease, causes blisters on the:
   a. cervix.
   b. external genitalia.
   c. vagina.
   d. all of the above areas.

2. The initial painful infection usually lasts:
   a. 1 week.   b. 2 weeks.   c. 4 weeks.   d. 6 weeks.

3. The herpes virus that is accountable for the majority of genital and perineal lesions is:
   a. Epstein-Barr virus
   b. cytomegalovirus
   c. herpes simplex, type 2
   d. varicella zoster

4. In order to acquire the infection, one must have close human contact in one of five ways. List five possible ways:

   _____, _____, _____,

   _____, and _____

5. Since there is no cure, list three antiviral agents that manage symptoms.

   _____, _____, and

   _____

6. The antiviral agent that can suppress symptoms and shorten the course of the infection is: _____.

7. List four probable nursing diagnoses for Paige.

   _____, _____,

   _____, and _____

CASE STUDY: Toxic Shock Syndrome

Irene, a 23-year-old woman, is admitted to the emergency department in shock with an elevated temperature. She is diagnosed as having TSS.

1. The nurse knows that TSS is a bacterial infection associated with the use of tampons. The bacterial toxin is believed to be:
   a. *Escherichia coli.*
   b. *Haemophilus influenzae.*
   c. *Staphylococcus aureus.*
   d. *Pseudomonas aeruginosa.*

2. The onset of TSS is characterized by the sudden appearance of:
   a. an elevated fever (up to 102°F).
   b. a red, macular rash.
   c. myalgia and dizziness.
   d. uncontrolled hypotension.

3. Signs associated with TSS include all of the following *except*:
   a. an elevated blood urea nitrogen level.
   b. a decreased bilirubin level.
   c. leukocytosis.
   d. oliguria.

4. Diagnostic evaluation is made from examination of cultures from:
   a. the blood and urine.
   b. the cervix.
   c. the vagina.
   d. all of the above areas.

5. A priority of medical management is:
   a. alleviating respiratory distress.
   b. treating the shock.
   c. controlling the infection.
   d. managing the emotional distress.

CASE STUDY: Pelvic Inflammatory Disease

Donna is a 26-year-old graduate student who has been sexually active with multiple partners for 5 years. Last year she experienced several incidences of cervicitis. She now believes she has PID.

1. Based on your knowledge of PID, you know that the inflammatory condition of the pelvic cavity may involve the following five areas: _____, _____, _____,

_____ and _____.

2. Choose six words to describe the characteristics of the infection: _____, _____,

_____, _____, _____ and _____.

3. The infection is caused by a:
   a. bacteria.
   b. fungus.
   c. parasite.
   d. virus.

4. Name the two most common causative organisms for PID.
   _____ and _____

5. List five disorders that can result from the PID infection.

   _____, _____, _____,

   _____, and _____

6. Name four localized symptoms of PID and six generalized symptoms.

Localized	*Generalized*
_____	_____
_____	_____
_____	_____
_____	_____
	_____
	_____

48

Assessment and Management of Patients With Breast Disorders

I. Interpretation, Completion, and Comparison

Multiple Choice. Read each question carefully. Circle your answer.

1. The optimal time for breast self-examination is usually beginning at the _____ day after menses.
  a. third
  b. fifth
  c. eighth
  d. tenth

2. The average percentage of women who perform breast self-examination is believed to be about:
  a. 15%.
  b. 25%.
  c. 40%.
  d. 80%.

3. Mammography can diagnose breast cancer before it is clinically palpable, meaning that the lump can be detected by x-ray when it is approximately_____ in size.
  a. 1 cm
  b. 1 mm
  c. 2 cm
  d. 1 m

4. As part of health teaching, the nurse needs to alert patients that mammography can yield a false-negative result in _____ instances out of 100.
  a. 5 to 10
  b. 10 to 15
  c. 15 to 20
  d. 20 to 25

5. Mammography should be used to annually screen women who are:
  a. younger than 35 years of age.
  b. between the ages of 35 and 40 years.
  c. between 40 and 50 years old.
  d. older than 50 years of age.

6. Characteristics of the lumps present in cystic disease of the breasts include all of the following *except*:
  a. a rapid increase and decrease in size.
  b. increased tenderness before menstruation.
  c. a painless or tender lump.
  d. skin dimpling and nipple retraction.

7. The risk of developing breast cancer is now 1 woman out of:
  a. 8.
  b. 20.
  c. 35.
  d. 50.

8. The current 5-year survival rate of breast cancer is:
   a. 60%.
   b. 75%.
   c. 88%.
   d. 98%.

9. Carcinoma in situ, a noninvasive form of cancer, has in incidence rate of:
   a. 5–10%
   b. 15–20%.
   c. 25–35%.
   d. 50–70%.

10. A 1998 clinical study yielded significant reduction in the incidence of breast cancer for those participants who took the chemopreventive agent:
   a. doxorubicin.
   b. methotrexate.
   c. raloxifen.
   d. tamoxifen.

11. The strongest factor (80% correlation) that influences the incidence of breast cancer is:
   a. chemical elements.
   b. environmental pollution.
   c. genetic predisposition.
   d. the number of menstrual cycles.

12. The chance of developing breast cancer doubles if:
   a. the woman had her first child after 30 years of age.
   b. the woman's mother had breast cancer.
   c. the woman was exposed to radiation after puberty.
   d. all of the above are true.

13. The majority of breast cancers occur in the:
   a. upper, inner quadrant.
   b. lower, inner quadrant.
   c. upper, outer quadrant.
   d. lower, outer quadrant.

14. Early clinical manifestations of breast carcinoma include all of the following *except*:
   a. a nontender lump.
   b. asymmetry of the breasts.
   c. nipple retraction.
   d. pain in the breast tissue.

15. A noninvasive breast tumor between 2 cm and 5 cm in size is classified as a stage:
   a. I.
   b. II.
   c. III.
   d. IV.

16. Carcinoma of the breast results from cell doubling. A cell that doubles every 60 days would become palpable after:
   a. 3 years.
   b. 5 years.
   c. 10 years.
   d. 15 years.

17. At diagnosis of breast carcinoma, the risk for presence of metastasis is about:
   a. 25%.
   b. 38%.
   c. 55%.
   d. 73%.

18. The most common site of distant metastasis for breast carcinoma is the:
   a. adrenals.
   b. bone.
   c. lungs.
   d. liver.

19. If the number of positive axillary lymph nodes is between five and six on biopsy, the risk for breast cancer recurrence is:
   a. less than 10%.
   b. 15%.
   c. 30%.
   d. greater than 50%.

20. A patient is scheduled for removal of her left breast and the axillary lymph nodes; the pectoralis minor muscle is to be left in place. This surgical intervention is called:
   a. an extended radical mastectomy.
   b. a modified radical mastectomy.
   c. a quadrantectomy.
   d. a simple mastectomy.

21. The most common hormonal method of intervention is the use of:
   a. Cytadren.
   b. diethylstilbestrol.
   c. Megace.
   d. tamoxifen.

22. Suggested postoperative positioning of the affected arm after surgical intervention (mastectomy) is:
   a. abduction to promote incisional healing.
   b. adduction to minimize trauma to sensitive tissue.
   c. elevation to promote lymphatic drainage.
   d. extension to facilitate isometric exercises.

23. Postmastectomy arm exercises facilitate the development of collateral circulation, which decreases lymphedema. Collateral circulation is usually developed within:
a. 1 month.
b. 3 months.
c. 5 months.
d. 8 to 10 months.

24. A patient with lymphedema in an arm should be advised to avoid:
a. blood pressure assessments in that arm.
b. injections or needles in that arm.
c. prolonged exposure of that arm to sunlight.
d. all of the above.

25. The most commonly encountered breast condition in the male is:
a. breast cancer.
b. mastitis.
c. gynecomastia.
d. cystic breast disease.

II. Critical Thinking Questions and Exercises

Clinical Situations

Read the following case study. Circle the correct answers.

CASE STUDY: Simple Mastectomy

Louise is 53 years old and single. The biopsy findings indicate that she has a malignancy in her breast. She is scheduled for a simple mastectomy.

1. Based on knowledge about the cause of breast cancer, the nurse knows that the highest incidence of this type of cancer is found:
a. among those who give birth to their first child after 35 years of age.
b. among those who have had multiple pregnancies.
c. in the unmarried woman who has not had children.
d. in the woman who has menopause after 50 years of age.

2. On examination, Louise's tumor is found in the anatomic area where tumors usually develop, the:
a. medial half of the breast.
b. nipple area.
c. posterior segment, inferior to the nipple.
d. upper, outer quadrant.

3. Louise is advised that if she chooses not to seek treatment, her life expectancy will be:
a. less than 1 year.
b. between 2 and 3 years.
c. about 5 years.
d. as long as 10 years.

4. The nurse can advise Louise that surgical management for her stage I cancer has a cure rate of:
a. 30%.
b. 50%.
c. 90%.
d. 100%.

Postoperatively, Louise returns to the clinical area and is alert and aware of her surroundings. She experiences moderate pain for the first 72 hours.

5. Postoperative care of the incision includes all of the following *except*:
a. applying cocoa butter to increase elasticity.
b. drying the area with slight friction to stimulate the circulation.
c. gently bathing the area with a nonabrasive soap.
d. massaging the area.

6. Louise's affected arm should be elevated on a pillow so that her:
a. entire arm is in a horizontal plane.
b. forearm is level with her heart.
c. wrist is higher than her elbow, which should be higher than her shoulder.
d. wrist is lower than her elbow so that circulation to her hand will not be decreased.

7. The nurse expects that Louise will be allowed out of bed in:
a. 1 to 2 days.
b. about 5 days.
c. about 1 week.
d. 1 to 2 weeks.

Identifying Patterns

Five figures of a woman performing breast self-examination follow. Start with the first figure and explain the activity associated with each step.

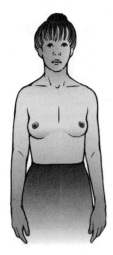

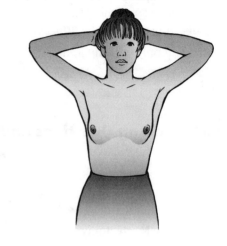

FIGURE 1

1. _____

2. _____

3. _____

FIGURE 2

1. _____

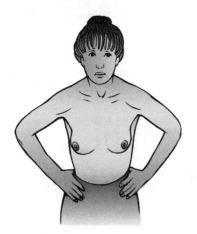

FIGURE 3

1. _____

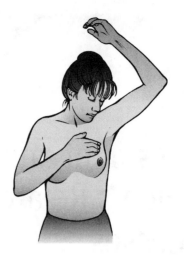

FIGURE 4

1. _____
2. _____
3. _____
4. _____
5. _____
6. _____

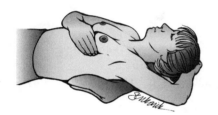

FIGURE 5

1. _____
2. _____
3. _____

49

Assessment and Management of Problems Related to Male Reproductive Processes

I. Interpretation, Completion, and Comparison

Multiple Choice. *Read each question carefully. Circle your answer.*

1. Health education for a patient with prostatitis includes all of the following *except*:
   a. avoiding drinks that increase prostatic secretions.
   b. forcing fluids to prevent urine from backing up and distending the bladder.
   c. taking several hot sitz baths daily.
   d. using antibiotic therapy for 10 to 14 days.

2. Enlargement of the prostate gland, benign prostatic hyperplasia, is usually associated with:
   a. dysuria.
   b. dilation of the ureters.
   c. hydronephrosis.
   d. all of the above.

3. The incidence of prostate cancer in the general male population is:
   a. 10%.   b. 20%.   c. 30%.   d. 50%.

4. As a cause of death in American men older than 55 years of age, cancer of the prostate ranks:
   a. first.
   b. second.
   c. third.
   d. fourth.

5. The racial group most likely to acquire and die from prostate cancer is:
   a. African Americans.
   b. Caucasians.
   c. Hispanics.
   d. Italians.

6. Prostatic cancer commonly metastasizes to the:
   a. bone.
   b. liver.
   c. lungs.
   d. brain.

7. The concentration of prostate-specific antigen (PSA) is proportional to the total prostatic mass. As a diagnostic tool, PSA would indicate all of the following *except*:
   a. local progression of the disease.
   b. patient responsiveness to cancer therapy.
   c. recurrence of prostate cancer.
   d. the presence of malignancy.

8. The closed surgical procedure used for a prostatectomy is a ____ approach.
   a. perineal
   b. suprapubic
   c. retropubic
   d. transurethral

9. The prostatectomy approach that is associated with a high incidence of impotency is:
   a. perineal.
   b. retropubic.
   c. suprapubic.
   d. transurethral.

10. Patients undergoing open surgical removal of the prostate seem to experience a high incidence of:
    a. paralytic ileus.
    b. pneumonia.
    c. impotence.
    d. all of the above.

11. In most instances, patients can be advised that sexual activity can resume, after a prostatectomy, in about:
    a. 4 weeks.
    b. 2 months.
    c. 10 weeks.
    d. 4 months.

12. An expected postoperative outcome of prostatectomy is light pink urine within:
    a. 24 hours.
    b. 48 hours.
    c. 3 days.
    d. 1 week.

13. During the 2 months it takes for the prostatic fossa to heal, the patient is advised not to:
    a. engage in strenuous exercise.
    b. perform the Valsalva maneuver.
    c. take long automobile rides.
    d. do all of the above.

14. In the 15- to 35-year-old age group, testicular cancer as a cause of death ranks:
    a. first.
    b. second.
    c. third.
    d. fourth.

15. Retroperitoneal lymphadenectomy after orchiectomy would probably lead to:
    a. altered libido.
    b. inability to have orgasm.
    c. infertility.
    d. all of the above.

16. One cause of infertility in men is a:
    a. hydrocele.
    b. varicocele.
    c. paraphimosis.
    d. phimosis.

17. Neonatal circumcision is an important protective measure against carcinoma of the:
    a. penis.
    b. testes.
    c. scrotum.
    d. urethra.

18. All of the following are true of priapism except that it:
    a. is a urologic emergency.
    b. may result in gangrene.
    c. is painless.
    d. may result in impotence.

Fill-In. *Read each statement carefully. Write your response in the space provided.*

1. Two specific tests used to diagnose prostate cancer are: _____ and _____.

2. List four medications associated with erectile dysfunction.

   _____, _____,

   _____, and _____

3. The most common isolated organism that causes prostatitis is: _____.

4. List five symptoms associated with prostatitis.

_____, _____, _____,

_____, and _____

5. List five symptoms found with benign prostatic hyperplasia (BPH).

_____, _____, _____,

_____, and _____

6. The most commonly used medication for estrogen therapy in the treatment of prostatic cancer is:_____.

7. Explain why low-dose heparin is usually given to patients undergoing prostatectomy.

_____

_____

8. Describe epididymitis and several of its common causes.

_____

_____

9. Define priapism and list its major symptoms.

_____

Matching. *Match the term listed in Column II with its description of disorders of the male reproductive system listed in Column I.*

Column I

1._____collection of fluid in the testes

2._____an obstructive complex characterized by increased urinary frequency

3._____constricted foreskin of the penis

4._____failure of the testes to descend into the scrotum

5._____inflammation of the testes

6._____abnormal dilation of the veins in the scrotum

7._____inflammation of the prostrate gland

8._____infection of the epididymis

Column II

a. cryptorchidism

b. epididymitis

c. hydrocele

d. orchitis

e. phimosis

f. prostatism

g. prostatitis

h. variocele

II. Critical Thinking Questions and Exercises

CASE STUDY: Prostatectomy

Read the following case study. Fill in the blanks or circle the correct answer.

Tom is a 65-year-old college administrator who is schedule for a prostatectomy.

1. Preoperatively, two objectives to determine readiness for surgery are: _____ and _____.

2. Prostatectomy must be performed before: _____

3. The most commonly performed surgical procedure that is carried out through endoscopy is:
   a. perineal approach.
   b. retropubic approach.
   c. suprapubic approach.
   d. transurethral approach.

4. List two possible postoperative complications of the transurethral resection of the prostate (TURP) approach.

_____ and _____

5. List four general postoperative complications of a prostatectomy.

_____,   _____,

_____, and   _____

5. Explain why impotence may result from a prostatectomy.

_____

6. List three possible preoperative nursing diagnoses:

_____,   _____, and   _____

7. Identify two nursing activities to help relieve postoperative bladder spasms.

_____ and _____

8. Explain why the patient is advised not to sit for prolonged periods of time immediately.

_____

9. Describe how you would teach a patient to do perineal exercises.

_____

_____

UNIT 11
Immunologic Function

50

Assessment of Immune Function

I. Interpretation, Completion, and Comparison

Multiple Choice. Read each question carefully. Circle your answer.

1. The immune system is essentially composed of:
   a. bone marrow.
   b. lymphoid tissue.
   c. white blood cells.
   d. all of the above components.

2. The primary production site of white blood cells involved in immunity is the:
   a. bone marrow.
   b. adenoids.
   c. thymus gland.
   d. spleen.

3. An example of biologic response modifiers that interfere with viruses is:
   a. bradykinin.
   b. eosinophils.
   c. granulocytes.
   d. interferon.

4. Granulocytes, which fight invasion by releasing histamine, do not include:
   a. basophils.
   b. eosinophils.
   c. lymphocytes.
   d. neutrophils.

5. The leukocytes that arrive first at a site where inflammation occurs are:
   a. B lymphocytes.
   b. cytotoxic T cells.
   c. helper T cells.
   d. neutrophils.

6. The body's first line of defense is the:
   a. antibody response.
   b. cellular immune response.
   c. phagocytic immune response.
   d. white blood cell response.

7. The primary cells responsible for recognition of foreign antigens are:
   a. leukocytes.
   b. lymphocytes.
   c. monocytes.
   d. reticulocytes.

8. Lymphocytes interfere with disease by picking up specific antigens from organisms to alter their function during the ____ stage of an immune response.
   a. effector
   b. proliferation
   c. recognition
   d. response

9. During the proliferation stage:
   a. antibody-producing plasma cells are produced.
   b. lymph nodes enlarge.
   c. lymphocytes rapidly increase.
   d. all of the above occur.

10. Antibodies are believed to be a type of:
   a. carbohydrate.
   b. fat.
   c. protein.
   d. sugar.

11. Cell-mediated immune responses are responsible for all of the following *except*:
   a. anaphylaxis.
   b. graft-versus-host reactions.
   c. transplant rejection.
   d. tumor destruction.

12. It is important to realize that cellular membrane damage results from all the following *except*:
   a. activation of complement.
   b. antibody-antigen binding.
   c. arrival of killer T cells.
   d. attraction of macrophages.

13. Effector T cells destroy foreign organisms by:
   a. altering the antigen's cell membrane.
   b. causing cellular lysis.
   c. producing lymphokines, which destroy invading organisms.
   d. all of the above mechanisms.

14. Interferon is a lymphokine that exerts its effect by:
   a. increasing vascular permeability.
   b. inhibiting the growth of certain antigenic cells.
   c. stopping the spread of viral infections.
   d. suppressing the movement of macrophages.

15. Complement acts by:
   a. attracting phagocytes to an antigen.
   b. destroying cells through destruction of the antigen's membrane.
   c. rendering the antigen vulnerable to phagocytosis.
   d. a combination of all of the above mechanisms.

Fill-In. *Read each statement carefully. Write your response in the space provided.*

1. List four ways that disorders of the immune system occur.

_____,   _____,

_____, and   _____

2. Distinguish between natural and acquired immunity.

Natural: _____

Acquired: _____

3. Explain what "complement" is and how it is formed.

_____

4. Name the two ways biologic response modifiers affect the immune response:

_____

_____

5. Explain what research has shown about the role of stem cells.

_____

_____

Matching. *Match the immunoglobulin listed in Column II with its associated immunoglobulin (Ig) activity listed in Column I. An answer may be used more than once.*

Column I

1.____ enhances phagocytosis

2.____ appears in intravascular serum

3.____ helps defend against parasites

4.____ activates complement system

5.____ protects against respiratory infections

6.____ influences B-lymphocyte differentiation

7.____ prevents absorption of antigens from food

Column II

a. IgA

b. IgD

c. IgE

d. IgG

e. IgM

Matching. *Match the immune system effect listed in Column II with its corresponding medication listed in Column I. An answer may be used more than once.*

Column I

1._____ cyclosporine

2._____ dactinomycin

3._____ indomethacin

4._____ methotrexate

5._____ mustagen

6._____ propylthiouracil

7._____ vancomycin

Column II

a. Agranulocytosis, leukopenia

b. Agranulocytosis, neutropenia

c. Leukopenia, aplastic bone marrow

d. Leukopenia, T-cell inhibition

e. Transient leukopenia

Unscramble *the letters to answer each statement.*

1. A protein subsance that responds to a specific antigen

Y N I D T O A B

2. Enzymatic proteins that destroy bacteria

T L P M N C E O E M

3. A substance that stimulates the production of antibodies

G I N T E A N

4. Lymphocytes that directly attack antigens

R P T E L H L E C L E S

5. Cells that engulf and destroy foreign bodies

O G T A E Y P C S H

6. Proteins formed when cells are exposed to foreign agents

F E O T N E S R I R N

51

Management of Patients With Immunodeficiency

I. Interpretation, Completion, and Comparison

Multiple Choice. Read each question carefully. Circle your answer.

1. Immunodeficiency disorders are caused by defects or deficiencies in:
a. the complement system.
b. B and T lymphocytes.
c. phagocytic cells.
d. all of the above.

2.. The cardinal symptoms of immunodeficiency are:
a. chronic diarrhea.
b. chronic or recurrent severe infections.
c. poor response to treatment of infections.
d. inclusive of all the above.

3. The nitroblue tetrazolium reductase (NTR) test is used to diagnose immunodeficiency disorders related to:
a. complement.
b. B lymphocytes.
c. T lymphocytes.
d. phagocytic cells.

4. More than 50% of individuals with ____ develop pernicious anemia.
a. Bruton disease
b. common variable immunodeficiency (CVID)
c. DiGeorge syndrome
d. Nezelaf syndrome

5. The most frequent presenting sign in patients with DiGeorge syndrome is:
a. chronic diarrhea.
b. hypocalcemia.
c. neutropenia.
d. pernicious anemia.

6. The primary cause of death for individuals with ataxia-telangiectasia is:
a. acute renal failure.
b. chronic lung disease.
c. neurologic dysfunction.
d. overwhelming infection.

7. The most common secondary immunodeficiency disorder is:
a. AIDS.
b. DAF.
c. CVID.
d. SCID.

8. The recommended dose of intravenous gamma globulin for a 60-kg man is ____ given monthly.
a. 15 g
b. 30 g
c. 45 g
d. 60 g

9. When gamma globulin is infused intravenously, the rate should not exceed:
   a. 1.5 mL/min.
   b. 3 mL/min.
   c. 6 mL/min.
   d. 10 mL/min.

10. The nurse knows to stop an infusion of gamma globulin if the patient experiences:
   a. flank pain.
   b. shaking chills.
   c. tightness in the chest.
   d. any or all of the above.

II. Critical Thinking Questions and Exercises

Identifying Patterns

For each group of clustered clues, write the corresponding immunodeficiency disorder.

Increased incidence of bacterial infections
Readily develops fungal infections from candida organism
Easily infected from herpes simplex
Afflicted with chronic eczematoid dermatitis

1. Disorder is: _____

There is disappearance of germinal centers from lymphatic tissue.
There is complete lack of antibody production.
It is associated with the most common immunodeficiency seen in childhood.
Disease onset occurs most often in the second decade of life.

2. Disorder is: _____

Lymphopenia is usually present.
Thymus gland fails to develop.
Chronic mucocutaneous candidiasis is an associated disorder.

3. Disorder is: _____

IgA deficiency is present in 40% of individuals.
T-cell deficiencies become more severe with age.
Neurologic symptoms usually occur before 5 years of age.

4. Disorder is: _____

It usually occurs as a result of underlying disease processes.
It frequently is caused by certain autoimmune disorders.
It may be caused by certain viruses.

5. Disorder is:

_____

Examining Associations

Read each analogy. Fill in the space provided with the best response. Explain the correlation.

1. Job's syndrome: phagocytic dysfunction:: Bruton's disease: _____

2. Colony-stimulating factor: HIE syndrome:: IV gamma globulin: _____

3. CVID: bacterial infections:: Ataxia-telangiectasia: _____

4. Angioneurotic edema: frequent episodes of edema::Paroxysmal nocturnal hemoglobinuria: _____

52

Assessment and Management of Patients With HIV and AIDS

I. Interpretation, Completion, and Comparison

Multiple Choice. Read each question carefully. Circle your answer.

1. The Centers for Disease Control and Prevention (CDC) initially and officially "defined" AIDS after 100 cases were reported in:
   a. 1978.
   b. 1982.
   c. 1986.
   d. 1991.

2. According to one study, the greatest number of reported HIV cases were due to:
   a. male homosexual contact.
   b. male injection drug use.
   c. female homosexual contact.
   d. female injection drug use.

3. The racial/ethnic group that has the highest rate of exposure due to injection drug use among men is:
   a. Caucasians.   b. Hispanics.   c. African Americans.   d. Asians.

4. Postexposure prophylaxis (PEP) medications should be started within _____ after exposure but no longer than _____ to offer any benefit.
   a. 2 hours; 72 hours
   b. 4 days; 7 days
   c. 1 week; 3 weeks
   d. 1 month; 2 months

5. Up to 85% of individuals infected with HIV will develop symptoms of AIDS within ____ years after infection.
   a. 3
   b. 6
   c. 10
   d. 15

6. Abnormal laboratory findings seen with AIDS include:
   a. decreased CD4 and T-cell count.
   b. +p24 antigen.
   c. positive ELISA test.
   d. all of the above.

7. One of the most frequent systemic side effects of anti-HIV drugs is:
   a. osteoporosis.
   b. hyperglycemia.
   c. lipodystrophy syndrome.
   d. pancreatitis.

8. The most common infection in persons with AIDS is:
   a. cytomegalovirus.
   b. Legionnaire's disease.
   c. *Mycobacterium tuberculosis.*
   d. *Pneumocystis carinii pneumonia.*

9. At least 90% of individuals with AIDS experience:
   a. anorexia.
   b. candidiasis.
   c. diarrhea.
   d. fungal infections.

10. The minimum number of daily calories recommended for a 70-kg individual with AIDS-related "wasting syndrome" is:
   a. 1500.
   b. 2000.
   c. 2800.
   d. 4000.

11. The minimum number of daily protein calories for a 70-kg individual with AIDS-related "wasting syndrome" is:
   a. 20.
   b. 35.
   c. 45.
   d. 60.

12. The most common malignancy seen with HIV infection is:
   a. carcinoma of the skin.
   b. Kaposi's sarcoma.
   c. pancreatic cancer.
   d. stomach cancer.

Fill-In. *Read each statement carefully. Write your response in the space provided.*

1. In the United States, five states have the largest number of reported AIDS cases (1999–2000). They are:

_____, _____, _____, _____ and _____.

2. The two major means of HIV transmission are: _____ and _____.

3. List five types of body fluids that can transmit HIV-1.

_____, _____, _____,

_____, and _____

4. HIV belongs to a group of viruses known as: _____.

5. List two of four selected laboratory tests used for diagnosing and tracking HIV: _____ and

_____.

6. Treatment decisions for HIV are based on three criteria: _____, _____ and _____.

7. The four goals of treatment are:

_____, _____,

_____, and _____

8. All anti-HIV drugs work in one of two ways: _____ or _____.

9. The initial manifestation of AIDS in more than 60% of patients is the appearance of _____.

10. A recommended chemotherapeutic agent for Kaposi's sarcoma is: _____.

Matching. *Match the AIDS-indicated category listed in Column II with its associated clinical condition listed in Column I. An answer may be used more than once.*

Column I

1._____histoplasmosis

2._____hairy leukoplakia

3._____Kaposi's sarcoma

4._____acute primary HIV infection

5._____pneumocystis carinii

6._____bacillary angiomatosis

7._____persistent generalized lymphadenopathy (PGL)

8._____extrapulmonary crytococcosis

Column II

a. Clinical Category A

b. Clinical Category B

c. Clinical Category C

II. Critical Thinking Questions and Exercises

Discussion and Analysis

1. Give specific examples of how health care providers can maintain "Standard Precautions" to prevent HIV transmission.

2. Describe the stage of HIV disease known as *primary infection.*

3. Describe the appearance of the cutaneous lesions seen with Kaposi's sarcoma.

Clinical Situations

Read the following case study. Fill in the blanks or circle the correct answer.

CASE STUDY: Acquired Immunodeficiency Syndrome

Brenden is a 39-year-old homosexual who has been recently diagnosed with AIDS.

1. On initial assessment, the nurse identifies two major potential risk factors associated with AIDS: _____ and _____.

2. As part of her assessment, the nurse checks Brenden for candidiasis. To do this, she would inspect Brenden's.
   a. heart.
   b. lungs.
   c. oral cavity.
   d. skin.

3. Assessment data indicated dehydration as evidenced by:
   a. bradycardia.
   b. hypertension.
   c. urine specific gravity greater than 1.025.
   d. urine output greater than 70 mL/hour.

4. The assessment data indicates five possible collaborative problems; list two. _____ and _____

5. The nurse advises Brenden to avoid certain foods that are bowel irritants to prevent diarrhea. She advises him not to eat:
   a. bland foods.
   b. cooked cereal.
   c. jello and pudding.
   d. popcorn.

6. To improve Brenden's nutritional status, the nurse would:
   a. encourage him to rest before eating.
   b. limit fluids 1 hour before meals.
   c. serve five to six small meals per day.
   d. do all of the above.

53

Assessment and Management of Patients With Allergic Disorders

I. Interpretation, Completion, and Comparison

Multiple Choice. Read each question carefully. Circle your answer.

1. The body's first line of defense against potential invaders is the:
   a. gastrointestinal tract.
   b. respiratory tract.
   c. skin.
   d. combination of all the above.

2. An example of an *incomplete protein antigen* that triggers an allergic response is:
   a. animal dander.
   b. horse serum.
   c. medications.
   d. pollen.

3. The classification of immunoglobulin (Ig) that occupies certain receptors on mast cells and produces an inflammatory response is:
   a. IgA.
   b. IgD.
   c. IgE.
   d. IgG.

4. Histamine acts on major organs by:
   a. contracting bronchial smooth muscle.
   b. dilating small venules.
   c. increasing gastric secretions.
   d. stimulating all of the above mechanisms.

5. A popular medication that has an affinity for H_1 receptors is:
   a. Benadryl.
   b. Prilosec.
   c. Tagamet.
   d. Zantac.

6. Hypersensitivity reactions follow reexposure and are classified by type of reaction. An anaphylactic reaction is usually identified as type:
   a. I.
   b. II.
   c. III.
   d. IV.

7. Delayed hypersensitivity (type IV) is said to have occurred when the inflammatory response to an allergen peaks within:
   a. 4 to 8 hours.
   b. 24 to 72 hours.
   c. 4 to 6 days.
   d. 1 to 2 weeks.

8. The nurse monitors the patient's eosinophil level. She suspects a definite allergic disorder with a value of _____ of the total leukocyte count.
   a. 1% to 3%   c. 5% to 10%
   b. 3% to 4%   d. 15% to 40%

9. Atopic disorders that result from an allergic response to an allergen include:
   a. allergic rhinitis.   c. bronchial asthma.
   b. atopic dermatitis   d. all of the above.

10. Pruritus and nasal congestion may be indicators of an impending anaphylactic reaction. These symptoms usually occur within _____ hours after exposure.
    a. 2   b. 6   c. 12   d. 24

11. When a patient is experiencing an allergic response, the nurse should initially assess the patient for:
    a. dyspnea, bronchospasm, and/or laryngeal   c. the presence and location of pruritus.
       edema.   d. the severity of cutaneous warmth and flushing.
    b. hypotension and tachycardia.

12. Allergic rhinitis is induced by:
    a. airborne pollens or molds.   c. parenteral medications.
    b. ingested foods.   d. topical creams or ointments.

13. Patients who are sensitive to ragweed should be advised that weed pollen begins to appear in:
    a. early spring.   c. summer.
    b. early fall.   d. midwinter.

14. A major side effect of antihistamines that requires accurate patient education is:
    a. dryness of the mouth.   c. palpitations.
    b. anorexia.   d. sedation.

15. An area of nursing concern when administering a sympathomimetic drug is the drug's ability to:
    a. cause bronchodilation.   c. dilate the muscular vasculature.
    b. constrict integumentary smooth muscle. d. do all of the above.

16. Injected allergens are used for "hyposensitization" and may produce systemic reactions that can be harmful. The medication that should be on hand in case of an adverse reaction is:
    a. Dramamine.   c. Phenergan hydrochloride.
    b. epinephrine.   d. Pyribenzamine.

17. For a 132-lb (60-kg) woman who is experiencing anaphylaxis, the nurse should immediately administer a minimum of:
    a. 2 mL of adrenaline, intramuscularly. c. 6 mL of adrenaline, intramuscularly.
    b. 4 mL of adrenaline, intramuscularly. d. 8 mL of adrenaline, intramuscularly.

18. The most serious manifestation of hereditary angioedema is:
    a. abdominal pain.   c. larnygeal edema.
    b. conjunctivitis.   d. urticaria.

19. One of the most severe food allergies is caused by:
    a. chocolate.   b. milk.   c. peanuts.   d. shimp.

Fill-In. *Read each statement carefully. Write your response in the space provided.*

1. Antibodies react with antigens by: _____, _____, _____ and

   _____.

2. An allergic reaction occurs when:

   _____

   _____

3. Prostaglandins are primary chemical mediators that respond to a stimulus by contracting smooth muscle and increasing capillary permeability. This response causes: _____

4. Type III hypersensitivity reactions involve the binding of antibodies to antigens, as occurs in the following two disorders: _____ and _____.

5. Two examples of a type IV hypersensitivity reaction are: _____ and _____.

6. The primary treatment available for latex allergy is: _____.

II. Critical Thinking Questions and Exercises

Discussion and Analysis

1. Briefly describe the physiologic response that causes an allergic reaction.

2. Explain the production and function of immunoglobulins.

3. Describe the clinical manifestations that occur with a severe anaphylactic reaction.

Clinical Situations

Read the following case study. Fill in the blanks or circle the correct answer.

CASE STUDY: Allergic Rhinitis

Chris is a 26-year-old contractor who specializes in finished basements. Because of his job, he is frequently working in environments where there are substances that stimulate an allergic reaction.

1. Based on assessment data, two likely nursing diagnoses would be:

   _____ and _____

2. Four probable patient goals would be:

   _____,   _____,

   _____, and   _____

3. The nurse advises Chris that his attacks may be preceded by the symptoms of:
   a. breathing difficulty.
   b. pruritus.
   c. tingling sensations.
   d. all of the above.

4. The nurse also advises him that other symptoms may be more alarming, such as:
   a. hoarseness.
   b. a rash or hives.
   c. wheezing.
   d. all of the above.

5. A teaching plan for Chris would include information about:
   a. reducing exposure to allergens.
   b. desensitization procedures.
   c. correct use of medications.
   d. all of the above.

6. The nurse tells Chris that if the physician recommends a series of inoculations for desensitization, he should expect to receive injections every:
   a. day for 30 days.
   b. week for 1 year.
   c. 2 to 4 weeks.
   d. month for 4 years.

54

Assessment and Management of Patients With Rheumatic Disorders

I. Interpretation, Completion, and Comparison

Multiple Choice. *Read each question carefully. Circle your answer.*

1. Joint swelling in rheumatic disease may be due to:
   a. bony overgrowth.
   b. fluid accumulation.
   c. hypertrophied synovium.
   d. all of the above.

2. The most common symptom of rheumatic disease that causes a patient to seek medical attention is:
   a. joint swelling.
   b. limited movement.
   c. fatigue.
   d. pain.

3. Synovial fluid from an inflamed joint is characteristically:
   a. clear and pale.
   b. milky, cloudy, and dark yellow.
   c. scanty in volume.
   d. straw-colored.

4. A serum study that is positive for the rheumatoid factor is:
   a. diagnostic for Sjögren's syndrome.
   b. diagnostic for systemic lupus erythematosus.
   c. specific for rheumatoid arthritis.
   d. suggestive of rheumatoid arthritis.

5. A disease-modifying antirheumatic drug (DMARD) that is successful in the treatment of rheumatoid arthritis yet has retinal eye changes as a side effect is:
   a. Imuran.
   b. Aralen.
   c. Plaquenil.
   d. Solganal.

6. Nonsteroidal anti-inflammatory drugs (NSAIDs) include all of the following *except*:
   a. Clinoril.
   b. Cytoxan.
   c. Motrin.
   d. Celebrex.

7. When a person with arthritis is temporarily confined to bed, the position recommended to prevent flexion deformities is:
   a. prone.
   b. semi-Fowler's.
   c. side-lying with pillows supporting the shoulders and legs.
   d. supine with pillows under the knees.

8. To immobilize an inflamed wrist, the nurse should splint the joint in a position of:
   a. slight dorsiflexion.
   b. extension.
   c. hyperextension.
   d. internal rotation.

9. In rheumatoid arthritis, the cartilage is replaced with fibrous connective tissue during the stage of synovial joint destruction known as:
   a. cartilage erosion.
   b. increased phagocytic production.
   c. lymphocyte infiltration.
   d. pannus formation.

10. The rheumatoid arthritis (RA) reaction produces enzymes that break down:
   a. collagen.
   b. elastin.
   c. hematopoietic tissue.
   d. strong supporting tissue.

11. In rheumatoid arthritis, the autoimmune reaction primarily occurs in the:
   a. joint tendons.
   b. cartilage.
   c. synovial tissue.
   d. interstitial space.

12. The diagnosis of rheumotoid arthritis is consistent with a:
   a. decreased C4 complement.
   b. decreased sedimentation rate.
   c. negative antinuclear antibody (ANA).
   d. positive C-reactive protein.

13. A characteristic cutaneous lesion, called the "butterfly rash," appears across the bridge of the nose in patients with:
   a. gout.
   b. rheumatoid arthritis.
   c. systemic sclerosis.
   d. systemic lupus erythematosus.

14. The single, most important medication for the treatment of systemic lupus erythematosus (SLE) is:
   a. immunosuppressants.
   b. corticosteroids.
   c. NSAIDs.
   d. salicylates.

15. Clinical manifestations of scleroderma include:
   a. decreased ventilation owing to lung scarring.
   b. dysphagia owing to hardening of the esophagus.
   c. dyspnea owing to fibrotic cardiac tissue.
   d. all of the above.

16. The most common type of connective tissue disease in the United States is:
   a. carpal tunnel syndrome.
   b. degenerative joint disease.
   c. fibrositis.
   d. polymyositis.

17. Pathophysiologic changes seen with osteoarthritis include:
   a. joint cartilage degeneration.
   b. the formation of bony spurs at the edges of the joint surfaces.
   c. narrowing of the joint space.
   d. all of the above changes.

18. The nurse knows that a patient diagnosed with a spondyloarthropathy would not have:
   a. ankylosing spondylitis.
   b. Raynaud's phenomenon.
   c. reactive arthritis.
   d. psoriatic arthritis.

19. With a diagnosis of gout, a nurse should expect to find:
   a. glucosuria.
   b. hyperuricemia.
   c. hypoproteinuria.
   d. ketonuria.

20. A purine-restricted diet is prescribed for a patient. The nurse should recommend:
   a. dairy products.
   b. organ meats.
   c. raw vegetables.
   d. shellfish.

Matching. *Match the clinical interpretation/laboratory significance listed in Column II with its associated test listed in Column I.*

Column I

1. _____uric acid

2. _____complement

3. _____rheumatoid factor

4. _____hematocrit

5. _____HLA-B27 antigen

6. _____antinuclear antibody (ANA)

Column II

a. A decrease can be seen in chronic inflammation.

b. A positive test is associated with SLE, RA, and Raynaud's disease.

c. An increase in this substance is seen with gout.

d. This protein substance is decreased in RA and SLE.

e. This is present in 80% of those who have rheumatoid arthritis.

f. This is present in 85% of those with ankylosing spondylitis.

II. Critical Thinking Questions and Exercises

Discussion and Analysis

1. Explain the difference between *exacerbation* and *remission*:

_____

2. Distinguish between the pathophysiology of inflammatory rheumatic disease and that of degenerative rheumatic disease.

_____

3. Discuss the physiologic rationale supporting the goals and strategies for the treatment of rheumatic diseases:

_____

Clinical Situations

Read the following case studies. Fill in the blanks or circle the correct answer.

CASE STUDY: Diffuse Connective Tissue Disease

June, a 33-year-old mother of two, has joint pain and stiffness, decreased mobility, and increased frequency of fatigue. She is depressed.

1. The physician immediately suspects a diagnosis of _____, a diffuse connective tissue disease which the nurse knows manifests itself primarily in women.
   a. polymyositis
   b. rheumatoid arthritis
   c. scleroderma
   d. systemic lupus erythematosus

2. On initial examination, the physician notes that Jane's knees are hot, swollen, and painful. The physician orders specific laboratory studies. The test result, which is not significant for a diagnosis of rheumatoid arthritis, is:
   a. a decreased red blood count.
   b. an elevated C4 complement component.
   c. an elevated erythrocyte sedimentation rate.
   d. a positive C-reactive protein.

3. The nurse also assesses the four systemic features usually found with rheumatoid arthritis:

   a. _____

   b. _____

   c. _____

   d. _____

4. Jane is scheduled for an arthrocentesis. The nurse advises her that her knee joint will be anesthetized locally and a fluid specimen will be obtained. There is no special preparation or precautions after the procedure. Jane is told that a positive finding would be joint fluid that:
   a. contains few inflammatory cells.
   b. does not contain leukocytes.
   c. is viscous and tan in color.
   d. will not form a mucin clot.

5. A positive diagnosis of rheumatoid arthritis results in a multidisciplinary approach to treatment. Jane's pharmacotherapy regimen includes several drug classifications. A popular, NSAID that may be prescribed is:
   a. Aralen.
   b. Imuran.
   c. Motrin.
   d. Ridaura.

6. If Jane experiences gastric irritation and/or ulceration, the physician may order a new class of NSAIDs called _____.

7. A low-dose corticosteroid regimen is begun for a short period. The nurse advises Jane to be aware of certain drug-induced side effects, such as:
   a. elevated blood pressure.
   b. gastric upset.
   c. weight gain.
   d. all of the above.

CASE STUDY: Systemic Lupus Erythematosus

Brooke is a 41-year-old mother of two teenagers who has had symptoms of joint tenderness for about 10 years. Lately she has noticed significant morning stiffness and a slight rash over the bridge of her nose and cheeks. Her physician suspects a diagnosis of SLE.

1. Before beginning the assessment, the nurse knows that the etiology of SLE is an altered immune regulation that can be caused by disturbances in: _____, _____, _____, and _____.

2. The altered immune response can be described as: _____.

3. The nurse is aware that the physician will do a complete cardiovascular assessment, checking the patient for _____, _____, and _____.

4. Blood testing will be ordered to determine the presence of: _____, _____, _____, and _____.

5. The nurse knows that the physician may order _____ medications for treating Brooke's symptoms, if they are considered mild.

6. As part of health teaching, the nurse reminds Brooke that possible cardiovascular complications require periodic screening for _____ and _____.

Interpreting Patterns

Review Fig. 54–1 in the text, which depicts the results of the inflammatory response in the knee joint, as well as Fig. 54-3, which shows the pathophysiology of rheumatoid arthritis. Outline in detail the series of related steps that lead to the inflammation, beginning with the antigen stimulus that activates monocytes and T-lymphocytes.

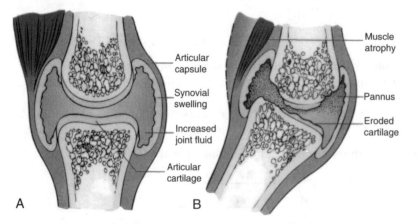

FIGURE 54–1 (A) Synovial swelling and fluid accumulation. (B) Pannus (a proliferation of synovial tissue), eroded articular cartilage, and joint space narrowing, all of which contribute to muscle atrophy and ankylosis (joint rigidity and immobility).

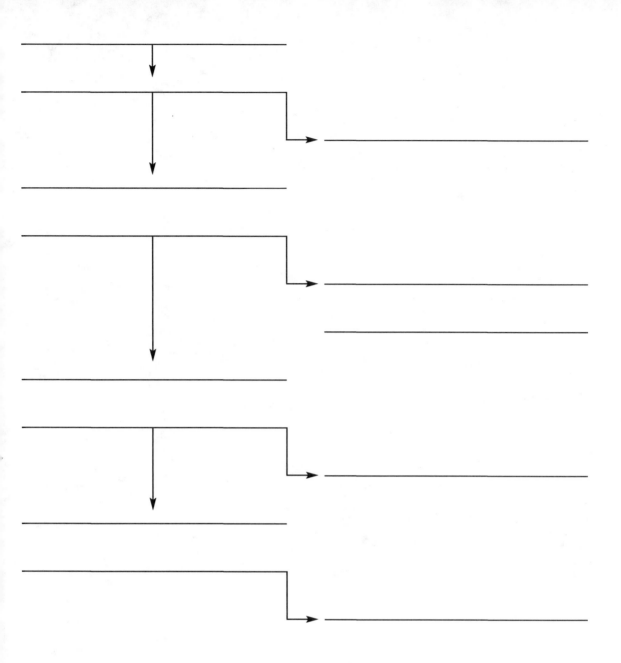

UNIT **12**
Integumentary Function

55

Assessment of Integumentary Function

I. Interpretation, Completion, and Comparison

Multiple Choice. Read each question carefully. Circle your answer.

1. For the average adult with a normal body temperature, a nurse needs to know that insensible water loss is approximately:
   a. 250 mL/day.
   b. 600 mL/day.
   c. 800 mL/day.
   d. 1000 mL/day.

2. When a nurse applies a cold towel to a patient's neck to reduce body heat, heat is reduced by:
   a. conduction.
   b. convection.
   c. evaporation.
   d. radiation.

3. Sweating, a process by which the body regulates heat loss, does not occur until the core body temperature exceeds the base level of:
   a. 24°C.
   b. 37°C.
   c. 43°C.
   d. 51°C.

4. In a dark-skinned person, color change that occurs in the presence of shock can be evidenced when the skin appears:
   a. ashen gray and dull.
   b. dusky blue.
   c. reddish pink.
   d. whitish pink.

5. Dark-skinned patients who have cherry-red nail beds, lips, and oral mucosa may be exhibiting signs of:
   a. anemia.
   b. carbon monoxide poisoning.
   c. polycythemia.
   d. shock.

6. A clinical example of a primary skin lesion known as a macule is:
   a. hives.
   b. impetigo.
   c. port-wine stains.
   d. psoriasis.

II. Critical Thinking Questions and Exercises

Analyzing Comparisons

Read each analogy. Fill in the space provided with the best response.

1. Keratin: skin hardening:: melanin: _____.
2. Bluish skin color: insufficient oxygenation:: yellow-green skin: _____.
3. Merkel cells: nervous system:: Langerhans cells: _____
4. Hirsutism: excessive hair growth:: _____: hair loss
5. Vitamin D deficiency: rickets:: vitamin C deficiency: _____.
6. Palpation: skin turgor:: _____ : vesicle.
7. Acne: a pustule:: psoriasis: _____.

Identifying Patterns

Consider the cutaneous manifestations of systemic disease listed in each grouping. Cluster the data to identify the skin manifestation.

Seen in systemic lupus erythematosus
Characterized by red, spidery lines
Appears in placques on the nose and ears
Seen on scales on the cheek area

1. _____

Appears as an ulcerated lesion
Is a painless chancre

2. _____

Seen in platelet disorders
Associated with vessel fragility
Characterized by purpura

3. _____

Occurs in infections
Seen with allergic reactions
Characteristic of drug reactions

4. _____

Present as macules, papules, plaques, or nodules
Lesions are visually multiple
Lesions are characteristically blue-red or dark brown
Seen in AIDS

5. _____

Identifying Pattersn

For each of the following eight primary or secondary lesions, document two defining characteristics.

1. Cherry angioma

   a. _____ b. _____

2. Crust

   a. _____ b. _____

3. Cyst

   a. _____ b. _____

4. Fissure

   a. _____ b. _____

5. Keloid

   a. _____ b. _____

6. Telangiectasis

   a. _____ b. _____

7. Petechia

   a. _____ b. _____

8. Spider Angioma

   a. _____ b. _____

Applying Concepts

For each pathophysiologic change in the skin that occurs with aging, list associated alterations in function.

1. Thinning of the dermis and epidermis at their junction (example)

   a. _____

   b. _____

   c. _____

   d. _____

2. Loss of subcutaneous tissue of elastin, fat, and collagen

   a. _____

   b. _____

   c. _____

3. Decreased cellular replacement

   a. _____

   b. _____

4. Decrease in the number and function of sweat and sebaceous glands

   a. _____

5. Reduced hormonal levels of androgens

   a. _____

56

Management of Patients With Dermatologic Problems

I. Interpretation, Completion, and Comparison

Multiple Choice. Read each question carefully. Circle your answer.

1. In the absence of infection or heavy discharge, chronic wounds should remain covered for:
   a. 6–12 hours.
   b. 12–24 hours.
   c. 24–36 hours.
   d. 48–72 hours.

2. Moisture-retentive dressings, more effective than wet compresses at removing exudate, should remain in place a minimum of:
   a. 3 hours.
   b. 6 hours.
   c. 12 hours.
   d. 18 hours.

3. A moisture-retentive dressing that promotes débridement and helps form granulation tissue is a _____ dressing.
   a. calcium alginate
   b. foam
   c. hydrocolloid
   d. hydrogel

4. Occlusive dressings applied to a dermatosis are used to:
   a. enhance the absorption of topical medications.
   b. improve hydration.
   c. increase the local skin temperature.
   d. do all of the above.

5. The nurse caring for a patient with an occlusive dressing knows to assess the skin every 12 hours for the potential complication of:
   a. local atrophy.
   b. striae.
   c. telangiectasia.
   d. all of the above.

6. The patient is advised to apply a suspension-type lotion to a dermatosis site. The nurse advises the patient that the lotion must be applied every ____ to be effective.
   a. hour
   b. 3 hours
   c. 12 hours
   d. day at the same time

7. The nurse knows to assess for the local side effect of _____ when corticosteroids are used for dermatologic conditions.
   - a. skin atropy
   - b. atriae
   - c. telangiectasia
   - d. all of the above

8. An example of a very potent corticosteroid used for treating a dermatologic condition is:
   - a. Aclovate
   - b. Aristocort
   - c. Temovate
   - d. Westcort

9. The most common symptom of pruritus is:
   - a. a rash.
   - b. itching.
   - c. flaking.
   - d. pain.

10. A nurse should assess all possible causes of pruritus, including the presence of endocrine disease, such as:
   - a. biliary cirrhosis.
   - b. hypothyroidism.
   - c. lymphoma.
   - d. multiple sclerosis.

11. Nurses should advise patients with pruritus to avoid all of the following *except*:
   - a. drying soaps.
   - b. emollient lubricants.
   - c. vigorous towel drying.
   - d. warm to hot water.

12. A systemic pharmacologic agent prescribed for nodular cystic acne is:
   - a. Accutane.
   - b. Benzoyl peroxide.
   - c. Retin-A.
   - d. Salicylic acid.

13. Management of follicular disorders includes all of the following *except*:
   - a. cleansing of the skin with an antibacterial soap to prevent spillage of bacteria to adjacent tissues.
   - b. rupture of the boil or pimple to release the pus.
   - c. systemic antibiotic therapy to treat the infection.
   - d. warm, moist compresses to increase resolution of the furuncle or carbuncle.

14. Herpes zoster (shingles) is:
   - a. a varicella-zoster viral infection related to chickenpox.
   - b. an inflammatory condition that produces vesicular eruptions along nerve pathways.
   - c. manifested by pain, itching, and tenderness.
   - d. characterized by all of the above.

15. The most common fungal infection that frequently affects young adults is:
   - a. tinea pedis.
   - b. tinea corporis.
   - c. tinea cruris.
   - d. tinea unguium.

16. Tinea capitis (ringworm of the scalp) can be identified by the presence of:
   - a. papules at the edges of inflamed patches.
   - b. circular areas of redness.
   - c. scaling and spots of baldness.
   - d. all of the above.

17. Patient education for the management of pediculosis capitis should include advising the patient to:
   - a. comb his or her hair with a fine-toothed comb dipped in vinegar to remove nits.
   - b. disinfect all combs and brushes.
   - c. wash his or her hair with a shampoo containing lindane (Kwell).
   - d. do all of the above.

18. A patient is complaining of severe itching that intensifies at night. The nurse decides to assess the skin using a magnifying glass and penlight to look for the "itch mite." The nurse suspects the skin condition known as:
   - a. contact dermatitis.
   - b. pediculosis.
   - c. scabies.
   - d. tinea corporis.

19. Psoriasis is an inflammatory dermatosis that results from:
   - a. a superficial infection with *Staphylococcus aureus*.
   - b. dermal abrasion.
   - c. epidermal proliferation.
   - d. excess deposition of subcutaneous fat.

20. The characteristic lesion of psoriasis is a:
   - a. circular patch covered with silver scales.
   - b. cluster of pustules.
   - c. group of raised vesicles.
   - d. pattern of bullae that rupture and form a scaly crust.

21. Exfoliate dermatitis is characterized by erythema and scaling and is associated with:
a. a loss of stratum corneum.
b. capillary leakage.
c. hypoproteinemia.
d. all of the above.

22. Nursing care for a patient with toxic epidermal necrolysis (TEN) should include:
a. inspection of the oral cavity.
b. assessment of urinary output.
c. application of topical skin agents.
d. all of the above actions.

23. The incidence of skin cancer in fair-skinned Americans is approximately:
a. 8%.
b. 12%.
c. 20%.
d. 35%.

24. The harmful effects of skin cancer may be severe by age:
a. 20 years.
b. 30 years.
b. 40 years.
d. 50 years.

25. The most lethal of all skin cancers is:
a. basal cell.
b. squamous cell.
c. malignant melanoma.
d. Kaposi's sarcoma.

26. Danger signals of melanoma include changes in a mole's:
a. color.
b. shape or outline.
c. size or surface.
d. all of the above.

27. The etiology of Kaposi's sarcoma is believed to be:
a. environmental.
b. genetic.
c. viral.
d. a combination of one or all of the above.

28. A living tissue transplant from the same person is known as:
a. an allograft.
b. an alloplastic implant.
c. an autograft.
d. a xenograft.

29. For a graft to "take,"
a. the area must be free of infection.
b. the recipient bed must have an adequate blood supply.
c. immobilization must be ensured.
d. all of the above conditions must be present.

Fill-In. *Read each statement carefully. Write your response in the space provided.*

1. Moisture-retentive dressings are very efficient at removing exudate because they:

_____.

2. Cytokines, a new advance in wound treatment, work by: _____.

3. A common nursing diagnosis for a patient with dermatosis would be: _____.

4. The most common skin condition in adolescents and young adults between the ages of 12 and 35 years is:

_____.

5. The most common primary bacterial skin infections are: _____ and _____.

6. Bullous impetigo, a deep-seated infection characterized by large, fluid-filled blisters, is caused by the

bacteria _____.

7. Two major complications of TEN and Stevens-Johnson syndrome (SJS) are: _____ and

_____.

8. The most common cancer in the United States is _____; the most common types of this

cancer are _____ and _____.

II. Critical Thinking Questions and Exercises

Discussion and Analysis

1. Explain the purpose and process of wet-to-dry dressings.
2. Discuss the advantages of moisture-retentive dressings over wet dressings.
3. Explain why a foul odor will be present when enzymatic débridement is used.

Clinical Applications

Read the following case studies. Fill in the blank spaces or circle the correct answer.

CASE STUDY: Acne Vulgaris

Brian is a 15-year-old who has been experiencing facial eruptions of acne for about a year. The numerous lesions are inflamed and present on the face and neck. He has tried many over-the-counter medications and nothing seems to help. His father had a history of severe acne when he was a teenager.

1. Based on knowledge of acne vulgaris, the nurse knows that the skin disorder is characterized by five types of lesions:

   _____,   _____,

   _____, _____, and   _____

2. The etiology of acne stems from:
   a. genetic factors.
   b. bacterial factors.
   c. hormonal factors.
   d. an interplay of all of the above.

3. Acne, most prevalent at puberty, is the direct result of oversecretion of the _____glands.
   a. exocrine   b. lacrimal   c. sebaceous   d. mucous

4. Explain the rationale for using benzoyl peroxide:

   _____

5. Explain the rationale for using synthetic vitamin A compounds (retinoids): _____

6. A common antibiotic that is frequently prescribed for treatment of acne is:
   a. terbutaline   b. tamoxifen   c. tetracycline   d. terfenadine

7. A common oral retinoid that is used for acne is:
   a. Accutane   b. Acne-Aid   c. Actinex   d. Adalat

8. Based on assessment data, identify two collaborative problems:

   _____ and _____

CASE STUDY: Malignant Melanoma

Steve is a 26-year-old professional baseball player for a Florida farm team. He spent many hours in the sun practicing between 9:00 AM and 4:00 PM. His V-neck uniform left little protection to his chest. Steve had a mole on his chest for 5 years. One day last October he noticed that the margins of the mole were elevated and palpable and the color had become darker. Since his father had malignant melanoma when he was 32 years old, Steve decided to see a physician.

1. Steve knows that malignant melanoma currently causes 2% of all cancers. Based on statistical predictions, the number of deaths in 10 years will be approximately:
   a. 2%.
   b. 4%.
   c. 5%.
   d. 10%.

2. On examination, the physician notes a circular lesion with irregular outer edges and a pinkish hue in the center. The physician suspected the lesion to be:
   a. an acral-lentiginous melanoma.
   b. a lentigo-maligna melanoma.
   c. a nodular melanoma.
   d. a superficial spreading melanoma.

3. The physician confirms the diagnosis by:
   a. complete blood count analysis.
   b. computed tomography.
   c. excisional biopsy.
   d. skin examination.

4. The lesion is greater than 14 mm in thickness and growing vertically. The physician knows that:
   a. dermal invasion is likely.
   b. the prognosis is favorable.
   c. metastasis is probable.
   d. peripheral growth will occur next.

5. The physician considers immunotherapy with a biologic response modifier such as:
   a. interferon alfa.
   b. BCG vaccine.
   c. *Cornebacterium parvum.*
   d. levamisole.

57

Management of Patients With Burn Injury

I. Interpretation, Completion, and Comparison

Multiple Choice. Read each question carefully. Circle your answer.

1. A full-thickness burn is:
   a. classified by the appearance of blisters.
   b. identified by the destruction of the entire dermis.
   c. not associated with edema formation.
   d. usually very painful because of exposed nerve endings.

2. With partial-thickness (second-degree) burns, skin regeneration begins to take place:
   a. within 7 days.
   b. in 2 to 4 weeks.
   c. after 2 months.
   d. between the third and sixth month.

3. Plasma seeps out into surrounding tissues after a burn. The greatest amount of fluid leaks out in:
   a. the first 2 hours.
   b. 4 to 8 hours.
   c. 12 hours.
   d. 24 to 36 hours.

4. As fluid is reabsorbed after injury, renal function maintains a diuresis for up to:
   a. 3 days.
   b. 1 week.
   c. 2 weeks.
   d. 1 month.

5. Fluid shifts during the first week of the acute phase of a burn injury that cause massive cell destruction result in:
   a. hypernatremia.
   b. hypokalemia.
   c. hyperkalemia.
   d. hypercalcemia.

6. An *unexpected* laboratory value during the fluid remobilization phase of a major burn is a:
   a. hematocrit of 45%.
   b. pH, 7.20; PaO_2, 38 mm Hg; and bicarbonate, 15 mEq/L.
   c. serum potassium of 3.2 mEq/L.
   d. serum sodium of 140 mEq/L.

7. Plasma leakage produces edema, which increases:
   a. circulating blood volume.
   b. the hematocrit level.
   c. systolic blood pressure.
   d. all of the above.

8. The leading cause of death in fire victims is believed to be:
   a. cardiac arrest.
   b. carbon monoxide intoxication.
   c. hypovolemic shock.
   d. septicemia.

9. A serious gastrointestinal disturbance that frequently occurs with a major burn is:
a. diverticulitis.
b. hematemesis.
c. paralytic ileus.
d. ulcerative colitis.

10. A child tips a pot of boiling water onto his bare legs. The mother should:
a. avoid touching the burned skin, and take the child to the nearest emergency department.
b. cover the child's legs with ice cubes secured with a towel.
c. immerse the child's legs in cool water.
d. liberally apply butter or shortening to the burned area.

11. A man suffers leg burns from spilled charcoal lighter fluid. His son extinguishes the flames. While waiting for an ambulance, the burn victim should:
a. have someone assist him into a bath of cool water, where he can wait for emergency personnel.
b. lie down, have someone cover him with a blanket, and cover his legs with petroleum jelly.
c. remove his burned pants so that the air can help cool the wound.
d. sit in a chair, elevate his legs, and have someone cut his pants off around the burned area.

12. As the first priority of care, a patient with a burn injury will initially need:
a. an airway established.
b. an indwelling catheter inserted.
c. fluids replaced.
d. pain medication administered.

13. Eyes that have been irritated or burned with a chemical should be flushed with cool, clean water:
a. immediately.
b. in 5 to 10 minutes.
c. after an eye examination.
d. after 24 hours.

14. Decreased urinary output during the first 48 hours of a major burn is secondary to all of the following *except*:
a. decreased adrenocortical activity.
b. hemolysis of red blood cells.
c. hypovolemia.
d. sodium retention.

15. Electrolyte changes in the first 48 hours of a major burn include:
a. base bicarbonate deficit.
b. hypernatremia.
c. hypokalemia.
d. all of the above.

16. The Evans formula for replacing fluid lost during the first 24 to 48 hours recommends the administration of:
a. colloids.
b. electrolytes.
c. glucose.
d. all of the above.

17. The most recent consensus formula for fluid replacement recommends that a balanced salt solution be administered in the first 24 hours of a burn in the range of 2 mL/kg/% of burn. A 176-lb (80-kg) man with a 30% burn should receive _____ in the first 8 hours.
a. 1200 mL
b. 2400 mL
c. 3600 mL
d. 4800 mL

18. One parameter of adequate fluid replacement is an hourly urinary output in the range of:
a. 10 to 30 mL.
b. 30 to 50 mL.
c. 80 to 120 mL.
d. 100 to 200 mL.

19. Fluid remobilization usually begins:
a. within the first 24 hours, when massive amounts of fluid are being administered intravenously.
b. after 48 hours, when fluid is being reabsorbed from the interstitial tissue.
c. after 1 week, when capillary permeability has returned to normal.
d. after 1 month, when scar tissue covers the wound and prevents evaporative fluid loss.

20. Wound cleansing and débridement usually begin when eschar begins to separate at:
a. 72 hours.
b. 1 week.
c. 1 ½ to 2 weeks.
d. 1 month.

21. Leukopenia within 48 hours is a side effect associated with the topical antibacterial agent:
a. cerium nitrate solution.
b. gentamicin sulfate.
c. sulfadiazine, silver (Silvadene).
d. mafenide (Sulfamylon).

22. After an occlusive dressing is applied to a burned foot, the foot should be placed in the position of:
a. adduction.
b. dorsiflexion.
c. external rotation.
d. plantar flexion.

23. Biologic dressings that use skin from living or recently deceased humans are known as:
a. autografts.
b. heterografts.
c. homografts.
d. xenografts.

24. The recommended route for administration of low-dose narcotics is:
a. intramuscular.
b. intravenous.
c. oral.
d. subcutaneous.

25. To meet his early nutritional demands for protein, a 198-lb (90-kg) burned patient will need to ingest a minimum of:
a. 90 g/day.
b. 110 g/day.
c. 180 g/day.
d. 270 g/day.

26. Early indicators of late-stage septic shock include all of the following *except:*
a. decreased pulse pressure.
b. a full, bounding pulse.
c. pale, cool skin.
d. renal failure.

Fill-In. Read each statement carefully. Write your response in the space provided.

1. The two age groups that are at high risk for burn injury are: _____ and _____ .

2. The majority of burn injuries occur: _____ .

3. Burn injuries are classified according to _____ and _____ .

4. List two pulmonary complications that occur secondary to inhalation injuries:

_____ and _____

5. The leading cause of death in themally injured patients is: _____ .

6. The analgesic of choice for acute burn pain is: _____ .

II. Critical Thinking Questions and Exercises

Discussion and Analysis

1. Explain why the survival rate for burn victims has increased significantly over the last 10 years.

2. Explain the pathophysiology of carbon mooxide poisoning.

3. Discuss why congestive heart failure is a potential complication of an acute burn.

Identifying Patterns

Complete the following flow chart illustrating the pathophysiologic sequence of reactions that result from a systemic response to a burn injury.

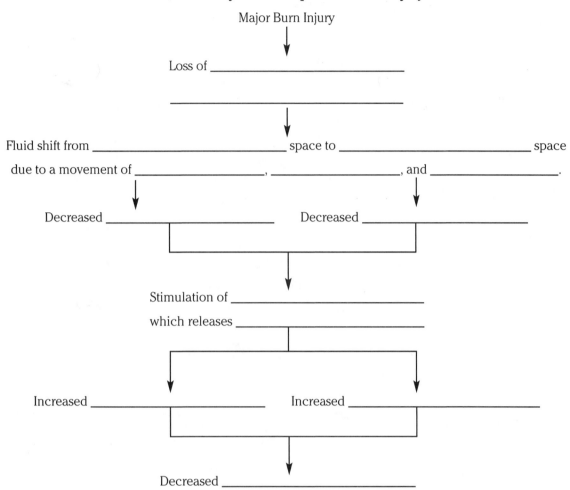

Flow Chart: Systemic Response to Burn Injury

Major Burn Injury

Loss of _____

_____

Fluid shift from _____ space to _____ space

due to a movement of _____, _____, and _____.

Decreased _____   Decreased _____

Stimulation of _____

which releases _____

Increased _____   Increased _____

Decreased _____

Clinical Situations

Develop a nursing care plan for each of the two situations below. For each nursing diagnosis, list goals, nursing actions, rationale, and expected outcomes.

Suggested Situations

1. Aimee, 9 months old, climbed onto a stove where an electric range was on high. Her pajamas caught fire, and she was burned over 60% of her body (excluding her face and neck) with second- and third-degree burns. Her mother managed to extinguish the flames and immerse her in a sink of cool water before emergency help arrived. Aimee was transported to a burn treatment center. There are two other preschool children in her family.

2. Brad, 12 years old, sustained full-thickness burns on his upper chest, face, and neck when he was trying to start a charcoal fire to prepare dinner for his father. His father sprayed him with water from a hose and took him to a hospital emergency department 3 miles away. On arrival Brad was semiconscious and in extreme respiratory distress. He and his divorced father live together.

UNIT 13
Sensorineural Function

58

Assessment and Management of Patients With Eye and Vision Disorders

I. Interpretation, Completion, and Comparison

Multiple Choice. Read each question carefully. Circle your answer.

1. Vision becomes less efficient with age, because aging is associated with:
   a. a decrease in pupil size.
   b. a slowing of accommodation.
   c. an increase in lens opaqueness.
   d. all of the above.

2. During a routine eye examination, a patient complains that she is unable to read road signs at a distance when driving her car. The physician knows to check for:
   a. astigmatism.
   b. anisometropia.
   c. myopia.
   d. presbyopia.

3. Legal blindness refers to visual acuity that is _____ or worse.
   a. 20/50
   b. 20/100
   c. 20/150
   d. 20/200

4. Increased ocular pressure is indicated by a reading of:
   a. 0 to 5 mm Hg.
   b. 6 to 10 mm Hg.
   c. 11 to 20 mm Hg.
   d. greater than 21 mm Hg.

5. A diagnostic clinical manifestation of glaucoma is:
   a. a significant loss of central vision.
   b. diminished acuity.
   c. pain associated with a purulent discharge.
   d. the presence of halos around lights.

6. When assessing the visual fields in acute glaucoma, the nurse would expect to find a:
   a. clear cornea.
   b. constricted pupil.
   c. marked blurring of vision.
   d. watery ocular discharge.

7. Pharmacotherapy for primary glaucoma that increases the outflow of aqueous humor would include all of the following *except:*
   a. α-adrenergic agonists.
   b. carbonic anhydrase inhibitors.
   c. β-blockers.
   d. miotics.

8. After cataract surgery, a patient is encouraged to:
   a. maintain bed rest for 1 week.
   b. lie on his or her stomach while sleeping.
   c. avoid bending his or her head below the waist.
   d. lift weights to increase muscle strength.

9. Clinical symptoms of a detached retina include:
   a. a sensation of floating particles.
   b. a definite area of blank vision.
   c. momentary flashes of light.
   d. all of the above.

10. The most common type of retinal detachment is:
   a. exudative.
   b. rhegmatogenous.
   c. traction.
   d. a combination of rhegmatogenous and traction.

11. The most common cause of visual loss in people older than 60 years of age is:
   a. macular degeneration.
   b. ocular trauma.
   c. retinal vascular disease.
   d. uveitis.

12. Chemical burns of the eye are treated with:
   a. local anesthetics and antibacterial drops for 24 to 36 hours.
   b. hot compresses applied at 15-minute intervals.
   c. flushing of the lids, conjunctiva, and cornea.
   d. cleansing of the conjunctiva with a small cotton-tipped applicator.

13. Acute conjunctivitis is associated with:
   a. blurred vision.
   b. elevated intraocular pressure.
   c. moderate to copious ocular discharge.
   d. severe pain.

14. The most common neoplasm of the eyelids is:
   a. basal cell carcinoma.
   b. a chalazion.
   c. xanthelasmas.
   d. squamous cell carcinoma.

15. Mydriatics and _____ are used in combination to dilate the patient's pupil.
   a. anti-infectives
   b. corticosteroids
   c. cyclopedics
   d. NSAIDs

16. The most common antifungal agent used to treat eye infections is:
   a. acyclovir
   b. amphotericin
   c. ganciclovir
   d. penicillin

Fill-In. *Read the statement carefully. Write your response in the space provided.*

1. List three leading causes of visual impairment:

_____, _____, and _____

2. The leading cause of irreversible blindness in the world is: _____.

3. Two significant changes in the optic nerve in glaucoma are: _____ and _____.

4. The most common laser surgeries for glaucoma are: _____ and _____.

5. The leading cause of blindness in the world is the presence of: _____.

6. An initial treatment for a splash injury to the eye would be: _____.

7. The most common microorganisms that cause conjuctivitis are: _____, _____,

and _____.

8. One of the most serious ocular consequences of diabetes mellitus is: _____.

Matching. *Match the characteristic or function of the eye listed in Column II with its associated structure listed in Column I.*

Column I

1._____ choroid

2._____ lens

3._____ pupil

4._____ retina

5._____ vitreous humor

6._____ cornea

7._____ sclera

8._____ iris

9._____ uvea

10._____ limbus

Column II

a. maintains the form of the eyeball

b. area where most of the blood vessels for the eye are located

c. degree of convexity modified by contraction and relaxation of the ciliary muscles

d. contractile membrane between the cornea and lens

e. transparent part of the fibrous coat of the eyeball

f. accommodates to the intensity of light by dilating or contracting

g. white part of the eye

h. the pigmented, vascular coating of the eye

i. the edge of the cornea where it joins the sclera

j. contains nerve endings that transmit visual impulses to the brain

Complete the following crossword puzzle using common ophthalmologic terms.

Crossword Puzzle

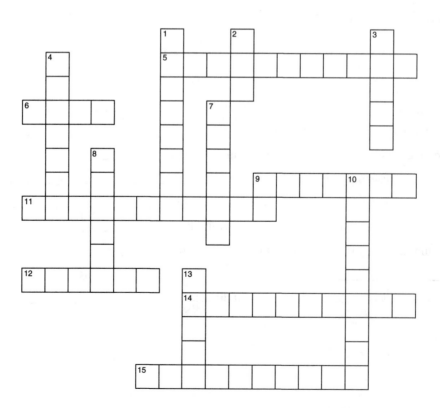

Down

1. Excessive production of tears
2. Another term for an external hordeolum
3. The term *oculus dexter* refers to the _____ eye
4. A term used to describe an inflammatory condition of the uveal tract
7. Another term for nearsightedness
8. An inflammatory condition affecting the iris
9. People who are photosensitive function better outdoors during this time of day
10. Inflammation of the cornea
13. A loss of cornea substance or tissue as a result of inflammation

Across

5. Abnormal sensitivity to light
6. The term *oculus sinister* refers to the _____ eye
9. Absence of the lens
11. Uneven curvature of the cornea
12. Drooping of the upper eyelid
14. A tear in the eye tissue
15. A condition in which one eye deviates from the object at which the person is looking

II. Critical Thinking Questions and Exercises

Identifying Patterns

Analyze the following clusters of information about disorders of the eyes and identify the specific disorder.

A chronic inflammation of the eyelid margins
Formation of scales and granulations on the eyelashes
White eyelashes may result from this condition
Staphylococcus aureus may be a primary infecting organism

1. _____

A superficial infection of the glands of the eyelids
Pain and swelling of the eyelids are characteristic signs
Warm, moist compresses on the eyelids facilitate healing
Topical sulfonamides may be prescribed

2. _____

Symptoms include hyperemia and edema of conjunctiva
Etiology may be bacterial, fungal, viral, or allergic
Lay person's term for condition is "pink-eye"

3. _____

Corneal edema is a common sign in this disorder
Ulceration and infection are associated with this disorder
Cycloplegics and mydriatics may be prescribed
Etiology is usually associated with trauma or compromise
Systemic or local defense mechanisms

4. _____

Characterized by an opacification of the lens
Usually associated with the aging process
Vision is clouded because light to the retina is blocked
Associated with compromised night vision

5. _____

Clinical Situations

Nursing Care Plan

Develop a nursing care plan based on the following clinical situation.

Elise is 65 years old and needs to have cataract surgery on her right eye. Elise lives with her daughter in a three-story house and has rheumatoid arthritis. She needs a cane to walk. Her daughter has a Down's syndrome child at home who requires constant care. Share your nursing care plan with your instructor for comments.

Nursing Diagnoses:

Goals	Nursing Actions	Rationale	Expected Outcomes

CASE STUDY: Cataract Surgery

Marcella is a 75-year-old single woman who has had progressive diminished vision and increased difficulty with night driving. Her physician suspects that Marcella has a cataract. He does a complete eye examination and history.

1. As part of an oral history, the physician tries to determine whether Marcella has any of the common factors that contribute to cataract development, such as: _____, _____, _____, and _____.

2. Marcella, during her history, told the physician that she was experiencing the three common symptoms found with cataracts: _____, _____, and _____.

3. On ophthalmic examination, the physician noted the major objective finding seen with cataracts: _____.

4. When assessing the need for surgery, the physician determined that Marcella's best corrected vision was worse than the minimal standard of:
   a. 20/15   b. 20/25   c. 20/35   d. 20/50

5. The physician decided to perform _____, the most preferred technique for cataract surgery.

6. The physician advised Marcella that there is a 25% chance that she may experience the common complication of:
   a. glucoma.   b. uveitis.   c. secondary membranes.   d. choroidal detachment.

7. Postoperatively, Marcella knows that she will need to wear an eye shield at night for about:
   a. 3 evenings.   b. 1 week.   c. 2 weeks.   d. 1 month.

59

Assessment and Management of Patients With Hearing and Balance Disorders

I. Interpretation, Completion, and Comparison

Multiple Choice. Read each question carefully. Circle your answer.

1. The organ of hearing is known as the:
   a. cochlea.
   b. eardrum.
   c. semicircular canal.
   d. stapes.

2. Mechanical vibrations are transformed into neural activity so that sounds can be differentiated by the:
   a. cochlea.
   b. organ of Corti.
   c. ossicles.
   d. semicircular canals.

3. To straighten the ear canal for examination, the nurse would grasp the auricle and pull it:
   a. backward.
   b. upward.
   c. slightly outward.
   d. in all of these directions.

4. A sensorineural (perceptive) hearing loss results from impairment of the:
   a. eighth cranial nerve.
   b. middle ear.
   c. outer ear.
   d. seventh cranial nerve.

5. The critical level of loudness that most people (without a hearing loss) are comfortable with is a decibel (dB) reading of:
   a. 15 dB.
   b. 30 dB.
   c. 45 dB.
   d. 60 dB.

6. Severe hearing loss is associated with a decibel loss in the range of:
   a. 25 to 40 dB.
   b. 40 to 55 dB.
   c. 70 to 90 dB.
   d. more than 90 dB.

7. A hearing loss that is a manifestation of an emotional disturbance is known as a ____ hearing loss.
   a. conductive
   b. functional
   c. mixed
   d. sensorineural

8. The minimum noise level known to cause noise-induced hearing loss, regardless of duration, is:
   a. 55–60 dB
   b. 65–70 dB
   c. 75–80 dB
   d. 85–90 dB

9. Hearing loss occurs in about ____ of those between 65 and 75 years of age.

a. 15%

b. 25%

c. 40%

d. 75%

10. Changes in the ear that occur with aging may include:

a. atrophy of the tympanic membrane.

b. increased hardness of the cerumen.

c. degeneration of cells at the base of the cochlea.

d. all of the above.

11. The most common fungus associated with ear infections is:

a. *Staphylococcus albus.*

b. *Staphylococcus aureus.*

c. *Aspergillus.*

d. *Pseudomonas.*

12. Nursing instructions for a patient suffering from external otitis should include the:

a. application of heat to the auricle.

b. avoidance of swimming.

c. ingestion of over-the-counter analgesics such as aspirin.

d. all of the above.

13. A symptom that is *not* usually found with acute otitis media is:

a. aural tenderness.

b. rhinitis.

c. otalgia.

d. otorrhea.

14. An incident of otitis media is usually associated with:

a. ear canal swelling.

b. discharge.

c. intense ear pain.

d. prominent localized tenderness.

15. A myringotomy is performed primarily to:

a. drain purulent fluid.

b. identify the infecting organism.

c. relieve tympanic membrane pressure.

d. accomplish all of the above.

16. A tympanoplasty, the most common procedure for chronic otitis media, is surgically performed to:

a. close a perforation.

b. prevent recurrent infection.

c. reestablish middle ear function.

d. accomplish all of the above.

17. Postoperative nursing assessment for a patient who has had a mastoidectomy should include observing for facial paralysis, which might indicate damage to the ____ cranial nerve.

a. first

b. fourth

c. seventh

d. tenth

18. A facial nerve neuroma is a tumor on the _____ cranial nerve.

a. third

b. fifth

c. seventh

d. eighth

19. A dietary modification for a patient with Meniere's disease would be:

a. a decrease in sodium intake to 200 mg daily.

b. fluid restriction to 2.0 L/day.

c. an increase in calcium to 1.0 g/day.

d. an increase in vitamin C to 1.5 g/day.

20. An acoustic neuroma is a benign tumor of the _____ cranial nerve:

a. fifth

b. sixth

c. seventh

d. eighth

II. Critical Thinking Questions and Exercises

Examining Associations

View Figure 59–1 below. For each anatomic area labeled, write the associated physiologic function.

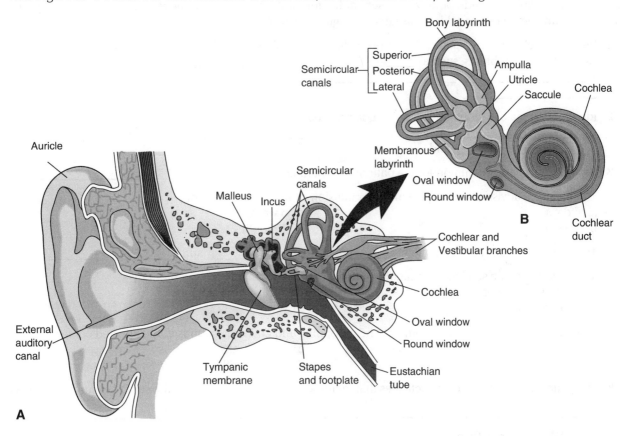

FIGURE 59-1 (*A*) Anatomy of the ear and (*B*) the inner ear.

1. Auricle _____

2. Malleus _____

3. Incus _____

4. Semicircular canals _____

5. Cochlea _____

6. Oval window _____

7. Round window _____

8. Eustachian tube _____

9. Stapes _____

10. Tympanic membrane _____

11. External auditory canal _____

Clinical Situations

Read the following case studies. Fill in the blanks or circle the correct answer.

CASE STUDY: Mastoid Surgery

Amber is a 73-year-old grandmother who is scheduled for mastoid surgery to remove a cholesteatoma, a cystlike sac filled with keratin debris, which was large enough to occlude the ear canal.

1. Preoperatively, the physician reviews the results of the audiogram and assesses for the presence of associated ear problems, such as:_____, _____, _____, _____, _____, _____, and _____.

2. Identify four major preoperative nursing goals for the patient:
   _____, _____,
   _____, and _____

3. Postoperatively, it is common for the patient to experience: _____.

4. The patient is advised that the postauricular incision should be kept dry for:
   a. 7 days.
   b. 2 weeks.
   c. 6 weeks.
   d. 1 month.

5. Two important signs of infection are: _____ and _____.

6. Manipulation of the semicircular canals during surgery may result in the symptom of:
   a. sharp, shooting pain.
   b. inner ear fullness.
   c. purulent drainage.
   d. vertigo.

7. The patient is advised that it is normal to hear popping and crackling sounds in the affected ear for about:
   a. 3 days.
   b. 1 week.
   c. 3 to 5 weeks.
   d. 2 to 4 months.

8. The patient is taught to prevent activities that increase intracranial pressure for 3 weeks after surgery, such as:
   _____, _____, and _____.

CASE STUDY: Menière's Disease

David is a 42-year-old lawyer who travels internationally. He has recently been diagnosed with Menière's disease.

1. The classic triad of symptoms that are diagnostic for Menière's disease are: _____, _____, and _____.

2. The basic pathophysiology causing the triad of symptoms listed in the previous question is:

   _____.

3. The most common and disrupting clinical symptom of this disease is: _____.

4. A diet for Menière's disease would include avoiding:
   a. bread.
   b. cheese.
   c. eggs.
   d. milk.

5. A popular medication prescribed to suppress the vestibular system is:
   a. Antivert.
   b. Lasix.
   c. Phenergan.
   d. Valium.

6. The most popular surgical procedure used to treat this disease is:
   a. endolymphatic sac decompression.
   b. labyrinthectomy.
   c. middle ear perfusion.
   d. vestibular nerve section.

UNIT 14
Neurologic Function

60

Assessment of Neurologic Function

I. Interpretation, Completion, and Comparison

Multiple Choice. Read each question carefully. Circle your answer.

1. A person's personality and judgment are controlled by that area of the brain known as the _____ lobe.
   a. frontal
   b. occipital
   c. parietal
   d. temporal

2. The lobe of the cerebral cortex that influences sensation is the _____ lobe.
   a. frontal
   b. occipital
   c. parietal
   d. temporal

3. Voluntary muscle control is governed by a vertical band of "motor cortex" located in the _____ lobe.
   a. frontal
   b. occipital
   c. parietal
   d. temporal

4. The sleep regulator and the site of the hunger center is known as the:
   a. hypothalamus.
   b. medulla oblongata.
   c. pituitary gland.
   d. thalamus.

5. The overall supervision of the autonomic nervous system is the function of the:
   a. cerebellum.
   b. hypothalamus.
   c. pons.
   d. temporal lobe of the cerebral cortex.

6. The "master gland" is also known as the _____ gland.
   a. adrenal
   b. thyroid
   c. pineal
   d. pituitary

7. The major receiving and communication center for afferent sensory nerves is the:
   a. medulla oblongata.
   b. pineal body.
   c. pituitary gland.
   d. thalamus.

8. The normal adult produces 125 to 150 mL of cerebrospinal fluid daily from the:
   a. ventricles.
   b. dura mater.
   c. circle of Willis.
   d. corpus callosum.

9. The spinal cord tapers off to a fibrous band of tissue at the level of the:
a. coccygeal nerve.
b. first lumbar vertebra.
c. lateral ventricle.
d. medulla oblongata.

10. The preganglionic fibers of the sympathetic neurons are located in those segments of the spinal cord identified as:
a. C1–T1.
b. C3–L1.
c. C8–L3.
d. T1–S5.

11. Parasympathetic impulses are mediated by the secretion of:
a. acetylcholine.
b. epinephrine.
c. norepinephrine.
d. all of the above.

12. Motor axons form pyramidal tracts that cross to the opposite side. This crossed pyramidal tract occurs in the brain in the area of the:
a. frontal cerebrum.
b. lateral portion of the cerebellum.
c. medulla oblongata.
d. pons.

13. The brain center responsible for balancing and coordination is the:
a. cerebellum.
b. second lumbar vertebra.
c. first sacral nerve.
d. sacrum.

14. The Romberg test is used to assess:
a. balance and coordination.
b. muscle strength.
c. biceps reflex.
d. muscle tone.

15. The Babinski response is used to assess:
a. muscle strength.
b. coordination.
c. central nervous system disease.
d. optical nerve damage.

16. Myelography with an oil-based medium requires the patient to lie ____ for 12 to 24 hours to reduce leakage of cerebrospinal fluid.
a. in high Fowler's position
b. in bed with head elevated 30 to 45 degrees
c. prone
d. recumbent

17. Patient preparation for electroencephalography includes omitting, for 24 hours before the test, all of the following *except*:
a. coffee and tea.
b. solid foods.
c. stimulants.
d. tranquilizers.

18. For a lumbar puncture, the nurse should assist the patient to flex his or her head and thighs while lying on the side so that the needle can be inserted between the:
a. fourth and fifth cervical vertebrae.
b. fifth and sixth thoracic vertebrae.
c. third and fourth lumbar vertebrae.
d. first and second sacral vertebrae.

Matching. Match the neurotransmitter listed in Column II with its definitive action listed in Column I

Column I

1. _____ γ-aminobutyric acid

2. _____ enkephalin

3. _____ norepinephrine

4. _____ dopamine

5. _____ acetylcholine

6. _____ serotonin

Column II

a. primarily excitatory; can produce vagal stimulation of heart

b. inhibits pain pathways and can control sleep

c. affects behavior, attention, and fine movement

d. excitatory response, mostly affecting moods

e. muscle and nerve inhibitory transmissions

f. excitatory; inhibits pain transmission

II. Critical Thinking Questions and Exercises

Examining Associations

Autonomic Nervous System

Write the effects produced by the parasympathetic and sympathetic nervous systems on each organ or tissue listed in Column I. Use the terms provided, and document in the space below. The answers for the first tissue are provided as an example.

Terms to be used
    acceleration
    constriction
    dilation
    inhibition
    increased motility
    secretion

Organ or Tissue	Parasympathetic Effect	Sympathetic Effect
a. bronchi	constriction	dilation
b. cerebral vessels		
c. coronary vessels		
d. heart		
e. iris of the eye		
f. salivary glands		
g. smooth muscle of		
(1) bladder wall		
(2) large intestine		
(3) small intestine		

Cranial Nerves

Next to each cranial nerve listed by number, write the appropriate corresponding terminology in Column I and a major associated function in Column II. The answers for the first cranial nerve are provided as an example.

Nerve No.	Column I	Column II
I	olfactory	smell
II		
III		
IV		
V		
VI		
VII		
VIII		
IX		

X _____   _____

XI _____   _____

XII _____   _____

Diagram of the Brain

View Figure 60–3 and list the major functions of each identified area.

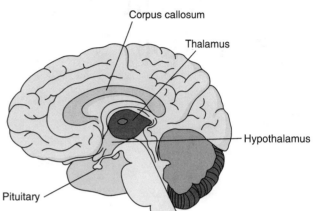

FIGURE 60–3 Medial view of the brain.

Thalamus	*Hypothalamus*	*Pituitary*
1. _____	1. _____	1. _____
2. _____	2. _____	2. _____
	3. _____	
	4. _____	
	5. _____	
	6. _____	
	7. _____	
	8. _____	

61

Management of Patients With Neurologic Dysfunction

I. Interpretation, Completion, and Comparison

Multiple Choice. Read each question carefully. Circle your answer.

1. Unconsciousness may have a _____ origin.
   a. neurologic
   b. metabolic
   c. toxicologic
   d. multisystem involvement

2. The first priority of treatment for a patient with altered level of consciousness is:
   a. assessment of pupillary light reflexes.
   b. determination of the cause.
   c. positioning to prevent complications.
   d. maintenance of a patent airway.

3. A nurse assesses the patient's level of consciousness using the Glasgow Coma Scale. The score of _____ indicates severe impairment of neurologic function.
   a. 3
   b. 6
   c. 9
   d. 12

4. The most severe neurologic impairments are evidenced by abnormal body posturing defined as:
   a. decerebrate.
   b. decorticate.
   c. flaccid.
   d. rigid.

5. The normal range of intracranial pressure (ICP) is:
   a. 5 to 8 mm Hg.
   b. 10 to 20 mm Hg.
   c. 20 to 30 mm Hg.
   d. 25 to 40 mm Hg.

6. Intracranial pressure can be increased by a:
   a. decrease in venous outflow.
   b. dilation of the cerebral blood vessels.
   c. rise in $PaCO_2$.
   d. change in all of the above.

7. Initial compensatory vital sign changes with increased ICP include all of the following *except*:
   a. a slow, bounding pulse.
   b. an increased systemic blood pressure.
   c. a decreased temperature.
   d. respiratory rate irregularities.

8. Irreversible neurologic dysfunction occurs when the cerebral perfusion pressure (CPP) is:
   a. less than 50 mm Hg.
   b. 60–80 mm Hg.
   c. 75–95 mm Hg.
   d. greater than 100 mm Hg.

9. A nurse knows that a patient experiencing Cushing's triad would *not* exhibit:
   a. bradycardia.
   b. bradypnea.
   c. hypertension.
   d. tachycardia.

10. The earliest sign of serious impairment of brain circulation related to increasing ICP is:
   a. a bounding pulse.
   b. bradycardia.
   c. hypertension.
   d. lethargy and stupor.

11. As ICP rises, the nurse knows that she may be asked to give _____, a commonly used osmotic diuretic.
   a. glycerin
   b. isosorbide
   c. mannitol
   d. urea

12. An indicator of compromised respiratory status significant enough to require mechanical ventilation for an average-weight adult patient with a neurologic dysfunction would be:
   a. an expiratory reserve volume of 1300 mL.
   b. an inspiratory capacity of 3000 mL.
   c. a residual volume of 1400 mL.
   d. a vital capacity of 1000 mL.

13. Nursing care activities for a patient with increased ICP would *not* include:
   a. assisting the patient with isometric exercises.
   b. avoiding activities that interfere with venous drainage of blood from the head.
   c. use of a cervical collar.
   d. teaching the patient to exhale when being turned (to avoid the Valsalva maneuver).

14. A nurse assessing urinary output as an indicator of diabetes insipidus knows that an hourly output of _____ over 2 hours may be a positive indicator.
   a. 50–100 mL/hour
   b. 100–150 mL/hour
   c. 150–200 mL/hour
   d. more than 200 mL/hour

15. Neurologic and neurosurgical approaches to pain relief would include:
   a. stimulation procedures.
   b. administration of intraspinal opiates.
   c. interruption of nerve tracts that conduct pain.
   d. all of the above mechanisms.

16. Postcraniotomy cerebral edema is at a maximum _____ after brain surgery.
   a. 6 hours
   b. 12 to 20 hours
   c. 24 to 72 hours
   d. 3 to 5 days

17. The majority of cases of epilepsy occur in those:
   a. younger than 20 years of age.
   b. 25–35 years of age.
   c. approximately 45 years of age.
   d. older than 60 years of age.

18. Long-term use of anti-seizure medication in women leads to an increased incidence of:
   a. anemia.
   b. osteoarthritis.
   c. osteoporosis.
   d. obesity.

19. Nursing care for a patient who is experiencing a convulsive seizure includes all of the following *except*:
   a. loosening constrictive clothing.
   b. opening the patient's jaw and inserting a mouth gag.
   c. positioning the patient on his or her side with head flexed forward.
   d. providing for privacy.

20. A seizure characterized by loss of consciousness and tonic spasms of the trunk and extremities, rapidly followed by repetitive generalized clonic jerking, is classified as a:
   a. focal seizure.
   b. generalized seizure.
   c. Jacksonian seizure.
   d. partial seizure.

21. Headaches classified as *primary* would include all of the following *except*:
   a. aneurysm.
   b. cluster.
   c. migrane.
   d. tension.

22. A popular drug used for the prevention of a migraine headache is:
   a. Cafergot.
   b. Inderal.
   c. Sansert.
   d. Seconal.

Fill-In. *Read each statement carefully. Write your response in the space provided.*

1. Potential collaborative problems for a patient with an altered level of consciousness would include:_____, _____, _____, _____, and _____.

2. List three major potential complications in a patient with a depressed level of consciousness: _____, _____, and _____

3. The earliest sign of increased ICP is: _____.

4. List three primary complications of increased ICP: _____, _____, and _____

5. List six treatment goals for the prompt management of increased ICP:

    _____, _____, _____,

    _____, _____, and _____

6. Name four ICP monitoring devices that a nurse may be asked to manage:

    _____, _____,

    _____, and _____

7. Name three complications of intracranial surgery:

    _____, _____, and _____

8. The leading cause of seizures in the elderly is: _____.

9. A major potential complication of epilepsy is: _____.

10. List six "triggers" known to cause migraine headaches:

    _____, _____, _____,

    _____, _____, and _____

Matching. *Match the neurologic dysfunction in Column II with its associated nursing interventions found in Column I. An answer may be used more than once.*

Column I

1._____ Assist with daily active or passive range of motion.

2._____ Elevate the head of the bed 30 degrees.

3._____ Institute a bowel-training program.

4._____ Maintain dorsiflexion to affected area.

5._____ Place the patient in a lateral position.

Column II

a. footdrop

b. incontinence

c. impaired cough reflex

d. keratitis

e. paralyzed diaphragm

f. paralyzed extremity

II. Critical Thinking Questions and Exercises

Discussion and Analysis

1. Describe some nursing interventions for maintaining the airway for a patient with an altered level of consciousness.

2. Explain the rationale for reducing body temperature in patients with cerebral disorders.

3. Describe the nursing management of a patient during a seizure

Interpreting Patterns

Complete the following analogies by inserting the word that reflects the association.

1. Craniotomy: surgery involving entry into the cranial vault:: Craniectomy: _____.

2. Cushing's response: increased arterial pressure in response to increased intracranial pressure:: Cushing's triad: _____.

3. Decerebration: extreme extension of the upper and lower extremities::_____: abnormal flexion of the upper extremities.

4. A primary headache: controllable localized pain:: Migraine headache: _____.

5. Ataxic breathing: random sequences of deep and shallow breaths:: Cheyne-Stokes breathing: _____.

Clinical Situations

Read the following case study. Develop a plan of care using the format shown below.

Miss Potter, a 32-year-old, single circus performer has been unconscious since she was admitted to the hospital 1 week ago after falling from a high wire. Her family must leave the area to travel with the circus and is expected to return in 2 months.

Nursing Diagnoses:

Goals	Nursing Actions	Rationale	Expected Outcomes

62

Management of Patients With Cerebrovascular Disorders

I. Interpretation, Completion, and Comparison

Multiple Choice. *Read each question carefully. Circle your answer.*

1. As a cause of death in the United States, stroke currently ranks:
   a. second.
   b. third.
   c. fourth.
   d. fifth.

2. The most common cause of cerebrovascular disease is:
   a. arteriosclerosis.
   b. embolism.
   c. hypertensive changes.
   d. vasospasm.

3. The majority of ischemic strokes are _____ in origin.
   a. cardiogenic embolic
   b. cryptogenic
   c. large artery thrombotic
   d. small artery thromotic

4. Approximately _____ of patients who experience a transient ischemic attack (TIA) will have a stroke within 3 years.
   a. 5%
   b. 20%
   c. 40%
   d. 80%

5. The degree of neurologic damage that occurs with an ischemic stroke depends on the:
   a. location of the lesion.
   b. size of the area of inadequate perfusion.
   c. amount of collateral blood flow.
   d. combination of the above factors.

6. The initial mortality rate for a stroke can be as high as:
   a. 10%.
   b. 20%.
   c. 30%.
   d. 50%.

7. The most common motor dysfunction of a stroke is:
   a. ataxia.
   b. diplopia.
   c. dysphagia.
   d. hemiplegia.

8. The initial diagnostic test for a stroke, usually performed in the Emergency Department, is a:
   a. 12-lead electrocardiogram.
   b. carotid ultrasound study.
   c. noncontrast computed tomogram.
   d. transcranial Doppler flow study.

9. To be effective, thrombolytic therapy must be given to a stroke patient within a timeframe of _____ hours after onset of the stroke.
   a. 3
   b. 6–12
   c. 18
   d. 24–48

10. An emergency room nurse understands that a 110-lb recent stroke victim will receive at least the minimum dose of recombinant tissue plasminogen activator (t-PA). The patient will receive a minimum of _____ of t-PA.
   a. 45 mg
   b. 60 mg
   c. 85 mg
   d. 100 mg

11. The most common side-effect of t-PA is:
   a. an allergic reaction.
   b. bleeding.
   c. severe vomiting.
   d. a second stroke in 6–12 hours.

12. Hemorrhagic stroke is primarily caused by:
   a. an embolus.
   b. a cerebral thrombus.
   c. a brain tumor.
   d. uncontrolled hypertension.

13. Most patients who suffer hemorrhagic strokes are placed in bed in the _____ position.
   a. high-Fowler's
   b. prone
   c. supine
   d. semi-Fowler's (head of bed at 30 degrees)

Fill-In. *Read each statement carefully. Write your response in the space provided.*

1. The primary cerebrovascular disorder in the United States is _____, recently given the term _____ to emphasize the urgency of its occurrence.

2. Four non-modifiable risk factors for stroke are:
   _____, _____,
   _____, and _____

3. Four classifications of stroke using the time course are:
   _____, _____,
   _____, and _____

4. Define the term *bruit:*_____.

5. The main surgical procedure for managing TIAs is: _____.

6. Two possible collaborative problems for a patient recovering from an ischemic stroke are:
   _____ and _____.

7. Hemorrhagic strokes are caused by bleeding into _____, _____, or _____.

8. Almost 50% of the mortality and morbidity associated with hemorrhagic stroke is due to:
   _____.

9. Immediate complications of a hemorrhagic stroke are: _____, _____, and
   _____.

Matching. *Match the clinical manifestations of specific neurologic deficits listed in Column II with its associated cause listed in Column I.*

Column I

1. _____ataxia

2. _____receptive aphasia

3. _____dysphagia

4. _____homonymous hemianopsia

5. _____loss of peripheral vision

6. _____expressive aphasia

7. _____diplopia

8. _____paresthesia

Column II

a. difficulty judging distances

b. unaware of the borders of objects

c. double vision

d. staggering, unsteady gait

e. difficulty in swallowing

f. difficulty with proprioception

g. unable to form words that are understandable

h. unable to comprehend the spoken word

II. Critical Thinking Questions and Exercises

Discussion and Analysis

1. Explain the pathophysiology of a brain attack.

2. Describe the focus of nursing interventions when helping a patient recover from an ischemic stroke.

Clinical Situations

Construct a nursing care plan for Mrs. Coe.

Mrs. Coe recently sustained an ischemic stroke. She is 41 years old and lives with her husband and three sons. Emphasize the rehabilitative phase, which should have begun with her diagnosis, and stress the retraining of her flaccid right upper and lower extremities. She also needs to be taught how to sit, stand, and walk with balance and how to use a wheelchair.

Nursing Diagnoses:

Goals	Nursing Actions	Rationale	Expected Outcomes

63

Management of Patients With Neurologic Trauma

I. Interpretation, Completion, and Comparison

Multiple Choice. *Read each question carefully. Circle your answer.*

1. All of the following statements about the occurrence of head injuries are correct *except*:
   a. Almost 70% of all victims are younger than 30 years of age.
   b. An estimated 100,000 persons die annually from these injuries.
   c. Motor vehicle crashes are the primary cause.
   d. The majority of injuries occur in females.

2. A cerebral hemorrhage located within the brain is classified as:
   a. an epidural hematoma.
   b. an extradural hematoma.
   c. an intracerebral hematoma.
   d. a subdural hematoma.

3. Comatose patients are mechanically ventilated to control intracranial pressure (ICP). Hypocapnia is a goal that can be achieved with a $PaCO_2$ in the range of:
   a. 10 to 25 mm Hg.
   b. 25 to 30 mm Hg.
   c. 30 to 35 mm Hg.
   d. 35 to 40 mm Hg.

4. The Glasgow Coma Scale is used to determine the level of consciousness. A score considered indicative of a coma is:
   a. 1.
   b. 3.
   c. 5.
   d. 7.

5. Assessing the level of consciousness is an important nursing measure postinjury. Signs of increasing ICP include:
   a. bradycardia.
   b. increased systolic blood pressure.
   c. widening pulse pressure.
   d. all of the above.

6. An indicator of elevated body temperature in a head-injured patient is:
   a. cerebral irritation from hemorrhage.
   b. damage to the hypothalamus.
   c. infection.
   d. all of the above.

7. To prevent decreased cerebral perfusion after brain injury, the nurse knows that cerebral perfusion pressure must be at a minimum reading of:

a. 15 mm Hg.

b. 30 mm Hg.

c. 50 mm Hg.

d. 70 mm Hg.

8. Cerebral edema and swelling that peaks ____ after the injury is a common cause of increased ICP.

a. 12 hours

b. 12 to 24 hours

c. 2 to 3 days

d. 7 days

9. Posttraumatic seizures that are classified as *late* occur more than ____ after the injury.

a. 48 hours

b. 72 hours

c. 4 to 6 days

d. 7 days

10. Most victims of spinal cord injury are:

a. 30 years of age or younger.

b. 30 to 40 years of age.

c. 40 to 50 years of age.

d. 50 years of age or older.

11. In the United States, the number of new spinal cord injuries each year averages approximately:

a. 5000 cases.

b. 11,000 cases.

c. 15,000 cases.

d. 25,000 cases.

12. The primary cause of spinal cord injuries is:

a. gunshot wounds.

b. industrial accidents.

c. sports activities.

d. motor vehicle crashes.

13. Spinal cord injury can be classified according to the area of spinal cord damage. Motor deficits in the upper rather than the lower extremities, usually due to edema in the cervical area, is classified as _____ syndrome.

a. anterior cord

b. Brown-Sequard

c. central cord

d. peripheral

14. Respiratory difficulty and paralysis of all four extremities occur with spinal cord injury:

a. above C4.

b. at C6.

c. at C7.

d. around C8.

15. High doses of this drug have been found to reduce swelling and disability if given within 8 hours of injury.

a. Mannitol

b. Methylprednisolone

c. Naloxone

d. Neomycin

16. Loss of autonomic nervous system function below the level of the lesion causes _____ shock.

a. cardiac

b. hypovolemic

c. septic

d. neurogenic

17. Recovery of vital organ functions resulting from spinal shock can take up to:

a. 4 months.

b. 12 months.

c. 2 years.

d. 4 years.

18. Orthostatic hypotension is a common problem for spinal cord injuries at the level of:

a. C4.

b. T7.

c. L4.

d. S1.

19. A common complication of immobility in a spinal cord injury is:

a. pressure ulcers.

b. deep vein thrombosis.

c. urinary tract infections.

d. pneumonia.

Fill-In. *Read each statement carefully. Write your response in the space provided.*

1. A characteristic sign of a basal skull fracture is:

_____

2. A brain injury can cause serious brain damage because:

_____

3. Five symptoms of postconcussion syndrome are:

_____, _____, _____,

_____, and _____

4. After concussion, a patient needs to know to seek medical attention if any of the following six symptoms occur:

_____, _____, _____,

_____, _____, and _____

5. The most serious brain injury that can develop within the cranial vault is a: _____.

6. Identify four signs of a rapidly expanding, acute subdural hematoma that would require immediate surgical intervention:

_____, _____,

_____, and _____

7. List five collaborative problems that a nurse should assess for a patient with a brain injury:

_____, _____, _____,

_____, and _____

8. Name the three criteria used to assess level of consciousness using the Glasgow Coma Scale:

_____, _____, and _____

9. Complications after traumatic head injuries can be classified according to: _____,

_____, and _____.

10. The five vertebrae most commonly involved in spinal cord injuries are the: _____,

_____, _____, _____, and _____ vertebrae.

11. List four common manifestations of pulmonary embolism:

_____, _____,

_____, and _____

12. Three potential complications that may develop in spinal cord injury are:

_____, _____, and _____

II. Critical Thinking Questions and Exercises

Discussion and Analysis

1. Discuss the frequency of head injuries in the United States.
2. Explain why the most important consideration in any head injury is whether the brain is injured.
3. Explain what the Uniform Determination of Brain Death Act regulates.
4. Discuss the nursing measures that an be used to control ICP in severely brain injured patients.

Clinical Situations

Read the following case studies. Develop a plan of care as indicated below.

CASE STUDY: Cervical Spine Injury

Develop a nursing care plan for Katie, an 11-year-old who suffered a cervical spine injury after diving into a swimming pool. Katie is in traction applied by Crutchfield tongs and is on a Stryker frame. She is the oldest of three children and has never been hospitalized before. Complete your care plan, and share it with your instructor for comments.

Nursing Diagnoses:

Goals	Nursing Actions	Rationale	Expected Outcomes

CASE STUDY: Paraplegia

Matthew, a 29-year-old Navy pilot, was recently injured in a training maneuver. Matthew is a paraplegic. He has been hospitalized for 1 week. He was recently married, and his wife is expecting their first child in 2 months. Emphasize the following areas in your nursing care plan: psychological support, weight-bearing activities, muscle exercises, mobilization, and sexual needs. Share your work with your clinical instructor.

Nursing Diagnoses:

Goals	Nursing Actions	Rationale	Expected Outcomes

64

Management of Patients With Neurologic Infections, Autoimmune Disorders, and Neuropathies

I. Interpretation, Completion, and Comparison

Multiple Choice. Read each question carefully. Circle your answer.

1. Identify the bacteria *not associated* with the cause of septic meningitis:
   a. *C. neoformans*
   b. *H. influenzae*
   c. *N. meningitidis*
   d. *S. pneumoniae*

2. The most severe form of meningitis is considered to be:
   a. bacterial.
   b. aseptic.
   c. septic.
   d. viral.

3. Bacterial meningitis alters intracranial physiology, causing:
   a. cerebral edema.
   b. increased permeability of the blood-brain barrier.
   c. raised intracranial pressure.
   d. all of the above changes.

4. A brain abscess is a collection of infectious material within the substance of the brain that is caused by:
   a. direct invasion of the brain.
   b. spread of infection from nearby sites.
   c. spread of infection by other organs.
   d. all of the above mechanisms.

5. A positive diagnosis of myasthenia gravis can be reached using the following test:
   a. anticholinesterase levels
   b. magnetic resonance imaging
   c. CAT scan
   d. electromyography

6. A surgical intervention that can cause substantial remission of myasthenia gravis is:
   a. esophagostomy.
   b. myomectomy.
   c. thymectomy.
   d. spleenectomy.

7. The initial neurologic symptom of Guillain-Barré syndrome is:
   a. absent tendon reflexes.
   b. dysrhythmias.
   c. paresthesia of the legs.
   d. transient hypertension.

8. Tic douloureux is a disorder of the _____ cranial nerve that is characterized by paroxysms of pain and burning sensations.

    a. third   c. seventh

    b. fifth   d. eighth

9. Bell's palsy is a disorder of the _____ cranial nerve that is characterized by weakness or paralysis of the facial muscles.

    a. third   c. seventh

    b. fifth   d. eighth

10. Tinnitus and vertigo are clinical manifestations of damage to the _____ cranial nerve.

    a. fourth   c. eighth

    b. sixth   d. tenth

Fill-In. Read each statement carefully. Write your response in the space provided.

1. List six signs of bacterial meningitis that a nurse should assess:

_____, _____, _____,

_____, _____, and _____

2. The most common cause of acute encephalitis in the United States is: _____. The medication of choice is: _____.

3. The diagnosis of Creutzfeldt-Jakob disease can now be made by the presence of: _____.

4. The primary pathology of multiple sclerosis is damage to the: _____.

5. List the three forms of multiple sclerosis based upon the frequency and progression of symptoms:

_____, _____, and _____

6. Myasthenia gravis is considered an autoimmune disease in which antibodies are directed against

_____.

7. The most common causes of peripheral neuropathy are: _____, _____, and

_____.

II. Critical Thinking Questions and Exercises

Discussion and Analysis

1. Explain how a nurse would assess for the Kernig sign and the Brudzinski sign in determining a diagnosis of bacterial meningitis.

2. Explain what "demyelination" refers to in reference to multiple sclerosis.

Clinical Situations

Read the following case study. Circle the correct answer.

CASE STUDY: Multiple Sclerosis

Toni, a 32-year-old mother of two, has had multiple sclerosis for 5 years. She is currently enrolled in a school of nursing. Her husband is supportive and helps with the care of their preschool sons. Toni has been admitted to the clinical area for diagnostic studies related to symptoms of visual disturbances.

1. The nurse is aware that multiple sclerosis is a progressive disease of the central nervous system characterized by:

    a. axon degeneration.   c. sclerosed patches of neural tissue.

    b. demyelination of the brain and the spinal cord.   d. all of the above.

2. During the physical assessment, the nurse recalls that the areas most frequently affected by multiple sclerosis are the:

a. lateral, third, and fourth ventricles.

b. optic nerve and chiasm.

c. pons, medulla, and cerebellar peduncles.

d. above areas.

3. During the nursing interview, Toni minimizes her visual problems, talks about remaining in school to attempt advanced degrees, requests information about full-time jobs in nursing, and mentions her desire to have several more children. The nurse recognizes Toni's emotional responses as being:

a. an example of inappropriate euphoria characteristic of the disease process.

b. a reflection of coping mechanisms used to deal with the exacerbation of her illness.

c. indicative of the remission phase of her chronic illness.

d. realistic for her current level of physical functioning.

4. Toni's disease process involves a sacral plexus. Assessment should include:

a. bladder problems or urinary tract infections.

b. bowel management.

c. sexual activity.

d. all of the above.

65

Management of Patients With Oncologic or Degenerative Neurologic Disorders

I. Interpretation, Completion, and Comparison

Multiple Choice. Read each question carefully. Circle your answer.

1. The highest incidence of brain tumors occurs _____ decade of life.
   a. earlier than the third
   b. in the third
   c. in the fourth
   d. between the fifth and second

2. The most frequently seen brain neoplasm is:
   a. an acoustic neuroma.
   b. an angioma.
   c. a glioma.
   d. a meningioma.

3. A patient is diagnosed with an intracerebral tumor. The nurse knows that the diagnosis may include all of the following *except*:
   a. astrocytoma.
   b. ependymoma.
   c. medulloblastoma.
   d. meningioma.

4. The most common benign encapsulated brain tumor (representing 20% of primary brain tumors) is:
   a. an angioma.
   b. a glioblastoma multiforme.
   c. a meningioma.
   d. a neuroma.

5. A nurse knows that a patient exhibiting seizure-like movements localized to one side of the body most likely has:
   a. a cerebellar tumor.
   b. a frontal lobe tumor.
   c. a motor cortex tumor.
   d. an occipital lobe tumor.

6. The most common tumor types seen in the elderly include all of the following *except*:
   a. anaplastic astrocytoma.
   b. cerebral metastasis from other sites.
   c. glioblastoma multiforme.
   d. medulloblastoma.

7. The majority of brain tumors are treated by:
   a. neurosurgery.
   b. chemotherapy.
   c. radioisotope implants.
   d. all of the above mechanisms.

8. Metastatic brain lesions occur in _____ of patients with cancer.
   a. 10%
   b. 20–30%
   c. 40%
   d. 50–70%

9. The median survival time for patients with brain lesion metastasis is _____ when radiation therapy is used.
   a. 3–6 months
   b. 9–12 months
   c. 18 months
   d. 24 months

10. Parkinsonian symptoms usually appear in the _____ decade of life.
   a. fourth
   b. fifth
   c. sixth
   d. seventh

11. The clinical manifestations of Parkinson's disease (bradykinesia, rigidity, and tremors) are directly related to a decreased level of:
   a. acetylcholine.
   b. dopamine.
   c. seratonin.
   d. phenylalanine.

12. An example of an anticholinergic agent effective in controlling the tremor of parkinsonism is:
   a. Requip.
   b. cycrimine.
   c. Symmetrel.
   d. Pemex.

13. Clinical manifestations of Huntington's disease include:
   a. abnormal involuntary movements (chorea).
   b. emotional disturbances.
   c. intellectual decline.
   d. all of the above.

14. The average time from onset to death for patients diagnosed with amyotropic lateral sclerosis (ALS) is:
   a. 3 years.
   b. 5–8 years.
   c. 10 years.
   d. 15–20 years.

15. The majority of lumbar disc herniations occur at the level of:
   a. L1–L2.
   b. L3–L4.
   c. L4–L5.
   d. S1–S2.

Fill-In. *Read each statement carefully. Write your response in the space provided.*

1. The majority of metastatic brain tumors occur in six areas:

_____, _____, _____,

_____, _____, and _____

2. Name the three most common signs of increased ICP:

_____, _____, and _____,

3. List three common focal or localized symptoms of a brain tumor:

_____, _____, and _____,

4. A spinal cord tumor located within the spinal cord is classified as: _____.

5. List five degenerative disorders of the central and peripheral nervous system:

_____, _____, _____,

_____, and _____

6. Identify at least four autonomic clinical manifestations of Parkinson's disease:

_____, _____,

_____, and _____

7. List the five chief symptoms of amyotrophic lateral sclerosis:

_____, _____, _____,

_____, and _____

8. Identify the common characteristics of muscular dystrophies: _____, _____, and _____.

9. Cervical disk herniation usually occurs at the _____ interspaces.

10. Identify two major collaborative problems for patients with a cervical discectomy: _____ and _____.

II. Critical Thinking Questions and Exercises

Discussion and Analysis

1. Discuss a variety of physiologic changes that result from the infiltration of tissue subsequent to the growth of a brain tumor.

2. Describe the various classifications of brain tumors based on their pathophysiology.

CASE STUDY: Parkinson's Disease

Charles is a 76-year-old retired professional golfer. He has recently been diagnosed as having Parkinson's disease.

1. The nurse knows that Parkinson's disease, a progressive neurologic disorder, is characterized by:
   a. bradykinesia.
   b. muscle rigidity.
   c. tremor.
   d. all of the above.

2. The nurse assesses for the characteristic movement of Parkinson's disease, which is:
   a. an exaggerated muscle flaccidity that leads to frequent falls.
   b. a hyperextension of the back and neck that alters normal movements.
   c. a pronation-supination of the hand and forearm that interferes with normal hand activities.
   d. a combination of all of the above.

3. Charles is started on chemotherapy which is aimed at restoring dopaminergic activities. An example of such a drug is:
   a. Artane.
   b. Benadryl.
   c. Elavil.
   d. Dopar.

4. Nutritional considerations as part of the nursing care plan would include all of the following *except*:
   a. The diet should be semisolid to facilitate the passage of food.
   b. Calcium should be avoided.
   c. The patient should be sitting in an upright position during feeding.
   d. Thick fluids should be encouraged to provide additional calories.

CASE STUDY: Huntington's Disease

Develop a nursing care plan for the patient described below.

Mike is a 49-year-old television producer who has been diagnosed as having Huntington's disease. He lives alone in a penthouse apartment and is extremely busy and successful in his business. He has no living relatives. He is experiencing uncontrollable movements and difficulties feeding himself. He recently started chemotherapy with haloperidol (Haldol). Share your care plan with your instructor for comments.

Nursing Diagnosis: Potential for accidental injury related to abnormal involuntary movements.

Goals	Nursing Actions	Rationale	Expected Outcomes

UNIT **15**
Musculoskeletal Function

66

Assessment of Musculoskeletal Function

I. Interpretation, Completion, and Comparison

Multiple Choice. *Read each question carefully. Circle your answer.*

1. The vertebrae can be classified as a type of:
   a. flat bone.
   b. irregular bone.
   c. long bone.
   d. short bone.

2. The sternum, a bone that is a site for hematopoiesis, is classified as a:
   a. flat bone.
   b. irregular bone.
   c. long bone.
   d. short bone.

3. The basic cells responsible only for the formation of bone matrix are:
   a. osteoblasts.
   b. osteoclasts.
   c. osteocytes.
   d. all of the above.

4. About 3 weeks after fracture, an internal bridge of fibrous material, cartilage, and immature bone joins bone fragments so that ossification can occur. The building of a "fracture bridge" occurs during the stage of bone healing known as:
   a. inflammation.
   b. cellular proliferation.
   c. callus formation.
   d. ossification.

5. The hip and shoulder are examples of diarthroses joints that are classified as:
   a. ball-and-socket types.
   b. hinge joints.
   c. pivot joints.
   d. saddle joints.

6. The primary energy source for muscle cells is:
   a. adenosine triphosphate (ATP).
   b. creatine phosphate.
   c. glucose.
   d. glycogen.

7. Isometric contraction of the vastus lateralis is part of the exercises known as:
   a. biceps-tightening exercises.
   b. triceps-resisting exercises.
   c. gluteal-setting exercises.
   d. quadriceps exercises.

8. Patient education for musculoskeletal conditions for the aging is based on the understanding that bone mass peaks at age _____, after which there is a gradual loss of bone.
   a. 20 years
   b. 35 years
   c. 40 years
   d. 50 years

9. By age 75 years, the average woman has lost about _____ of cancellous bone and is susceptible to bone fractures.

a. 15%   c. 60%
b. 40%   d. 75%

10. The removal of synovial fluid from a joint is called:

a. arthrectomy.   c. arthrography.
b. arthrocentesis.   d. arthroscopy.

Matching. *Match the range-of-motion term listed in Column II with its associated description listed in Column I.*

Column I

1.____ pulling down toward the midline of the body

2.____ the act of turning the foot inward

3.____ the opposite movement of flexion

4.____ turning around on an axis

5.____ turning the palms down

6.____ pulling the jaw forward

7.____ moving away from the midline

8.____ conelike circular movement

9.____ turning the palm up

10.____ turning the foot outward

Column II

a. supination

b. extension

c. circumduction

d. abduction

e. protraction

f. eversion

g. pronation

h. adduction

i. inversion

j. rotation

Fill-In. *Read each statement carefully. Write the best response in the space provided.*

1. List several general functions of the musculoskeletal system.

_____

_____

2. The approximate percentage of total body calcium present in the bones is: _____.

3. In the human body, there are _____ bones.

4. The growth plate is also called the _____ located at the end of long bones.

5. Red bone marrow is located in the shaft of four long and flat bones: _____, _____,

_____ and _____.

6. Explain how vitamin D helps to regulate the balance between bone formation and resorption.

_____

_____

7. The major hormonal regulators of calcium homeostasis are:

_____.

8. Ossification for major adult long bone fractures can take up to:_____.

9. The term used to describe the grating, crackling sound heard over irregular joint surfaces like the knee is:

_____

Unscramble *the letters to answer each statement.*

1. The fibrous membrane that covers the bone

   E O P T R M E S U I

2. These connect muscles to muscles

   A N S I G M L T E

3. The contractile unit of skeletal muscle

   O E S E A R M R C

4. These attach muscles to bone

   N T S O E D N

5. Loss of bone mass common in postmenopausal women

   I S S T P O O R E O O S

6. A lateral curving deviation of the spine

   L S O S O S I I C

7. Excessive fluid within a joint capsule

   N E O F I F S U

8. Aspiration of a joint to obtain synovial fluid

   S A I R E T T H N R E O C

67

Musculoskeletal Care Modalities

I. Interpretation, Completion, and Comparison

Multiple Choice. Read each question carefully. Circle your answer.

1. Choose the *incorrect* statement about the traditional plaster cast. After a plaster cast has been set, it:
   a. will take 1 to 3 days to dry.
   b. may be dented with pressure from the fingers of the hands when being moved.
   c. should be covered with a blanket to promote quick drying.
   d. will not have maximum strength until it is dry.

2. A patient with an arm cast complains of pain. The nurse should do all of the following *except*:
   a. assess the fingers for color and temperature.
   b. administer a prescribed analgesic to promote comfort and allay anxiety.
   c. suspect that the patient may have a pressure sore.
   d. determine the exact site of the pain.

3. The nurse who assesses bone fracture pain expects the patient to describe the pain as:
   a. a dull, deep, boring ache.
   b. sharp and piercing.
   c. similar to "muscle cramps."
   d. sore and aching.

4. The nurse suspects "compartment syndrome" for a casted extremity. She would assess for characteristic symptoms such as:
   a. decreased sensory function.
   b. excruciating pain.
   c. loss of motion.
   d. all of the above.

5. The nurse knows to assess the patient in an arm cast for possible pressure ulcers in the following area:
   a. lateral malleolus.
   b. olecranon.
   c. radial styloid.
   d. ulna styloid.

6. After removal of a cast, the patient needs to be instructed to do all of the following *except*:
   a. apply an emollient lotion to soften the skin.
   b. control swelling with elastic bandages, as directed.
   c. gradually resume activities and exercise.
   d. use friction to remove dead surface skin by rubbing the area with a towel.

7. A common pressure problem area for a long leg cast is the:
   a. dorsalis pedis.
   b. peroneal nerve.
   c. popliteal artery.
   d. posterior tibialis.

8. The nurse assesses for peroneal nerve injury by checking the patient's casted leg for the primary symptom of:
a. burning.
b. numbness.
c. tingling.
d. all of the above indicators.

9. The nurse is very concerned about the potential debilitating complication of peroneal nerve injury, which is:
a. permanent paresthesis.
b. footdrop.
c. deep vein thrombosis.
d. infection.

10. Choose the *incorrect* statement about turning a patient in a hip spica cast.
a. A minimum of three persons are needed so that the cast can be adequately supported by their palms.
b. Points over body pressure areas need to be supported to prevent the cast from cracking.
c. The abduction bar should be used to ensure that the lower extremity can be moved as a unit.
d. The patient should be encouraged to use the trapeze or side rail during repositioning.

11. Skin traction is usually limited to a weight between:
a. 1 to 3 lb.
b. 4 to 8 lb.
c. 10 to 12 lb.
d. 13 to 15 lb.

12. A patient in pelvic traction needs his or her circulatory status assessed. The nurse should check for a positive (+) Homans' sign by asking the patient to:
a. extend both hands while the nurse compares the volume of both radial pulses.
b. extend each leg and dorsiflex each foot to determine if pain or tenderness is present in the lower leg.
c. plantar flex both feet while the nurse performs the blanch test on all of the patient's toes.
d. squeeze the nurse's hands with his or her hands to evaluate any difference in strength.

13. Nursing assessment of a patient in traction should include:
a. lung sounds and bowel sounds.
b. circulation, sensation, and motion of the extremities in traction.
c. the patient's level of anxiety and apprehension.
d. all of the above interventions.

14. The nurse expects that up to _____ of weight can be used for a patient in skeletal traction.
a. 10 lb
b. 25 lb
c. 40 lb
d. 60 lb

15. When a patient is in continuous skeletal leg traction, it is important for the nurse to remember to do all of the following *except*:
a. encourage the patient to use the trapeze bar.
b. maintain adequate countertraction.
c. remove the weights when pulling the patient up in bed to prevent unnecessary pulling on the fracture site.
d. use a fracture bedpan to prevent soiling and to maintain patient comfort.

16. Patients with a hip and knee replacement begin ambulation with a walker or crutches _____ after surgery.
a. 24 hours
b. 72 hours
c. 1 week
d. 2 to 3 weeks

17. An artificial joint for total hip replacement involves an implant that consists of:
a. an acetabular socket.
b. a femoral shaft.
c. a spherical ball.
d. all of the above.

18. The recommended leg position to prevent prosthesis dislocation after a total hip replacement is:
a. abduction.
b. adduction.
c. flexion.
d. internal rotation.

19. Postoperatively a patient with a total hip replacement is allowed to turn:
    a. 45 degrees onto his or her unoperated side if the affected hip is kept abducted.
    b. from the prone to the supine position only, and the patient must keep the affected hip extended and abducted.
    c. to any comfortable position as long as the affected leg is extended.
    d. to the operative side if his or her affected hip remains extended.

20. The nurse caring for a postoperative hip-replacement patient knows that the incidence of deep vein thrombosis is as high as _____ within the first week after surgery.
    a. 35%
    b. 50%
    c. 70%
    d. 90%

21. One of the most dangerous of all postoperative complications is:
    a. atelectasis.
    b. hypovolemia.
    c. pulmonary embolism.
    d. urinary tract infection.

22. After a total hip replacement, stair climbing and stooping are to be avoided for:
    a. 1 to 3 months.
    b. 3 to 4 months
    c. 6 months.
    d. 8 to 9 months.

23. After a total hip replacement, the patient is usually able to resume daily activities after:
    a. 3 months.
    b. 6 months.
    c. 9 months.
    d. 1 year.

24. Preoperative nursing measures that are appropriate for an orthopedic patient should include:
    a. encouraging fluids to prevent a urinary tract infection.
    b. teaching isometric exercises and encouraging active range of motion.
    c. discouraging smoking to improve respiratory function.
    d. all of the above interventions.

25. Postoperative nursing concerns when caring for an orthopedic patient should include:
    a. determining that the patient's pain is controlled by administering prescribed analgesics.
    b. observing for signs of shock, such as hypotension and tachycardia.
    c. preventing infection by using aseptic technique when giving wound care.
    d. all of the above interventions.

Fill-In. *Read each statement carefully. Write your response in the space provided.*

1. List four purposes for applying a cast:

    _____, _____,

    _____, and _____.

2. The advantages of a fiberglass cast compared to a plaster cast are:

    _____

3. Unrelieved pain for a patient in a cast must be *immediately reported* to avoid four possible and serious potential problems:

    _____, _____,

    _____, and _____

4. Name several indicators of neurovascular status that the nurse should assess to determine circulatory status for a casted extremity.

    _____

    _____

5. List several danger signs of possible circulatory constriction for a casted extremity:

_____

6. List three major complications of a casted extremity:

_____, _____, and _____

7. Name four purposes for traction application:

_____, _____,

_____, and _____

8. List three examples of skin or running traction:

_____, _____, and _____

9. A nursing goal for a patient with skeletal traction is to avoid infection and the development of _____ at the site of pin insertion.

10. Name four possible complications of a total knee replacement:

_____, _____,

_____, and _____

II. Critical Thinking Questions and Exercises

Clinical Situations

Discussion and Analysis

1. Discuss three potential collaborative problems for a patient with a cast.
2. Discuss the major nursing goals for a patient with a cast.
3. Describe the complication, *compartment syndrome*, and its recommended treatment.
4. Describe the serious complication, *Volkmann's contracture*.
5. Discuss the major nursing goals for a patient in traction.

Read the following case studies. Fill in the blanks or circle the correct answer.

CASE STUDY: Buck's Traction

Bernadette is a 32-year-old bank secretary who was admitted to the hospital for unilateral Buck's extension traction to the left leg after a hip injury. Bernadette is the single parent of three children younger than 12 years of age.

1. Based on her knowledge of running traction, the nurse knows to expect that:
   a. the patient's leg will be flat on the bed to allow for a straight pulling force.
   b. the patient's leg will be flexed at the knee to allow for mobility without disruption of the pulling force.
   c. the traction will be applied directly to the bony skeleton to maintain a constant pulling force.
   d. the traction will allow the patient's leg to be suspended off the bed so that no further damage can occur to the hip.

2. The nurse knows that countertraction must be considered whenever traction is applied. Countertraction for Buck's traction is provided by: _____ and _____.

3. In preparing the patient's skin for Buck's traction application, the nurse knows that it is necessary to:

_____ and _____.

4. The nurse makes certain that the weights applied will not exceed:

a. 2 lb.

b. 4 lb.

c. 6 lb.

d. 8 lb.

5. The nurse consistently assesses neurovascular status when traction is in place. List seven indicators that the nurse would evaluate.

_____

_____

6. On assessment, the nurse notes a positive Homans' sign. Explain what this means.

_____

CASE STUDY: Total Hip Replacement

Tom is a 62-year-old athletic coach at a high school. Sports activities, especially baseball, have been the focus of his energies since he was in high school and college. Because of prior hip joint injuries and degenerative joint disease, he is scheduled for a total hip replacement.

1. Preoperatively, the nurse assesses the status of the cardiovascular system based on the knowledge that mortality for patients over 60 years is directly related to the complications of: _____ and

_____.

2. As part of preoperative teaching, the nurse makes the patient aware of four major potential complications of hip replacement:

a. _____

b. _____

c. _____

d. _____

3. Based on the knowledge that limited hip flexion decreases hip prosthesis dislocation, the nurse knows to:

a. keep the patient flat in bed with the leg extended.

b. gatch the knees to decrease the effect of pulling force on the hip.

c. raise the head of the bed between 30 and 45 degrees.

d. maintain the patient in semi-Fowler's position.

4. The nurse teaches Tom how to minimize hip extension during transfers and while sitting. The nurse should encourage him to:

a. rotate the hip inward slightly during sitting to prevent pressure on the external border of the hip.

b. hyperextend the leg during transfers so the hip socket will not "pop out."

c. maintain adduction and flexion when moving around to minimize strain at the surgical site.

d. always pivot on the unoperated leg to protect the operated leg from unnecessary work.

5. A dislocated prosthesis is evidenced by any of the following five indicators:

_____, _____, _____,

_____, and _____

6. In assessing postoperative wound drainage, the nurse knows that Tom's drainage of _____ in the first 24 hours is within normal range.

a. 150 mL

b. 350 mL

c. 600 mL

d. 1000 mL

7. The nurse is careful to assess for evidence of deep vein thrombosis (3% mortality), which occurs in approximately _____ of patients.

a. 20% to 30%

b. 45% to 70%

c. 75% to 85%

d. more than 85%

68

Management of Patients With Musculoskeletal Disorders

I. Interpretation, Completion, and Comparison

Multiple Choice. Read each question carefully. Circle your answer.

1. The intervertebral disks that are subject to the greatest mechanical stress and greatest degenerative changes are:
   a. C3 to C4.
   b. L1 to L2.
   c. L2 to L3.
   d. L4 to L5.

2. Back pain is classified as "chronic" when the pain lasts longer than _____ without improvement.
   a. 4 weeks
   b. 3 months
   c. 6 months
   d. 1 year

3. The best position to ease low back pain is:
   a. high Fowler's to allow for maximum hip flexion.
   b. supine with the knees slightly flexed and the head of the bed elevated 30 degrees.
   c. prone with a pillow under the shoulders.
   d. supine with the bed flat and a firm mattress in place.

4. When lifting objects, patients with low back pain should be encouraged to maximize the use of the:
   a. gastrocnemius.
   b. latissimus dorsi.
   c. quadriceps.
   d. rectus adominis.

5. The nurse should encourage a patient with low back pain to do all of the following *except*:
   a. lie prone with legs slightly elevated.
   b. strengthen abdominal muscles.
   c. avoid prolonged sitting or walking.
   d. maintain appropriate weight.

6. Carpal tunnel syndrome is a neuropathy characterized by:
   a. bursitis and tendonitis.
   b. flexion contracture of the fourth and fifth fingers.
   c. median nerve compression at the wrist.
   d. pannus formation in the shoulder.

7. The term for onychocryptosis, a common foot condition, is:
   a. callus.
   b. bunion.
   c. flatfoot.
   d. ingrown toenail.

8. An overgrowth of the horny layer of epidermis on the foot is called a:

  a. bunion.

  b. clawfoot.

  c. corn.

  d. hammer toe.

9. The average 75-year-old woman with osteoporosis has lost about _____ of her cortical bone.

  a. 5%

  b. 10%

  c. 25%

  d. 40%

10. The estimated intake of calcium to prevent bone loss for a postmenapausal woman is _____ mg/day. The actual intake is about _____ mg/day.

  a. 600/200

  b. 900/300

  c. 1200/400

  d. 1500/600

11. Bone formation is enhanced by:

  a. calcium intake.

  b. muscular activity.

  c. weight-bearing.

  d. all of the above.

12. The most common symptoms of osteomalacia are:

  a. bone fractures and kyphosis.

  b. bone pain and tenderness.

  c. muscle weakness and spasms.

  d. softened and compressed vertebrae.

13. Most cases of osteomyelitis are caused by:

  a. *Proteus.*

  b. *Pseudomonas.*

  c. *Salmonella.*

  d. *Staphylococcus aureus.*

14. Signs and symptoms of osteomyelitis may include all of the following *except*:

  a. pain, erythema, and fever.

  b. leukopenia, swelling, and purulent drainage.

  c. elevated erythrocyte sedimentation rate and increased white blood cell count.

  d. positive wound cultures and localized discomfort.

15. The specific treatment for chronic osteomyelitis would probably be:

  a. antibiotic therapy.

  b. drainage of localized foci of infection.

  c. immobilization.

  d. surgical removal of the sequestrum.

16. The most common benign bone tumor is:

  a. an enchondroma.

  b. a giant cell tumor.

  c. an osteochondroma.

  d. an osteoid osteoma.

17. The multiple myeloma tumor has its origin and principal location in the:

  a. bone marrow.

  b. liver.

  c. lymph nodes.

  d. spleen.

18. Appropriate nursing actions when caring for a patient with a primary malignant bone tumor would include all of the following *except*:

  a. allowing the patient to independently plan his or her daily routine.

  b. estimating the size and location of the mass daily by vigorously palpating the affected area.

  c. assuring the patient receiving chemotherapy that alopecia, if it occurs, is temporary.

  d. encouraging range-of-motion exercises to prevent atrophy of unaffected muscles.

Fill-In. Read each statement carefully. Write the best response in the space provided.

1. Identify at least five causes of acute low back pain.

_____,   _____,   _____,

_____, and   _____

2. List four nursing diagnoses for a patient undergoing foot surgery.

_____

_____

_____

_____

3. Two significant characteristics of osteoporosis are: _____ and _____.

4. The onset of osteoporosis begins in the _____ decade of life, when bone mass peaks and then begins to decline.

5. Explain the effects of the following on the development of age-related osteoporosis:
   a. Calcitonin: _____
   b. Estrogen: _____
   c. Parathyroid hormone: _____

6. Using a bone mineral density (BMD) score, *osteoporosis* is present if the score is ____ standard deviations (SD) below the young adult mean score; *osteopenia* is diagnosed if the score is _____ below the SD.

7. The primary deficit in osteomalacia is: _____.

II. Critical Thinking Questions and Exercises

Applying Concepts

Review the pictures of common foot deformities found in Figure 68–6 of the text and complete the exercises.

1. Identify each foot ailment and list the associated clinical manifestations.

2. For each ailment, list associated nursing diagnoses.

3. From each diagnosis, draft a nursing plan of care.

4. Broadly explain the medical/surgical management for each ailment.

Clinical Situations

Read the following case study. Fill in the blanks or circle the correct answer.

CASE STUDY: Osteoporosis

Emily is a 49-year-old administrative assistant at a community college who has just been diagnosed with osteoporosis. The physician has asked you to answer some of Emily's questions and explain the physician's directions for her level of activity and her nutritional needs.

1. Emily asks the nurse to explain why she is losing her bone mass. The nurse's explanation is based on the physiologic rationale that bone mass loss occurs when _____.

2. What two reasons could the nurse use to explain why women develop osteoporosis more frequently than men: _____ and _____.

3. The nurse advises Emily that about _____ of Caucasian women older than 50 years of age have some degree of osteoporosis.
   a. 10%
   b. 25%
   c. 50%
   d. 80%

4. The nurse advises Emily that the development of osteoporosis is significantly dependent on:
   a. decreased estrogen, which inhibits bone breakdown.
   b. increased calcitonin, which enhances bone resorption.
   c. increased vitamin D use, which interferes with calcium use.
   d. increased parathyroid hormone, which decreases with aging.

5. Part of Emily's teaching plan includes nutritional information about dietary calcium and vitamin D. The nurse advises Emily that she needs _____ mg of calcium a day.

a. 500

b. 1000

c. 1200

d. 1500

6. Emily is told that her x-ray results indicated bone radiolucency. The nurse knows that Emily has probably already exhibited _____ demineralization.

a. 5%

b. 10%

c. 20%

d. 30%

69

Management of Patients With Musculoskeletal Trauma

I. Interpretation, Completion, and Comparison

Multiple Choice. Read each question carefully. Circle your answer.

1. A muscle tear that is microscopic and due to overuse is called a:
a. contusion.
b. dislocation.
c. sprain.
d. strain.

2. The acute inflammatory stage of a strain or sprain usually lasts:
a. less than 24 hours.
b. between 24 and 48 hours.
c. about 72 hours.
d. at least 1 week.

3. After arthroscopic surgery for a rotator cuff tear, a patient can usually resume full activity in:
a. 3 to 4 weeks.
b. 8 weeks.
c. 3 to 4 months.
d. 6 to 12 months.

4. A patient who has a menisectemy by arthroscopic surgery needs to know that normal athletic activities can usually be resumed after:
a. 2 weeks.
b. 3 weeks.
c. 2 months.
d. 6 months.

5. An open fracture with extensive soft tissue damage is classified as a grade _____ fracture.
a. I
b. II
c. III
d. IV

6. Emergency management of a fracture should include:
a. covering the area with a clean dressing, if the fracture is open.
b. immobilizing the affected site.
c. splinting the injured limb.
d. all of the above nursing interventions.

7. The most serious complication of an open fracture is:
a. infection.
b. muscle atrophy caused by loss of supporting bone structure.
c. necrosis of adjacent soft tissue caused by blood loss.
d. nerve damage.

8. Shock, as an immediate complication of fractures, is usually classified as:
a. cardiogenic.
b. hypovolemic.
c. neurogenic.
d. septicemic.

9. As a complication of fractures, fat emboli:
a. represent the major cause of death in fracture patients.
b. result in symptoms of decreased mental alertness.
c. may compromise the patient's respiratory status, necessitating ventilator support.
d. are characterized by all of the above.

10. The onset of symptoms for *fat embolism syndrome,* after a fracture, occurs:
a. within 1 to 3 days.
b. 1 to 2 weeks after the fracture is set.
c. about 4 weeks after the bone fragments solidify.
d. immediately after the fracture heals, when activity begins.

11. The femur fracture that commonly leads to avascular necrosis or nonunion because of an abundant supply of blood vessels in the area is a fracture of the:
a. condylar area.
b. neck.
c. shaft.
d. trochanteric region.

12. Patients who experience a fracture of the humeral neck are advised that healing will take an average of _____ weeks, with restricted vigorous activity for an additional _____ weeks.
a. 6; 2
b. 10; 4
c. 10; 6
d. 16; 2

13. After an arm fracture, pendulum exercises are begun:
a. as soon as tolerated.
b. in 2 to 3 weeks, when callus ossification prevents easy movements of bony fragments.
c. in about 4 to 5 weeks, after new bone is well established.
d. in 2 to 3 months, after normal activities are resumed.

14. The most serious complication of a supracondylar fracture of the humerus is:
a. hemarthrosis.
b. paresthesia.
c. malunion.
d. Volkmann's ischemic contracture.

15. The two most serious complications of pelvic fractures are:
a. paresthesias and ischemia.
b. hemorrhage and shock.
c. paralytic ileus and a lacerated urethra.
d. thrombophlebitis and infection.

16. Nursing assessment for a pelvic fracture includes:
a. checking the urine for hematuria.
b. palpating peripheral pulses in both lower extremities.
c. testing the stool for occult blood.
d. all of the above.

17. An acetabular fracture of the femur involves the:
a. neck of the femur.
b. shaft of the femur.
c. supracondylar area of the femur.
d. trochanteric region of the femur.

18. The most common complication of a hip fracture in the elderly is:
a. avascular necrosis.
b. infection.
c. nonunion.
d. pneumonia.

19. An immediate nursing concern for a patient who has suffered a femoral shaft fracture is assessment for:
a. hypovolemic shock.
b. infection.
c. knee and hip dislocation.
d. pain resulting from muscle spasm.

20. The longest immobilization time necessary for fracture union occurs with a fracture of the:
a. intratrochanteric area of the femur.
b. midshaft of the humerus.
c. pelvis.
d. tibial shaft.

21. The major indicator of lower extremity amputation is:
    a. congenital deformity.
    b. malignant tumor.
    c. peripheral vascular disease.
    d. trauma.

22. A nurse can foster a positive self-image in a patient who has had an amputation by all of the following *except*:
    a. encouraging the patient to care for the residual limb.
    b. allowing the expression of grief.
    c. introducing the patient to local amputee support groups.
    d. encouraging family and friends to refrain from visiting temporarily because this may increase the patient's embarrassment.

Matching. Match the type of fracture in Column II with its descriptive terminology listed in Column I.

Part I

Column I

1.____ A break occurs across the entire section of the bone.

2.____ A fragment of the bone is pulled off by a ligament or tendon.

3.____ Bone is splintered into several fragments.

4.____ One side of a bone is broken and the other side is bent.

Column II

a. avulsion

b. comminuted

c. complete

d. epiphyseal

e. greenstick

Part II

Column I

1.____ A fracture occurs at an angle across the bone.

2.____ Fragments are driven inward.

3.____ The fractured bone is compressed by another bone.

4.____ The fracture extends through the skin.

Column II

a. compressed

b. depressed

c. oblique

d. open

e. pathologic

Fill-In. Read each statement carefully. Write your response in the space provided.

1. Those with open fractures risk three major complications:

_____,   _____, and   _____

2. List three *early* complications of fractures and three *delayed* complications:

Early: _____

Delayed: _____

3. Treatment of early shock in fractures consists of four activities:

_____,   _____,

_____, and   _____

4. Explain the concept *compartment syndrome:* _____

5. List three early and serious complications associated with bed rest and reduced skeletal muscle contractions for a patient with an open fracture:

_____,   _____, and   _____

6. The most common fracture of the distal radius is: _____.

II. Critical Thinking Questions and Exercises

Identifying Patterns

1. A strain: a microscropic muscle tear:: a sprain: _____.

2. A dislocation: lack of contact between the articular surfaces of bones:: _____: partial dislocation of associated joint structures.

3. Closed reduction: the alignment of bone fragments into opposition:: open reduction: _____.

4. Delayed union: delayed healing due to infection or poor nutrition:: nonunion: _____.

5. Autograft: donor to donor tissue:: _____: tissue from donor or other.

6. Intracapsula fracture: neck of the femur:: extracapsular fracture: _____.

Clinical Situations

Read the following case study. Circle the correct answers.

CASE STUDY: Above-the-Knee Amputation

William, a 70-year-old Catholic priest, lives in a center city rectory. He is scheduled to have an above-the-knee amputation of his left leg because of peripheral vascular disease.

1. Preoperatively the nurse knows that the circulatory status of the affected limb should be evaluated by assessing for:
   a. color and temperature.
   b. palpable pulses.
   c. positioning responses.
   d. all of the above.

2. The level of William's amputation was determined after assessing:
   a. the circulatory status of the affected limb.
   b. the type of prosthesis to be used.
   c. William's ability to understand and use the prosthetic device.
   d. all of the above.

3. Preoperatively the nurse needs to assist William in exercising the muscles needed for crutch walking. The major muscle to be strengthened is the:
   a. pectoralis major.
   b. gastrocnemius.
   c. quadriceps femoris.
   d. triceps brachii.

4. Postoperatively, William experiences phantom limb sensations. The most appropriate nursing response is to:
   a. agree with his statements, recognizing that he is expressing a psychological need.
   b. consistently stress the absence of the lower leg.
   c. disagree with him and reorient him to reality.
   d. keep him as active as possible and encourage self-expression.

5. William's amputation is treated with a soft compression dressing. Nursing care would include all of the following *except*:
   a. keeping the residual limb slightly elevated on a pillow to decrease edema.
   b. monitoring vital signs to detect any indication of bleeding.
   c. placing the residual limb in an extended position, with brief periods of elevation.
   d. keeping a tourniquet nearby in case of hemorrhage.

6. Preprosthetic nursing care should attempt to avoid any problem that can delay prosthetic fitting, such as:

a. abduction deformities of the hip.

b. flexion deformities.

c. nonshrinkage of the residual limb.

d. all of the above.

7. The nurse who is preparing to apply a bandage to William's residual limb knows that she should:

a. anchor the bandage on the posterior surface of the residual limb.

b. begin the vertical turns on the anterior surface of the residual limb.

c. maintain the residual limb in a position of flexion while bandaging.

d. use circular turns that run in a horizontal plane from the proximal to the distal segment.

8. The nurse teaches William to massage his residual limb to:

a. decrease local tenderness.

b. improve vascularity.

c. mobilize the scar.

d. accomplish all of the above.

UNIT 16
Other Acute Problems

70

Management of Patients With Infectious Diseases

I. Interpretation, Completion, and Comparison

Multiple Choice. Read each question carefully. Circle your answer.

1. It is recommended that the measles, mumps, and rubella (MMR) vaccine should be initially given to children at age:
   a. 2 months.
   b. 6 months.
   c. 12–15 months.
   d. 18–24 months.

2. Chickenpox and herpes zoster are both caused by the same viral agent:
   a. *Clostridium difficile*
   b. *Shigella*
   c. *Plasmodium vivax*
   d. *Varicella zoster*

3. Each year nosocomial infections affect about _____ patients.
   a. 250,000
   b. 500,000
   c. 1 million
   d. 2 million

4. The single most important means of preventing the spread of infection is:
   a. antibiotic therapy.
   b. gowning and gloving.
   c. hand washing.
   d. isolation measures.

5. The bacterium with significant nosocomial potential that is gram-positive, spore-forming, and highly resistant to antimicrobial therapy is:
   a. *Clostridium difficile*.
   b. methicillin-resistant *Staphylococcus aureus* (MRSA).
   c. *Staphylococcus aureus*.
   d. vancomycin-resistant enterococcus (VRE).

6. MRSA is a common nosocomial infection caused by _____, the most frequently occurring pathogen identified with this disorder.
   a. *Escherichia coli*
   b. *Proteus*
   c. *Pseudomonas aeruginosa*
   d. *Staphylococcus aureus*

7. A gram-positive organism that is less virulent than a gram-negative organism is:
   a. *Escherichia coli*.
   b. *Pseudomonas aeruginosa*.
   c. *Proteus*.
   d. *Staphylococcus aureus*.

8. Choose the *incorrect* statement about West Nile virus infection.

a. It was first seen in the United States in 1999.

b. It is caused by an infected mosquito.

c. It is treated successfully by intravenous antibiotics if diagnosed within 72 hours after symptoms onset.

d. Its symptoms are similar to those of meningitis.

9. A person diagnosed with Legionnaire's disease would have a primary infection in his or her:

a. bloodstream.

b. central nervous system.

c. gastrointestinal tract.

d. lungs.

10. The most common viral cause of diarrhea in children is:

a. *Campylobacter.*

b. *Shigella.*

c. *rotavirus.*

d. *Salmonella.*

11. The antibiotic of choice for Legionnaire's disease is:

a. Biaxin.

b. Ilotycin.

c. Levaquin.

d. Zithromax.

12. A common bacterial cause of diarrhea that has been linked to the ingestion of undercooked beef is:

a. *Escherichia coli.*

b. *Campylobacter.*

c. *Salmonella.*

d. *Shigella.*

13. The rehydration goal for a 70-kg patient who has moderate dehydration would be _____ over 4 hours.

a. 3000 mL

b. 5000 mL

c. 7000 mL

d. 9000 mL

14. Acquired immunodeficiency syndrome (AIDS) is a:

a. condition of unknown cause.

b. disorder of immunoregulation.

c. syndrome associated with high mortality.

d. condition consistent with all of the above.

15. The transmission route for human immunodeficiency virus (HIV) is through:

a. contaminated blood.

b. semen and vaginal secretions.

c. maternal-fetal blood.

d. all of the above.

16. Latent syphilitic lesions may still be treated with penicillin G benzathine for up to:

a. 2 to 3 months.

b. 3 to 6 months.

c. 6 to 9 months.

d. 1 year.

17. A chancre initially appears 2 to 3 weeks after inoculation with the spirochete, *Treponema pallidum*, in the sexually transmitted disease known as:

a. chlamydia.

b. gonorrhea.

c. HIV/AIDS.

d. syphilis.

18. Gonorrhea is a sexually transmitted infection that involves the mucosal surface of the:

a. genitourinary tract.

b. pharynx.

c. rectum.

d. all of the above.

19. The primary site for gonorrhea in women is the:

a. urethra.

b. kidney.

c. vagina.

d. uterine cervix.

20. The most deadly microorganism used as a biowarfare agent is _____, which has a mortality rate of 90%:

a. anthrax

b. Ebola virus

c. plague

d. smallpox

Fill-In. Read each statement carefully. Write your response in the space provided.

1. List at least six infectious diseases that have been controlled by successful vaccine programs:

_____, _____, _____,

_____, _____, and _____

2. It is recommended that immunosuppressed adults be vaccinated for: _____, _____, and _____.

3. Preferred alternate antibiotics for MRSA are: _____ and _____.

4. Normal skin flora usually consists of two organisms: _____ and _____.

5. According to the Centers for DIsease Control and Prevention(CDC), there are five emerging infectious diseases that have increased in the past two decades:

_____, _____, _____,

_____, and _____

6. Lyme disease is most prevalent in the _____ and _____ sections of the country.

7. It is estimated that about _____ people in the United States are currently infected with HIV-1.

8. The most common infectious diseases in the world are _____ diseases.

9. List five conditions classified as sexually transmitted diseases.

_____, _____, _____,

_____, and _____

Matching. Match the disease or condition listed in Column II with its associated causative organism listed in Column I.

Column I

1. _____varicella zoster
2. _____*Neisseria gonorrhoeae*
3. _____hepatitis B virus
4. _____*Staphylococcus aureus*
5. _____Epstein-Barr virus
6. _____*Salmonella* species
7. _____*Streptococcus pneumoniae*
8. _____*Microsporum* species

Column II

a. chickenpox
b. *bloodborne hepatitis*
c. diarrheal disease
d. *gonorrhea*
e. impetigo
f. *mononucleosis*
g. pneumococcal pneumonia
h. ringworm

II. Critical Thinking Questions and Exercises

Examining Associations and Applying Concepts

Examine Figure 70–1 below. For each of the six links in the infection cycle, describe specific nursing interventions that can be used to break transmission. The first entry is filled in as an example.

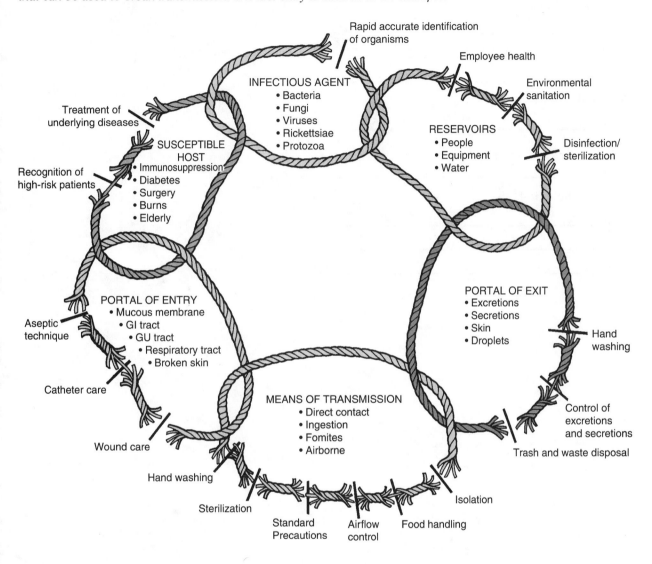

1. **Infectious Agent**

   a. Educate patient about immunization

   b. _____

   c. _____

2. **Reservoirs**

   a. _____

   b. _____

   c. _____

3. Portal of Exit

    a. _____

    b. _____

    c. _____

4. Means of Transmission

    a. _____

    b. _____

    c. _____

5. Portal of Entry

    a. _____

    b. _____

    c. _____

6. Susceptible Host

    a. _____

    b. _____

    c. _____

71

Emergency Nursing

I. Interpretation, Completion, and Comparison

Multiple Choice. Read each question carefully. Circle your answer.

1. A triage nurse in the emergency department determines that a patient with dyspnea and dehydration is not in a life-threatening situation. The triage category that the nurse would choose is:
   a. delayed.
   b. emergent.
   c. immediate.
   d. urgent.

2. A nurse at the scene of an industrial explosion uses "field triage" to categorize victims for treatment. A patient in need of emergent care would be tagged using the color:
   a. blue.
   b. green.
   c. red.
   d. yellow.

3. In the United States, the elderly, who are major consumers of emergency health care, account for about _____ million visits to the emergency room annually.
   a. 20
   b. 50
   c. 100
   d. 150

4. John, 16 years old, is brought to the emergency department after a vehicular accident. He is pronounced dead on arrival (DOA). When his parents arrive at the hospital, the nurse should:
   a. ask them to sit in the waiting room until she can spend time alone with them.
   b. speak to both parents together and encourage them to support each other and express their emotions freely.
   c. speak to one parent at a time in a private setting so that each can ventilate feelings of loss without upsetting the other.
   d. ask the emergency physician to medicate the parents so that they can handle their son's unexpected death quietly and without hysteria.

5. The first priority in treating any patient in the emergency department is:
   a. controlling hemorrhage.
   b. establishing an airway.
   c. obtaining consent for treatment.
   d. restoring cardiac output.

6. An oropharyngeal airway should be inserted:
   a. at an angle of 90 degrees.
   b. upside down and then rotated 180 degrees.
   c. with the concave portion touching the posterior pharynx.
   d. with the convex portion facing upward.

7. Clinical indicators for emergency endotracheal intubation include:
   a. airway obstruction.
   b. respiratory arrest.
   c. respiratory insufficiency.
   d. all of the above.

8. The initial nursing measure for the control of hemorrhage caused by trauma is to:
   a. apply a tourniquet.
   b. apply firm pressure over the involved area or artery.
   c. elevate the injured part.
   d. immobilize the area to control blood loss.

9. Indicators of hypovolemic shock associated with internal bleeding include all of the following *except*:
   a. bradycardia.
   b. cool, moist skin.
   c. hypotension.
   d. thirst.

10. The most common cause of shock in emergency situations is:
   a. cardiac failure.
   b. decreased arterial resistance.
   c. hypovolemia.
   d. septicemia.

11. The leading cause of death in children and adults younger than 44 years of age is:
   a. cancer.
   b. drowning.
   c. pneumonia.
   d. trauma.

12. Nursing measures for a penetrating abdominal injury would include:
   a. assessing for manifestations of hemorrhage.
   b. covering any protruding viscera with sterile dressings soaked in normal saline solution.
   c. looking for any associated chest injuries.
   d. all of the above actions.

13. A patient has experienced blunt abdominal trauma from a motor vehicle crash. The nurses assesses the patient with the knowledge that the most frequently injured solid abdominal organ is the:
   a. duodenum.
   b. large bowel.
   c. liver.
   d. spleen.

14. Nursing management for a crushing lower extremity wound includes:
   a. applying a clean dressing to protect the wound.
   b. elevating the site to limit the accumulation of fluid in the interstitial spaces.
   c. splinting the wound in a position of rest to prevent motion.
   d. all of the above measures.

15. Identify the sequence of medical or nursing management for a patient who experiences multiple injuries.
   a. Assess for head injuries, control hemorrhage, establish an airway, prevent hypovolemic shock.
   b. Control hemorrhage, prevent hypovolemic shock, establish an airway, assess for head injuries.
   c. Establish an airway, control hemorrhage, prevent hypovolemic shock, assess for head injuries.
   d. Prevent hypovolemic shock, assess for head injuries, establish an airway, control hemorrhage.

16. Nursing measures for an extremity fracture would include:
   a. assessing for manifestations of shock.
   b. immobilizing the fracture site.
   c. palpating peripheral pulses.
   d. all of the above actions.

17. Progressive deterioration of body systems occurs when hypothermia lowers the body temperature to:
   a. 98°F.
   b. 97°F.
   c. 96°F.
   d. 95°F.

18. Near-drowning is the third leading cause of unintentional death and occurs in about _____ of children younger than 4 years of age.
   a. 10%
   b. 25%
   c. 40%
   d. 75%

19. Approximately _____ million women experience domestic violence every year.
   a. 1
   b. 2
   c. 3
   d. 4

20. Rose, a 19-year-old student, has been sexually assaulted. When assisting with the physical examination, the nurse should do all of the following *except:*

a. have the patient shower or wash the perineal area before the examination.

b. assess and document any bruises and lacerations.

c. record a history of the event, using the patient's own words.

d. label all torn or bloody clothes and place each item in a separate brown bag so that any evidence can be given to the police.

Fill-In. *Read each question carefully. Write your response in the space provided.*

1. Name two viruses of major concern that could be released as part of biological warfare:

_____ and _____

2. Emergency room personnel are at increased risk for exposure to communicable disease through blood or body fluids because of the number of people infected with _____ and _____.

3. A patient with a foreign body airway obstruction demonstrates the inability to: _____, _____ or _____.

4. Describe the appearance of a wound classified as a *hematoma:*

_____

5. Identify three major components of injury prevention that a nurse can actively participate in:

_____, _____, and _____

6. An easy and immediate treatment for an ingested poison that is not caustic is _____, which immediately induces vomiting.

II. Critical Thinking Questions and Exercises

Discussion and Analysis

1. Nursing activities in the emergency room are based on objectives that are principle-centered and prioritized. Discuss the expected sequence of nursing activities used when assessing and treating patients in the emergency room.

2. Describe the five stages of crisis that families experience when a loved one is admitted to the emergency room.

3. Explain why lactated Ringer's solution is initially useful as fluid replacement for a patient experiencing hypovolemic shock.

Applying Concepts

For each of the following situations, identify a nursing action with supporting rationale.

Condition	Action		Rationale
Heimlich maneuver for standing or sitting conscious patient	a. _____		_____
	b. _____		_____
	c. _____		_____
Heimlich maneuver with patient lying unconscious	a. _____		_____
	b. _____		_____
	c. _____		_____

Finger sweep

a. _____ _____

b. _____ _____

c. _____ _____

Chest thrusts with conscious patient
standing or sitting

a. _____ _____

b. _____ _____

c. _____ _____

Chest thrusts with patient lying (unconscious)

a. _____ _____

b. _____ _____

c. _____ _____

Clinical Situations

For each of the following situations, supply nursing diagnoses, nursing interventions, and supporting rationales for intervention.

1. Consider a patient who has experienced blunt, abdominal trauma. Formulate nursing diagnoses and nursing interventions for the patient in the emergency department. Cite a rationale for each nursing action. List interventions in order of priority.

2. List the emergency nursing measures you would carry out if you were present when someone experienced an anaphylactic reaction to a bee sting. Formulate nursing diagnoses, list nursing interventions, and cite supporting rationales for your actions.

3. Ann is admitted to the emergency department because she ingested approximately 30 diet capsules 1 hour before admission. The nurse is to assist with gastric lavage. State nursing diagnoses, with nursing interventions and supporting rationale for each action.

Fill-In. *Read each question and write the answers in the spaces provided.*

4. List specific nursing interventions that can be used for drug abuse with each of the following drugs. It is assumed that the patient is presenting to the emergency department for treatment.

Drug	*Nursing Interventions*
a. Cocaine	_____
b. Dexedrine	_____
c. Valium	_____
d. Aspirin	_____

5. Compare nursing actions for psychiatric emergencies in dealing with the following patients.

Psychiatric Patients	*Nursing Actions*
a. An overactive patient	_____
b. A violent patient	_____
c. A depressed patient	_____
d. A suicidal patient	_____

72

Terrorism, Mass Casualty, and Disaster Nursing

I. Interpretation, Completion, and Comparison

Multiple Choice. Read each question carefully. Circle the correct answer.

1. Disasters are assigned level designations based on the anticipated level of response needed. A disaster that requires statewide and federal assistance would be classified as:
   a. Level I.
   b. Level II.
   c. Level III.
   d. Level IV.

2. The National Medical Response Team for Weapons of Mass Destruction is a sub-branch of the:
   a. Department of Health and Human Services.
   b. Department of Justice.
   c. Federal Emergency Management Agency.
   d. National Disaster Medical System.

3. The NATO triage system uses color-coded tagging to identify severity of injuries. A patient with survivable but life-threatening injuries (i.e., incomplete amputation) would be color-tagged with:
   a. black.
   b. green.
   c. red.
   d. yellow.

4. A triaged patient, with a significant injury that can wait several hours for treatment, would be assigned:
   a. Priority 1.
   b. Priority 2.
   c. Priority 3.
   d. Priority 4.

5. A triaged patient with psychological disturbances would be color-tagged with:
   a. black.
   b. green.
   c. red.
   d. yellow.

6. Those patients in a disaster who are unlikely to survive are triaged as:
   a. Priority 1.
   b. Priority 2.
   c. Priority 3.
   d. Priority 4.

7. The Environmental Protection Agency has identified four categories of personal protection equipment for health care workers in response to biological, chemical, or radiation exposure. The highest level of respiratory protection that includes a self-contained breathing apparatus and a chemical resistant suit is:
   a. Level A.
   b. Level B.
   c. Level C.
   d. Level D.

8. The most severe form of anthrax exposure is through:
   a. skin contact.
   b. inhalation.
   c. ingestion.
   d. open wounds or sores.

9. An example of a chemical agent that acts by inhibiting cholinesterase is a:
   a. nerve agent.
   b. blood agent.
   c. corrosive acid.
   d. vesicant.

10. The type of chemical agents that *do not* act within seconds (latency period) are:
    a. cyanide-based.
    b. sulfur mustards.
    c. nerve agents.
    d. vesicants.

11. An example of the *most toxic* chemical agent in existence is:
    a. chlorine.
    b. cyanide.
    c. mustard nitrogen.
    d. sarin.

12. There are five phases of radiation exposure related to the dose, exposure, and degree of radiation penetration. The phase characterized by decreasing amounts of leukocytes and lymphocytes is the:
    a. prodromal phase.
    b. latent phase.
    c. illness phase.
    d. recovery phase.

Fill-In. Complete each statement by filling in the blank space.

1. An example of a biological weapon of mass destruction is _____; an example of a chemical weapon of mass destruction is _____.

2. Two federal agencies that provide disaster assistance are the _____ and the _____.

3. Only four states in the country have locations for Disaster Medical Assistance Teams. These states are _____, _____, _____ and _____.

4. Describe the Incident Command System: _____

5. Identify five factors that influence an individual's response to disaster: _____, _____, _____, _____ and _____.

6. Distinguish between the terms *defusing* and *debriefing* as they relate to the Critical Incident Stress Management process: _____

7. Two biological agents *most likely* to be used during a terrorist attack are _____ and _____.

8. Exposure to anthrax, without clinical signs and symptoms of the disease, requires a 60-day treatment with one of two antibiotics: _____ or _____.

9. Smallpox has a case fatality rate of _____ percent.

10. Explain how pulmonary chemical agents (i.e., phosgene) act: _____

II. Critical Thinking Questions and Exercises

Discussion and Analysis

1. Explain why patients who are most critically ill, with a high mortality rate, would be assigned a low triage priority in a disaster situation.

2. Discuss some of the cultural variables that health care providers need to consider in any disaster situation where a large number of diverse religious and ethnic groups of patients need to be treated.

3. Describe common behavioral responses seen in victims of mass disaster.

4. Select one of three ethical theories (utilitarianism, beneficence, justice) and apply its constructs to solving ethical conflicts in a disaster situation.